SURVIVING INTEN

T0250642

Volume Editors:

Derek C. Angus,
MD, MPH, FCCM, FCCP
Associate Professor and Vice Chair
for Research
Department of Critical Care Medicine
University of Pittsburgh
Pittsburgh, Pennsylvania, USA

Jean Carlet, MD
Head of the Intensive Care Unit
Coordinator of the Intensive Care,
Anesthesiology and
Emergency Department
Fondation Hôpital St. Joseph
Paris, France

Series Editor:

Jean-Louis Vincent, MD, PhD, FCCM, FCCP
Head, Department of Intensive Care
Erasme University Hospital
Brussels, Belgium

With 40 Figures and 45 Tables

Springer

Derek C. Angus, MD, MPH, FCCM, FCCP
Associate Professor and Vice Chair for Research
Department of Critical Care Medicine
University of Pittsburgh
3550 Terrace Street
Pittsburgh, PA 15261
USA

Jean Carlet, MD
Head of the Intensive Care Unit
Coordinator of the Intensive Care,
Anaesthesiology and Emergency Department
Fondation Hôpital St Joseph
185 rue Raymond Losserand
75674 Paris Cedex 14
France

Series Editor
Jean-Louis Vincent, MD, PhD, FCCM, FCCP
Head, Department of Intensive Care
Erasme University Hospital
Route de Lennik 808
B-1070 Brussels
Belgium

Library of Congress Cataloging-in-Publication Data
Bibliographic information published by die Deutsche Bibliothek
Die Deutsche Bibliothek lists this publication in the Deutsche Nationalbibliografie:
detailed bibliographic data is availabie in the Internet at <http://dnb.ddb.de>

Printed on acid-free paper.

Hardcover edition © 2003 Springer-Verlag Berlin Heidelberg
Softcover edition © 2004 Springer-Verlag Berlin Heidelberg

Production managed by ProEdit GmbH Heidelberg, Germany
Typeset by am-productions GmbH, Wiesloch, Germany
Printed and bound by Mercedes-Druck, Berlin, Germany
Printed in Germany

9 8 7 6 5 4 3 2 1

ISSN 1610-4056
ISBN 3-540-44149-2   SPIN 10891461

Springer-Verlag New York Berlin Heidelberg
A member of BertelsmannSpringer Science + Business Media GmbH

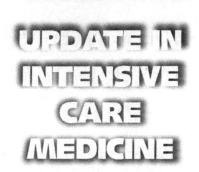

Series Editor: Jean-Louis Vincent

Springer
New York
Berlin
Heidelberg
Hong Kong
London
Milan
Paris
Tokyo

UPDATE IN INTENSIVE CARE MEDICINE

Series Editor: Jean-Louis Vincent

Contents

Improving Methods to Capture Long-term Outcomes in Clinical Studies

Approaches to Improve Long-term Outcomes

List of Contributors

Angus D.C.
Associate Professor
Dept of Critical Care Medicine
University of Pittsburgh
604 Scaife Hall
200 Lothrop Street
Pittsburgh, PA 15213
USA

Azoulay E.
Staff Intensivist
Dept of Intensive Care Medicine
Hôpital Saint-Louis
1 avenue Claude Vellefaux
75475 Paris Cedex 10
France

Bion J.
Reader in Intensive Care Medicine
University Dept of Anaesthesia
and Intensive Care Medicine
N5 Queen Elizabeth Hospital
Birmingham B15 2TH
UK

Black N.
Professor of Health Services Research
Health Services Research Unit
Dept of Public Health and Policy
London School of Hygiene and Tropical
Medicine
Keppel Street
London WC1 7HT
UK

Bottomley A.
Head
Quality of Life Unit
EORTC Data Center
Av. E. Mounier 83, Box 11
1200 Brussels
Belgium

Brett S.
Consultant
Dept of Anesthesia and Intensive Care
Hammersmith Hospital
Du Cane Road
London W12 0HS
UK

Brun-Buisson C.
Professor
Dept of Intensive Care
Hôpital Henri Mondor
94010 Créteil
France

Carlet J.
Staff Intensivist
Dept of Intensive Care
Fondation-Hôpital Saint-Joseph
75674 Paris Cedex 14
France

Cook D.J.
Professor of Medicine and Clinical
Epidemiology and Biostatistics
Academic Chair, Critical Care
McMaster University
Hamilton
Ontario L8N 4AG
Canada

Curtis J.R.
Associate Professor of Medicine
Dept of Pulmonary and Critical Care
Medicine
Harborview Medical Center
Box 359762
325 Ninth Avenue
Seattle WA 98104-2499
USA

Dodek P.
Physician Leader, Intensive Care Unit
Chair, Critical Care Working Group
Center for Health Evaluation and Out-
come Sciences
St. Paul's Hospital
1081 Burrard St.
Vancouver BC V6Z 1Y6
Canada

Ely E.W.
Associate Professor of Medicine
Allergy, Pulmonary and Critical Care
Health Services Research Center
Vanderbilt University School of Medi-
cine
Medical Center East 6109
Nashville TN 37232-8300
USA

Garrouste-Orgeas M.
Staff Intensivist
Dept of Intensive Care
Fondation-Hôpital Saint-Joseph
75674 Paris Cedex 14
France

Graham R.
Clinical Fellow
Dept of Pediatrics
Children's Hospital
300 Longwood Avenue
Boston MA 02115
USA

Grasso S.
Staff Intensivist
Dept of Intensive Care and Intensive
Care Medicine
Ospedale DiVenere
Bari
Italy

Guidet B.
Staff Intensivist
Dept of Intensive Care
Hôpital St Antoine
184 Rue du Faubourg
75012 Paris
France

Hall J.B.
Professor of Medicine, Anesthesia and
Critical Care
Section of Pulmonary and Critical Care
Medicine
MC 6026
University of Chicago
5841 S. Maryland Avenue
Chicago IL 60637
USA

Hart G.K.
Deputy Director
Dept of Intensive Care
Austin and Repatriation Medical Centre
Heidelberg
Victoria
Australia

Hartleib M.
Chief Medical Resident
Dept of Medicine
Sunnybrook & Women's College Health
Sciences Center
2075 Bayview Ave, Suite D474
Toronto
Ontario M4N 3M5
Canada

Herridge M.S.
Assistant Professor of Medicine
Dept of Respiratory and Critical Care
Medicine
University of Toronto Health Network
EN10-212
200 Elizabeth Street
Toronto ON M5G 2C4
Canada

Holzmueller C.G.
Research Administrative Coordinator
Dept of Anesthesiology and Critical
Care Medicine
The Johns Hopkins University School of
Medicine
600 N. Wolfe Street, Meyer 295
Baltimore MD 21287-7294
USA

Hopkins R.O.
Assistant Professor
Psychology Dept and Neuroscience
Center
1122 SWKT
Brigham Young University
Provo UT 84602
USA

Jenkinson C.
Deputy Director
Health Services Research Unit
Institute of Health Sciences
Old Road
Oxford OX3 7LF
UK

Kalassian K.G.
Assistant Professor
Dept of Critical Care Medicine
University of Pittsburgh
200 Lothrop Street
Pittsburgh PA 15261
USA

Keenan S.P.
Medical Director
Intensive Care Unit
Royal Columbian Hospital
103-250 Keary Street
New Westminster BC V3L 5E7
Canada

Khan Z.
Consultant and Honorary Senior Lecturer
Dept of Anaesthesia and Intensive Care
Medicine,
City Hospital
N5 Queen Elizabeth Hospital
Birmingham B15 2TH
UK

Kress J.
Assistant Professor of Medicine
Section of Pulmonary and Critical Care
Medicine
MC 6026
University of Chicago
5841 S. Maryland Avenue
Chicago IL 60637
USA

Levin P.D.
Attending Physician
Dept of Anesthesiology and Critical
Care Medicine
Hebrew University Medical Center
The Hebrews University
Jerusalem 91120
Israel

Levy M.M.
Associate Professor of Medicine
Medical Intensive Care Unit
Rhode Island Hospital
593 Eddy Street
Main Building, 7th Floor
Providence, RI 02903
USA

Mascia L.
Assistant Professor
University of Turin
Anesthesiology and Intensive Care Section
Ospedale S. Giovanni Battista
Corso Dogliotti 14
10126 Turin
Italy

Matos R..
Staff Intensivist
Dept of Intensive Care
Hospital de St. António dos Capuchos
Alameda de St. António dos Capuchos
1150 Lisbon
Portugal

McMullin J.
Assistant Professor of Medicine
Dept of Medicine
St. Joseph's Hospital
50 Charlton Avenue East
Hamilton
Ontario L8N 4AG
Canada

Metnitz P.G.H.
Professor
Dept of Anesthesiology and Intensive
Care Medicine
University Hospital of Vienna
Währinger Gürtel 18-20
1090 Vienna
Austria

Moreau D.
Staff Intensivist
Dept of Intensive Care Medicine
Hôpital Saint-Louis
1 avenue Claude Vellefaux
75475 Paris Cedex 10
France

Moreno R.
Staff Intensivist
Dept of Intensive Care
Hospital de St. António dos Capuchos
Alameda de St. António dos Capuchos
1150 Lisbon
Portugal

Pochard F.
Staff Intensivist
Dept of Intensive Care
Hôpital Saint-Louis
1 avenue Claude Vellefaux
75475 Paris Cedex 10
France

Pronovost P.
Associate Professor
Dept of Anesthesiology and Critical
Care Medicine, Surgery and Health Pol-
icy & Management
The Johns Hopkins University School of
Medicine
600 N. Wolfe Street, Meyer 295
Baltimore MD 21287-7294
USA

Randolph A.G.
Associate Director
Dept of Pediatrics
Children's Hospital
300 Longwood Avenue
Boston, MA 02115
USA

Ranieri V.M.
Professor of Anesthesia and Critical
Care Medicine
Dept of Anesthesiology
Ospedale S. Giovanni Battista
Corso Dogliotti 14
10126 Turin
Italy

Rowan K.M.
Director
Intensive Care National Audit and Re-
search Center
Tavistock House
Tavistock Square
London WC1H 9HR
UK

Rubenfeld G.D.
Division of Pulmonary and Critical Care
Medicine
Harborview Medical Center
University of Washington
Box 359762
325 9th Ave
Seattle WA 98104-2499
USA

Sibbald W.J.
Professor of Critical Care Medicine
Dept of Medicine
Sunnybrook & Women's College Health
Sciences Center
2075 Bayview Ave, Suite D474
Toronto
Ontario M4N 3M5
Canada

Sprung C.L.
Director, General Intensive Care Unit
Dept of Anesthesiology and Critical
Care Medicine
Hadassah University Medical Center
PO Box 12000
Jerusalem 91120
Israel

Sukantarat K.T.
Research Associate
Dept of Surgery
Faculty of Medicine
Imperial College
Chelsea & Westminster Hospital
369 Fulham Road
London SW10 9NH
UK

Van Glabbeke M.
Assistant Director
EORTC Data Center
Av. E. Mounier 83, Box 11
1200 Brussels
Belgium

van Hout B.A.
Professor of Medical Technology
Assessment
Julius Center for Health Sciences
and Primary Care
University Medical Center Utrecht
PO Box 86060
3508 AB Utrecht
The Netherlands

Vincent J.L.
Head
Dept of Intensive Care
Erasme Hospital
Free University of Brussels
Route de Lennik 808
1170 Brussels
Belgium

Wu A.
Associate Professor Health Policy &
Management
Dept of Anesthesiology and Critical
Care Medicine
The Johns Hopkins University School
of Medicine
600 N. Wolfe Street, Meyer 295
Baltimore MD 21287-7294
USA

Common Abbreviations

AIDS	Acquired immunodeficiency syndrome
ALI	Acute lung injury
APACHE	Acute physiology and chronic health evaluation
ARDS	Acute respiratory distress syndrome
CEA	Cost-effectiveness analysis
CNS	Central nervous system
COPD	Chronic obstructive pulmonary disease
GCS	Glasgow coma scale
HAD	Hospital anxiety and depression scale
HRQL	Health-related quality of life
HUI	Health utilities index
ICU	Intensive care unit
QALY	Quality-adjusted life year
RCT	Randomized controlled trial
SAPS	Simplified acute physiology score
SF-36	Short Form 36
SIP	Sickness impact profile
TISS	Therapeutic intervention scoring system

Natural History of Critical Illness

Survival as an Outcome for ICU Patients

S. P. Keenan and P. Dodek

Introduction

Why is 'survival' an important outcome? As intensive care unit (ICU) clinicians, it is important for us to obtain a clear understanding of the natural history of the critical illness we treat. While we would like to know how long a patient is likely to stay in the ICU or hospital, their probable future functional status and quality of life, the likelihood of their surviving their critical illness is of paramount interest. Understanding the impact of critical illnesses on survival allows us to share this information with patients and family and guide resource allocation more appropriately. The time interval over which a patient remains at increased risk of death varies among the critical illnesses we treat. For example, patients who become septic have a greater than expected mortality for a number of months beyond the onset of illness [1, 2], while patients surviving overdoses or multiple trauma have shorter time intervals of increased risk. Understanding the time intervals of risk can guide the design of interventional trials. These trials would ideally include a follow-up period that is comparable to the time interval of risk.

Survival is also the most important outcome we have in benchmarking ICU practice. While randomized controlled trials (RCTs) remain the gold standard for identifying effective new technology, benchmarking outcomes among a network of ICUs may reveal differences in survival. Further scrutiny will determine whether these differences are likely real and, if so, related differences in practice may be isolated. Global implementation of these best practices using a systematic approach has the potential to improve overall outcome.

In this chapter, we will briefly address short-term survival (all time-intervals up to ICU survival) for patients admitted to the ICU. Our main focus, however, will be survival beyond the ICU stay. What happens to patients after they are discharged from the ICU? How likely are they to survive their hospital stay or return to the ICU, and what happens once they leave hospital? To address these questions we searched the published literature using MEDLINE and the keywords 'intensive care units' or 'critical care' and 'survival' or 'mortality' or 'outcome'. We also searched 'related articles' for those citations considered most relevant. While RCTs add information and are remarkable in their survival intervals chosen, we have focused primarily on observational studies as they are less likely to be affected by the selection bias of many RCTs. As future chapters of this volume will be devoted exclusively to the natural history of elderly and pediatric critically ill populations we did not include studies specifically dealing with these patient populations.

Short-term Mortality

Mortality for patients admitted to the ICU is high compared to that for patients cared for in non-critical care units. While the literature on short-term outcomes during ICU stay is too vast to review in detail, three important issues emerge. First, the time interval selected for short-term mortality varies. The selection of intervals as low as 10 [3] to 14-days [4–7] for RCTs has been rationalized on the basis that either the therapy will only influence outcome during the period in which it is being applied (prone positioning) or that the disease process of interest (sepsis or ventilator associated pneumonia) has an attributable mortality that is restricted to the first 14-days. While it is true that for patients with sepsis most attributable mortality occurs early, studies have clearly demonstrated that the impact of sepsis on mortality extends well beyond the first 2 weeks [1, 2], suggesting that selection of a 14-day endpoint may be misleading for sepsis trials. Similarly, selecting a time interval for analysis of mortality to reflect the time interval during which the new treatment or technology is applied is potentially concerning. It is possible that such treatments may just delay death, an outcome that is clearly not desirable. The more commonly used 28-day endpoint in RCTs appears to be more reasonable but still does not fully address the longer-term impact of critical illness. In designing a RCT, one is faced with a trade-off in choosing the time interval for mortality. On the one hand, sensitivity is increased by choosing a shorter time interval to measure the effect of a new technology on survival, a period during which death is more likely to arise from the disease process of interest. As the time interval for study is extended, deaths will be increasingly due to factors other than the disease process of interest, this added 'noise' making it more difficult to demonstrate a true 'signal'. On the other hand, patients are most interested in surviving an event, in this case ICU stay and, more importantly, hospitalization (see Fig. 1).

Second, ICU survival appears to be improving over time despite the fact that advances in medicine have resulted in a greater population of sicker, immunosuppressed patients at risk of critical illness and an increasing proportion of our population being elderly. This improvement in outcome has been well documented. For example, a marked reduction was found in the mortality for the control groups of two trials on patients with acute respiratory distress syndrome (ARDS) of extracorporeal oxygenation [8] and extracorporeal carbon dioxide removal [9], with similar inclusion criteria, published 15 years apart (9 % versus 39 %, respectively). Similarly, the Seattle group demonstrated a reduction in mortality for patients with ARDS over time within their center in a carefully conducted study using similar definitions of ARDS over a 10-year period [10]. Finally, a number of recent landmark studies have demonstrated efficacy of treatments for sepsis [11], ARDS [12], and sedation protocols [13, 14] that establish new benchmarks for short-term outcome.

Lastly, despite this promising trend, there is evidence suggesting that some patient groups may not benefit from life support measures despite the apparent

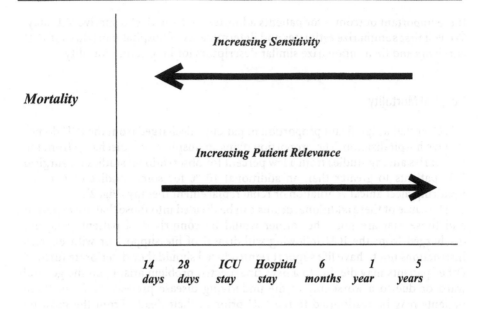

Fig. 1. This figure illustrates the potential trade-off facing designers of a randomized controlled trial in choosing their interval for survival.

need for such measures for immediate survival. For example, there has been an ongoing evaluation of the potential usefulness of ICU admission for patients who have human immunodeficiency virus (HIV) infection. This has become necessary as the introduction of new treatment regimens has radically altered their long-term outcome. While once considered poor candidates for ICU care, a case-by-case approach is warranted in these groups [15, 16]. Patients with underlying malignancies are a heterogeneous group but subpopulations such as patients who develop respiratory failure after bone marrow transplant remain a group with extremely high short-term mortality [17, 18]. Finally, there are other disease processes that appear to have such a poor short-term outcome that serious consideration should be given to avoiding ICU admission in these patients. For example, patients who have idiopathic pulmonary fibrosis who require mechanical ventilation have a very high hospital mortality [19–21]. We need more data on the outcomes, both short and longer-term, for these and other patient groups that may not benefit from ICU admission.

Long-term Mortality

If my patient were to survive her ICU stay, what is the probability that she will die before leaving hospital? If she survives hospitalization, what is the probability that she will die by 6 months, one year, or longer? Less literature exists that describes these important outcomes for patients admitted to the ICU who survive ICU stay. We will first summarize estimates and determinants of hospital mortality for ICU survivors and then summarize similar descriptors for long-term mortality.

Hospital Mortality

It is clear that a significant proportion of patients discharged from the ICU do not survive hospitalization. The proportion dying in hospital after discharge from the ICU varies among studies from a few percent for observational studies on surgical ICU patients to greater than an additional 10 % for some studies of patients requiring mechanical ventilation or renal replacement therapy (Fig. 2).

The cause of these additional deaths can be divided into those that are expected and those that are not. The former would be comprised of patients who are discharged from the ICU following withdrawal of life support or with express instructions not to have life support reintroduced should they deteriorate further. Other patients may die due to a new, unexpected problem arising on the general ward or due to a worsening of the underlying disease process. Some of these patients may be readmitted to the ICU prior to their death. From the growing literature addressing readmission to the ICU [22–30], well summarized in a review by Rosenberg and Watts [31], patients are readmitted to ICU for the same reason as their initial admission from 19 to 53 % of the time. Readmission rates vary from 4 to 14 % and these patients have prolonged length of stay and marked increase in hospital mortality (1.5 to 10 times that of other ICU patients).

Mortality after Hospitalization

Survival beyond hospitalization for patients requiring an admission to the ICU is an outcome of utmost importance to patients and family. The literature addressing

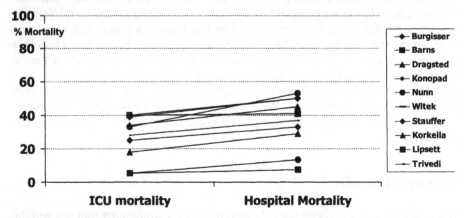

Fig. 2. This figure summarizes the respective ICU and hospital mortality for a representative group of cohort studies that also provided follow-up beyond hospitalization.

long-term survival is comprised of three different study designs. The most common are observational studies describing survival of a single cohort of ICU patients after hospitalization over time without a comparison group. In some studies, variables that distinguish survivors from non-survivors have been determined, most often using univariable analysis, less frequently reporting the more robust use of multivariable analysis. The population studied may either be consecutive patients admitted to a specific ICU, most often a general ICU, or a subset of ICU patients. Table 1 demonstrates wide variation in outcome among studies of 'general' ICU populations with a one-year mortality ranging from 18 to 56 % [32–50].

These studies vary in time of publication, country of origin and number of centers, most being single-centers while one study includes all ICU admissions in a specific health care region [50].

While these single-cohort observational studies provide insight into the apparently poor long-term prognosis of ICU patients who survive hospitalization, they include the expected high hospital mortality rate and do not account for this by comparing survival over time beyond hospitalization to a control group. To address this, a second study design adopted by a number of investigators includes a comparison of survival rates between their patient cohort and the general population [38], matched for age and gender [42, 44, 49, 50]. In the first of these studies, conducted over one-year at a single center, Zaren and Bergstrom found that survival beyond hospitalization, one-year after admission, was 96% of that predicted by comparing it to the general population [38]. However, four subsequent studies, most larger, and two multi-centered, have all documented a significantly greater long-term mortality among ICU patients compared to the general population matched for age and gender [40, 42, 47, 48]. Niskanen and colleagues reported a 5-year mortality rate for 12,180 patients admitted to 25 ICUs in Finland in 1987 that was 3.3 times that of Finland's general population [44]. They also noted that the difference between survival curves occurred over the first 2 years with the curves paralleling each other beyond that. Flaaten and Kvale also found that survival beyond 2 years after hospitalization paralleled that of the general population of Norway [49]. In a single center study in Glasgow, enrolling all patients over 4 years, Ridley and Plenderleith [42] found that the survival curve for ICU patients was significantly worse than that for an age and gender-matched general population. In this study, however, survival curves did not parallel each other until the fourth year. We also found that patients who required ICU admission fared worse than the general population in a study of all ICU admissions during a 3-year period in British Columbia [50]. This difference in survival persists over the three years of follow-up data available to us, although the ratio of observed to expected deaths declined from 6.47 during the first year to 3.10 in the third (Fig. 3).

Patients who require ICU admission differ from the general population, having more co-morbid disease on average prior to their acute event. As such, one would expect their outcome to be worse than that of the general population even without hospital admission. To understand the effect that exposure to an ICU has on long-term outcome, one should choose a comparison group more similar to those patients requiring ICU admission than the general population. The final study design found in the literature uses other hospitalized patients as controls. Parno and associates compared 2-year survival rates between 558 ICU patients and 124

Table 1. Long-term outcome (mortality) of general ICU population

Study	Patients	ICU	Hospital	3 months	6 months	1-yr	2-yrs	3-yrs	4-yrs	5-yrs	12-yrs
Thibault et al. (1980) [32]	2693		10 %			25 %*					
Parno et al. (1982) [33]	558		17.3 %				35.6 %				
Le Gall et al. (1982) [34]	228	34 %	33 %		50 %	51 %		50 %			
Burgisser et al. (1982) [35]	330	25 %	7.5 %				15.1 %				
Bams et al. (1985) [36]	238	5.4 %			39 %	42 %					
Jacobs et al. (1988) [37]	313	24 %				42 %					
Zaren et al. (1989) [38]	980	9.6 %				26.4 %					
Dragsted et al. (1989) [39]	1308	18 %	29 %			44 %					
Mundt et al. (1989) [40]	1545				6 %**						
Ridley et al. (1990) [41]	513	24 %				35 %	48 %	43 %	45 %	47 %	
Ridley et al. (1994) [42]	1168						38 %				
Konopad et al. (1995) [43]	504	5.4 %	13.5 %		21 %	25 %	30 %	32 %	33 %	33 %	
Niskanen et al. (1996) [44]	12,180	10 %				28 %	30 %	33 %			
Capuzzo et al. (1996) [45]	260					17.6 %					
Short et al. (1999) [46]	2268		35 %		41 %	56 %					
Eddleston et al. (2000) [47]	370	29 %		39 %		43 %					
Pettila et al. (2000) [48]	591	15 %			30 %	36 %	37 %				
Flaatten et al. (2001) [49]	219					34 %					58 %
Keenan et al. (2002) [50]	27,103	14 %			28 %	24 %	28 %	32 %			

* the "cumulative mortality over a mean of 15 months of follow-up"

** 200 patients lost to follow-up

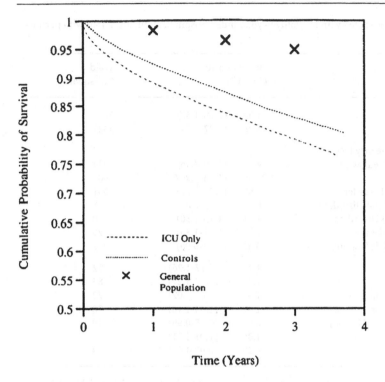

Fig. 3. Unadjusted survival curves for 2 groups of patients surviving hospitalization, one of which was admitted to the ICU during their stay. For comparison, yearly survival for a sample of the general population, adjusted for age and gender has been included (from [50] with permission).

non-ICU patients and while the 2-year mortality was considerably worse for the ICU group (35.6 versus 14.8 %), this was due largely to higher in-hospital mortality [51]. In fact, survival after hospital discharge was very similar, 83.3 versus 89.1 % at 2 years for ICU and non-ICU patients, respectively [51]. In our retrospective study of all ICU admissions in the province of British Columbia, we compared mortality after hospital discharge of ICU patients to that in a random sample of patients who required hospitalization but were not admitted to the ICU [50]. From Figure 3 it is clear that, while the unadjusted survival curve for ICU patients who survived to hospital discharge appears less favorable than that of the control group of hospitalized non-ICU patients, both groups fared considerably worse than a general population, matched for age and gender. Furthermore, after controlling for other prognostic factors we found that the difference in long-term mortality between ICU patients and hospitalized, non-ICU patients, bordered on negligible (see Table 2). This would suggest that after controlling for hospitalization, the difference in long-term mortality between ICU patients and the general population is due more to whatever leads patients to be hospitalized rather than admitted to the ICU.

Table 2. Factors associated with mortality beyond index hospitalization. From [50] with permission

Variable	Hazard Ratio (95% CI)		Wald Chi-square *
Age (per decade)	1.60	(1.58-1.62)	5093
Comorbidity	1.28	(1.27-1.29)	3321
Major Clinical Category (MCC)			
Lymphoma/Leukemia	4.00	(3.59-4.46)	624
HIV	20.99	(16.46-26.77)	602
Respiratory Disorders	1.63	(1.54-1.71)	331
Musculoskeletal Disorders	0.75	(0.69-0.81)	54
Neurological Disorders	1.21	(1.13-1.30)	30
Blood Disorders	1.56	(1.31-1.85)	25
Burns/Multiple Trauma	0.65	(0.47-0.90)	7
Sex (M vs F)	1.22	(1.17-1.26)	92
ICU admission	1.21	(1.17-1.27)	85
Prior Hospital admission	1.02	(1.01-1.02)	72
Prior ICU admission	1.07	(1.04-1.10)	20
Median Income (per $10,000)	0.99	(0.98-0.99)	19
Residence (urban vs rural)	1.06	(1.01-1.11)	5
Tier (1 to 7) **	0.99	(0.97-1.00)	4

* As all p <0.001, the Wald Chi-square has been reported to illustrate which variables are most significant
** The negative coefficient denotes that there is a decreased risk of death after discharge from hospital in patients who were admitted to ICUs at higher Tier number hospitals which are actually smaller hospitals, i.e., a given ICU patient is more likely to survive after hospital discharge from a smaller hospital.

Studies of general ICU populations like those in Table 1 provide average estimates for long-term mortality. Trying to prognosticate for an individual patient from these studies is more difficult. It is possible to make more precise estimates by considering additional variables that have been shown within these studies to influence mortality. These factors can be divided into patient or non-patient related variables. The patient-related variable that has been most consistently demonstrated to have a major influence on long-term mortality is age (Tables 3 and 4). As the effect of age on outcome is the subject of another chapter in this volume, we will not address it further here. In addition to age, male gender, worse pre-morbid functional status, greater degree of co-morbid disease, organ dysfunction and severity of illness during hospitalization, and reason for ICU admission (diagnosis) are among those demonstrated to increase long-term mortality in specific studies (Tables 3 and 4).

In our recent study, we identified increasing age, male gender, number of prior hospitalizations, major clinical category (diagnosis) and, to a lesser degree, socio-economic factors to be associated with mortality after an index hospitalization [50].

Table 3. Factors associated with poorer long-term survival using univariate analysis

Study	N	Age	Male gender	Comorbidity	Diagnosis	Severity of illness	Organ dysfunction	Pre-morbid functional status
Nunn et al. (1979) [52]	100	✓			✓			
Le Gall et al. (1982) [34]	228	✓						✓	✓
Parno et al. (1984) [51]	558	✓			✓			
Witek et al. (1985) [53]	100	✓						
Spicher et al. 1987) [55]	240	✓						✓
Dragsted et al. (1989) [39]	1308	✓						
Ridley et al. (1990) [41]	513	✓			✓	✓		
Stauffer et al. (1993) [58]	383	✓			✓			
Capuzzo et al. (1996) [45]	260				✓			
Carson et al. (1999) [60]	133	✓						✓
Short et al. (1999) [46]	2268	✓				✓		

Table 4. Factors associated with poorer long-term survival using multivariate analysis

Study	N	Age	Male gender	Comorbidity	Diagnostic group	Severity of illness
Ridley et al.* (1990) [41]	513	✓				✓
Niskanen et al.* (1996) [44]	12,180	✓	✓	✓	✓	
Keenan et al.* (2002) [50]	27,103	✓	✓		✓	

Major clinical categories associated with the highest long-term mortality included patients with HIV, lymphoma, leukemia, other blood disorders, respiratory disorders, or neurological disorders while multiple trauma or burn patients surviving to hospital discharge had a relatively low long-term mortality [50]. Of interest, while non-HIV infection was associated with a marked increased hospital mortality, it was not associated with mortality after the index hospitalization. These findings are consistent with that described by Niskanen and colleagues [44] who reported the highest long-term mortality for patients with cancer and a relatively high mortality for patients with cardiovascular, respiratory or gastroenterological diseases. Diagnostic categories that represent chronic progressive disorders, malignant or otherwise, appear to be those that are of greatest importance in determining a poor long-term outcome regardless of whether patients are admitted to the ICU or not. In contrast, patients admitted to the ICU because of an acute, self-limiting process such as drug overdose, accidental acute intoxication, or multiple trauma, who survive their hospitalization generally have a good recovery with little impact on long-term outcome arising as a result of their admission. Sepsis is an interesting entity as it appears that there is an ongoing increased mortality for a number of years despite the acute nature of this disease process [1, 2].

Differences in patient-related variables also explain some of the differences in mortality rates evident among studies. Lower mortality rates tend to be recorded by large multi-center studies that include ICUs of varying size that likely reflect a population with an average lower severity of illness and degree of organ dysfunction than single center studies at tertiary care centers. Case-mix may also vary among studies and the influence of this factor is clearly demonstrated in the higher mortality levels seen in patients requiring mechanical ventilation [52–60] (Table 5) or specific subgroups such as septic patients or bone marrow transplant patients who require ICU admission [1, 15, 17, 18, 61–78] (Table 6). From studies on chronic obstructive pulmonary disease (COPD), however, it is clear that factors other than diagnosis are of importance, including the stage of disease and severity of the exacerbation, particularly whether mechanical ventilation is required or not [71–78].

Variables that are independent of patients include ICU structure (available technology and personnel) and ICU model used (organizational factors, including the use of clinical practice guidelines and degree of training of attending staff). As these variables are potentially easier to modify than patient-related variables, there has been growing interest in determining whether these variables affect outcome. In the case of guidelines or protocols, there is an expanding literature demonstrating a positive effect on short-term outcomes [14, 15, 79–81], but relatively little on long-term outcomes. In addition, there are few published data on the effect of differences in ICU structure. The possible exception may be the use of non-invasive ventilation in patients with COPD. Two studies, using historical controls have demonstrated that COPD patients who presented with an acute exacerbation and who were treated with non-invasive positive pressure ventilation had a better 1-year survival rate than those who do not receive non-invasive ventilation [76, 77]. Admission policies to ICU that may be related to availability of ICU or other high-dependency beds may also explain some of the differences found among studies.

Table 5. Long-term outcome (mortality) of patients receiving mechanical ventilation

Study	Patients*	ICU	Hospital	3 months	6 months	1-yr	2-yrs	3-yrs	4-yrs	5-yrs	12-yrs
Nunn et al. (1979) [52]	100 > 4 hours	33%	53%					70%			
Davis et al. (1980) [53]	100 > 48 hrs		56%				72%				
Schmidt et al. (1983) [54]	137 > 48 hrs		64%			70%		72%			
Witek et al. (1985) [55]	100	40%	50%			67%					
Spicher et al. (1987) [56]	250 > 10 days		61%			71%	77%				
Gracey et al. (1992) [57]	104 > 29 days		42%			61%		68%			
Stauffer et al. (1993) [58]	383 > 1 hour	39%	50%			70%					
Douglas et al. (1997) [59]	57 > 5 days		44%		58%						
Carson et al. (1999) [60]	133 LTAC**		50%			77%					

* number of patients and minimal duration of mechanical ventilation
** LTAC long-term acute care hospitals providing care for prolonged critical illness

Table 6. Long-term outcome (mortality) of specific ICU patient groups

Study	Patients	ICU	Hospital	3 months	6 months	1-yr	2-yrs	3-yrs	4-yrs	5-yrs	12-yrs
Frutiger et al. (1991) [61]	233 severe trauma		18 %				24 %				
Crawford et al. (1992) [18]	348 ventilated BMT patients		96 %		97 %						
Huaringa et al. (2000) [17]	60 ventilated BMT patients	82 %			95 %						
Staudinger et al. (2000) [62]	414 cancer patients	47 %				77 %					
Sasse et al. (1995) [63]	153 septic patients		51 %		65 %	72 %					
Quartin et al. (1997) [1]	1505 septic patients / 607 sepsis / 674 severe sepsis / 224 septic shock					46 % / 71 % / 80 %					
Trouillet et al. (1996) [64]	116 cardiac surgery & organ failure	23.3 %									31 %#
Bashour et al. (2000) [65]	142 Cardiac surgery > 20 days ICU		33 %					64 %*			
Nickas et al. (2000) [15]	394 HIV patients		37 %			73 %	82 %	87 %	89 %		
Korkeila et al. (2000) [66]	62 RRT	34 %	45 %		55 %					65 %	
Lipsett et al. (2000) [67]	128 SICU pts > 6 days in ICU	40 %	41 %		54 %						
Trivedi et al. (2001) [68]	186 medical patients	28 %	37 %			41 %					

Table 6. (Continued)

Study	Patients	ICU	Hospital	3 months	6 months	1-yr	2-yrs	3-yrs	4-yrs	5-yrs	12-yrs
Schelling et al. (1998) [69]	192 ARDS	38 %				54 %					
Davidson et al. (1999) [70]	207 ARDS due to Sepsis (119) Trauma (88)		30 % 43 % 14 %	34 %							
Gottlieb et al. (1973) [71]	30 COPD					70 %					
Martin et al. (1982) [72]	36 COPD						28 %				
Menzies et al. * (1989) [73]	95 COPD					62 %					
Seneff et al. (1995) [74]	362 COPD		24 %	42 %	48 %	52 %					
Connors et al. (1996) [75]	1,106 COPD		11 %		33 %	42 %	49 %				
Confalonieri et al. (1996) [76] CMV NPPV	24 COPD 24 COPD		25 % 18 %		46 % 29 %	50 % 29 %					
Vitacca et al. (1996) [77] CMV NPPV	29 COPD 30 COPD	26 % 23 %		48 % 23 %		63 % 30 %					
Costello et al. (1997) [78]	85 COPD		20 %			39 %	54 %			73 %	

* over median follow-up of 30.6 months, # mean follow-up 81 months (range 70–93 months), CMV – conventional mechanical ventilation, NPPV – noninvasive positive pressure ventilation, RRT – renal replacement therapy, COPD – chronic obstructive pulmonary disease, ARDS – acute respiratory distress syndrome, BMT – bone marrow transplant

Conclusion

Patients admitted to the ICU have a high short-term mortality rate compared to patients who receive alternate levels of care. Over time there has been an improvement in survival as a result of both the introduction of innovative pharmacological and technological therapies and the improved organization of delivery of care. Survival after discharge from the ICU depends upon a number of patient factors; age, premorbid co-morbidity and diagnosis are the most important. While it is clear that ICU patients who survive hospitalization have a higher long-term mortality than the general population, it appears that this is not related so much to their ICU admission but rather to their need for hospitalization.

The studies and trials that have added to the literature on survival of ICU patients in general have high internal validity, describing an endpoint that is easily measured in a well-defined group of patients. However, there is a greater problem with external validity, or how others may try to use the results from these studies in their own setting; this arises from the heterogeneity of patients included that exists among studies. There is a need for large, multi-center, multi-national, prospective studies on *a priori* defined homogeneous populations of ICU patients. Data collected would include not only baseline demographics and severity of illness but also specific information on ICU and hospital interventions, complications, length of stay and discharge destination. These large cohorts would provide more useful information for families and clinicians. While this may appear daunting at first blush, the burgeoning field of informatics has provided the technology to proceed and groups such as Project IMPACT, sponsored by the Society of Critical Care Medicine in the United States, as well as ICNARC (Intensive Care National Audit and Research Center) in the United Kingdom are already collecting large amounts of data on many ICUs prospectively. With time, we will hopefully have the data on long-term survival, and more importantly associated quality of life, to be able to confidently discuss long-term prognosis with our patients and their families and make informed decisions regarding the institution, continuation, and withdrawal of life support measures.

References

1. Quartin AA, Schein RMH, Kett DH, et al (1997) Magnitude and duration of the effect of sepsis on survival. JAMA 277:1058–1063
2. Perl TM, Dvorak L, Hwang T, et al (1995) Long-term survival and function after suspected gram-negative sepsis. JAMA 274:338–345
3. Gattinoni L, Tognoni G, Pesenti A, et al (2001) Effect of prone positioning on the survival of patients with acute respiratory failure. N Engl J Med 345:568–573
4. McCloskey RV, Straube RC, Sanders C, et al (1994) Treatment of septic shock with human monoclonal antibody HA-1A. Ann Intern Med 121:1–5
5. Angus DC, Birmingham MC, Balk RA, et al (2000) E5 murine monoclonal antiendotoxin antibody in gram-negative sepsis. JAMA 283:1723–1730
6. Fagon J, Chastre J, Wolff M, et al (2000) Invasive and noninvasive strategies for management of suspected ventilator-associated pneumonia. Ann Intern Med 132:621–630

7. Reeves JH, Butt WW, Shann F, et al (1999) Continuous plasma filtration in sepsis syndrome. Crit Care Med 27:2096–2104
8. Zapol WM, Snider MT, Hill JD, et al (1979) Extracoporeal membrane oxygenation in severe acute respiratory failure. JAMA 242:2193–2196
9. Morris AH, Wallace CJ, Menlove RL, et al (1994) Randomized clinical trial of pressure-controlled inverse ratio ventilation and extracorporeal CO_2 removal for adult respiratory distress syndrome. Am J Respir Crit Care Med 149:295–305
10. Milberg JA, Davis DR, Steinberg KP, Hudson LD (1995) Improved survival of patients with acute respiratory distress syndrome: 1983–1993. JAMA 273:306–309
11. Bernard GR, Vincent JL, Laterre PF, et al (2001) Efficacy and safety of recombinant human activated protein C for severe sepsis. N Engl J Med 344:699–709
12. The Acute Respiratory Distress Syndrome Network (2000) Ventilation with lower tidal volumes as compared with traditional tidal volumes for acute lung injury and the acute respiratory distress syndrome. N Engl J Med 342:1301–1308
13. Brook AD, Ahrens TS, Schaiff R, et al (1999) Effect of nursing-implemented sedation protocol on the duration of mechanical ventilation. Crit Care Med 27:2609–2615
14. Kress PJ, Pohlman RN, OConnor MF, Hall JB (2000) Daily interruption of sedative infusions in critically ill patients undergoing mechanical ventilation. N Engl J Med 342:1471–1477
15. Nickas G, Wachter RM (2000) Outcomes of intensive care for patients with human immunodeficiency virus infection. Arch Intern Med 160:541–547
16. Afessa B, Green B. (2000) Clinical course, prognostic factors, and outcome prediction for HIV patients in the ICU. Chest 118:138–145
17. Huaringa AJ, Leyve FJ, Giralt SA, et al (2000) Outcome of bone marrow transplantation patients requiring mechanical ventilation Crit Care Med 28:1014–1017
18. Crawford SW, Peterson FB (1992) Long-term survival from respiratory failure after marrow transplantation for malignancy. Am Rev Respir Dis 145:510–514
19. Stern J, Mal H, Groussard O, et al (2001) Prognosis of patients with advanced idiopathic pulmonary fibrosis requiring mechanical ventilation for acute respiratory failure. Chest 120:213–219
20. Blivet S, Philit F, Sab JM, et al (2001) Outcome of patients with idiopathic pulmonary fibrosis admitted to the ICU for respiratory failure. Chest 120:209–212
21. Fumeaux T, Rothmeier C, Jolliet P (2001) Outcome of mechanical ventilation for acute respiratory failure in patients with pulmonary fibrosis. Intensive Care Med 27:1868–1874
22. Baigelman W, Katz R, Geary G (1983) Patient readmission to critical care units during the same hospitalization at a community teaching hospital. Intensive Care Med 9:253–256
23. Franklin C, Jackson D (1983) Discharge decision-making in a medical ICU: characteristics of unexpected readmissions. Crit Care Med 11:61–66
24. Snow W, Bergin KT, Horrigan TP (1985) Readmission of patients to the surgical intensive care unit: patient profiles and possibilities for prevention. Crit Care Med 13:961–964
25. Rubins HB, Moskowitz MA (1988) Discharge decision-making in a medical intensive care unit: identifying patients at high risk of unexpected death or unit readmission. Am J Med 84:863–869
26. Durbin CG, Kopel RF (1993) A case-control study of patients readmitted to the intensive care unit. Crit Care Med 21:1547–1553
27. Kirby EG, Durbin CG (1996) Establishment of a respiratory assessment team is associated with decreased mortality in patients re-admitted to the ICU. Respir Care 41:903–907
28. Cooper GS, Sirio CA, Rotondi AJ, et al (1999) Are readmissions to the intensive care unit a useful measure of hospital performance? Med Care 37:399–408
29. Chen LM, Martin CM, Keenan SP, et al (1998) Patients readmitted to the intensive care unit during the same hospitalization: clinical features and outcomes. Crit Care Med 26:1834–1841
30. Rosenberg AL, Hofer TP, Hayward RA, et al (2001) Who bounces back? Physiologic and other predictors of intensive care unit readmission. Crit Care Med 29:511–518
31. Rosenberg AL, Watts C (2000) Patients readmitted to ICUs: a systematic review of risk factors and outcomes. Chest 118:492–502

32. Thibault GE, Mulley AG, Barnett GO, et al (1980) Medical intensive care: indications, interventions, and outcomes. N Engl J Med 302:938–942
33. Parno JR, Teres D, Lemeshow S, Brown RB (1982) Hospital charges and long-term survival of ICU versus non-ICU patients. Crit Care Med 10:569–574
34. Le Gall JR, Brun-Buisson C, Trunet P, Latournerie J, Chantereau S, Rapin M (1982) Influence of age, previous health status, and severity of acute illness on outcome from intensive care. Crit Care Med 10:575–577
35. Burgisser C, Ritz R (1982) Follow-up of intensive medical care patients. Schweiz Med Wochenschr 112:1283–1286
36. Bams JL, Miranda DR (1985) Outcome and costs of intensive care: a follow-up study on 238 ICU-patients. Intensive Care Med 11:234–241
37. Jacobs CJ, van der Vliet JA, van Roozendaal MR, van der Linden CJ (1988) Mortality and quality of life after intensive care for critical illness. Intensive Care Med 14:217–220
38. Zaren B, Bergstrom R (1989) Survival compared to the general population and changes in health status among intensive care patients. Acta Anaesthesiol Scand 33:6–12
39. Dragsted L, Qvist J (1989) Outcome from intensive care. III. A 5-year study of 1308 patients: activity levels. Eur J Anaesthesiol 6:385–396
40. Mundt DJ, Gage RW, Lemeshow S, Pastides H, Teres D, Avrunin JS (1989) Intensive care unit patient follow-up: mortality, functional status, and return to work at six months. Arch Intern Med 149:68–72
41. Ridley S, Jackson R, Findlay J, Wallace P (1990) Long term survival after intensive care. Br Med J 301:1127–1130
42. Ridley S, Plenderleith L (1994) Survival after intensive care. Anaesthesia 49:933–935
43. Konopad E, Noseworthy TW, Johnston R, Shustack A, Grace M (1995) Quality of life measures before and one year after admission to an intensive care unit. Crit Care Med 23:1653–1659
44. Niskanen M, Kari A, Halonen P for the Finnish ICU Study Group (1996) Five-year survival after intensive care: comparison of 12,180 patients with the general population. Crit Care Med 24:1962–1967
45. Capuzzo M, Bianconi M, Contu P, Pavoni V, Gritti G (1996) Survival and quality of life after intensive care. Intensive Care Med 22:947–953
46. Short TG, Buckely TA, Rowbottom MY, Wong E, Oh TE (1999) Long-term outcome and functional health status following intensive care in Hong Kong. Crit Care Med 27:51–57
47. Eddleston JM, White P, Guthrie E (2000) Survival, morbidity, and quality of life after discharge from intensive care. Crit Care Med 28:2293–2299
48. Pettila V, Kaarlola A, Makelainen A (2000) Health-related quality of life of multiple organ dysfunction patients one year after intensive care. Intensive Care Med 26:1473–1479
49. Flaaten H, Kvale R (2001) Survival and quality of life 12 years after ICU: a comparison with the general Norwegian population. Intensive Care Med 27:1005–1011
50. Keenan SP, Dodek P, Chan K, et al (2002) Intensive care unit admission has minimal impact on long-term mortality. Crit Care Med 30:501–507
51. Parno JR, Teres D, Lemeshow S, Brown RB, Avrunin JS (1984) Two-year outcome of adult intensive care patients. Med Care 22:167–176
52. Nunn JF, Milledge JS, Singaraya J (1979) Survival of patients ventilated in an intensive care unit. Br Med J 1:1525–1527
53. Davis H, Lefrak SS, Miller D, Malt S (1980) Prolonged mechanically assisted ventilation: an analysis of outcome and charges. JAMA 243:43–45
54. Schmidt CD, Elliott CG, Carmelli D, et al (1983) Prolonged mechanical ventilation for respiratory failure: a cost-benefit analysis. Crit Care Med 11:407–411
55. Witek TJ, Schachter EN, Dean NL, Beck GJ (1985) Mechanically assisted ventilation in a community hospital: immediate outcome, hospital charges, and follow-up of patients. Arch Intern Med 145:235–239
56. Spicher JE, White DP (1987) Outcome and function following prolonged mechanical ventilation. Arch Intern Med 147:421–425

57. Gracey DR, Naessens JM, Krishan I, Marsh HM (1992) Hospital and posthospital survival in patients mechanically ventilated for more than 29 days. Chest 101:211–214
58. Stauffer JL, Fayter NA, Graves B, Cromb M, Lynch JC, Goebel P (1993) Survival following mechanical ventilation for acute respiratory failure in adult men. Chest 104:1222–1229
59. Douglas SL, Daly BJ, Brennan PF, Harris S, Nochomovitz M, Dyer MA (1997) Outcomes of long-term ventilator patients: a descriptive study. Am J Crit Care 6:99–105
60. Carson SS, Bach PB, Brzozowski L, Leff A (1999) Outcomes after long-term acute care: an analysis of 133 mechanically ventilated patients. Am J Respir Crit Care Med 159:1568–1573
61. Frutiger A, Ryf C, Bilat C, et al (1991) Five years follow-up of severely injured ICU patients. J Trauma 31:1216–1225
62. Staudinger T, Stoiser B, Mullner M, et al (2000) Outcome and prognostic factors in critically ill cancer patients admitted to the intensive care unit. Crit Care Med 28:1322–1328
63. Sasse KC, Nauenberg E, Long A, Anton B, Tucker HJ, Teh-wei H (1995) Long-term survival after intensive care unit admission with sepsis. Crit Care Med 23:1040–1047
64. Trouillet JL, Scheimberg A, Vuagnat A, Fagon JY, Chastre J, Gilert C (1996) Long-term outcome and quality of life of patients requiring multidisciplinary intensive care unit admission after cardiac operations. J Thorac Cardiovasc Surg 112:926–934
65. Bashour CA, Yared JP, Ryan TA, et al (2000) Long-term survival and functional capacity in cardiac surgery patients after prolonged intensive care. Crit Care Med 28:3847–3853
66. Korkeila M, Ruokonen E, Takala J (2000) Cost of care, long-term prognosis and quality of life in patients requiring renal replacement therapy during intensive care. Intensive Care Med 26:1824–1831
67. Lipsett AP, Swoboda SM, Dickerson J, et al (2000) Survival and functional outcome after prolonged intensive care unit stay. Ann Surg 231:262–268
68. Trivedi M, Ridley SA (2001) Intermediate outcome of medical patients after intensive care. Anaesthesia 56:841–146
69. Schelling G, Stoll C, Haller M, et al (1998) Health-related quality of life and posttraumatic stress disorder in survivors of the acute respiratory distress syndrome. Crit Care Med 26:651–659
70. Davidson TA, Rubenfeld GD, Caldwell ES, Hudson LD, Steinberg KP (1999) The effect of acute respiratory distress syndrome on long-term survival. Am J Respir Crit Care Med 160:1838–1842
71. Gottlieb LS, Balchum OJ (1973) Course of chronic obstructive pulmonary disease following first onset of respiratory failure. Chest 63:5–8
72. Martin TR, Lewis SW, Albert RK (1982) The prognosis of patients with chronic obstructive pulmonary disease after hospitalization for acute respiratory failure. Chest 82:310–314
73. Menzies R, Gibbons W, Goldberg P (1989) Determinants of weaning and survival among patients with COPD who require mechanical ventilation for acute respiratory failure. Chest 95:398–405
74. Seneff MG, Wagner DP, Wagner RP, Zimmerman JE, Knaus WA (1995) Hospital and 1-year survival of patients admitted to intensive care units with acute exacebation of chronic obstructive pulmonary disease. JAMA 274:1852–1857
75. Connors AF, Dawson NV, Thomas C, et al (1996) Outcomes following acute exacerbation of severe chronic obstructive lung disease. Am J Respir Crit Care Med 154:959–967
76. Confalonieri M, Parigi P, Scartabellati A, et al (1996) Noninvasive mechanical ventilation improves the immediate and long-term outcome of COPD patients with acute respiratory failure. Eur Respir J 9:422–430
77. Vitacca M, Clini E, Rubini F, Nava S, Foglio K, Ambrosino N (1996) Non-invasive mechanical ventilation in severe chronic obstructive lung disease and acute respiratory failure: short- and long-term prognosis. Intensive Care Med 22:94–100
78. Costello R, Deegan P, Fitzpatrick M, McNicholas WT (1997) Reversible hypercapnia in chronic obstructive pulmonary disease: a distinct pattern of respiratory failure with a favorable prognosis. Am J Med 1997; 103:239–244

79. Ely EW, Baker AM, Dunagan DP, et al (1996) Effect on the duration of mechanical ventilation of identifying patients capable of breathing spontaneously. N Engl J Med 335:1864–1869
80. Kollef MH, Shapiro SD, Silver P, et al (1997) A randomized, controlled trial of protocol-directed versus physician-directed weaning from mechanical ventilation. Crit Care Med 25:567–574
81. Marelich GP, Murin S, Battistella F, et al (2000) Protocol weaning of mechanical ventilation in medical and surgical patients by respiratory care practitioners and nurses: effect on weaning time and incidence of ventilator-associated pneumonia. Chest 118:459–467

Morbidity and Functional Limitation in Survivors of ARDS

M.S. Herridge

Introduction

The study of morbidity in survivors of critical illness is complex. The complexity resides in the multifactorial nature of morbidity, the individuality of host response to a similar insult, and the reality that morbidity is dynamic and therefore changes over time. The challenge in studying and improving morbidity is to identify homogeneous populations of survivors of critical illness, characterize in detail the nature of their morbidity, and understand those factors that predict and modify that disability. To better characterize this dysfunction, we need to devise a method of measuring morbidity that is objective, comprehensive, quantitative, and functionally relevant, and to establish the post-intensive care unit (ICU) time interval in which disability stabilizes. Once these predictors of disability have been identified, an intervention, likely a multidisciplinary intervention, needs to be tested to determine if this morbidity can be ameliorated.

A theoretical construct of the determinants and modifiers of morbidity is presented in Figure 1. This model is proposed as a framework to better characterize the factors that influence outcome so that appropriate interventions may be initiated. This model will likely be most effective when applied within a relatively homogeneous population of critically ill patients. Premorbid health status is of central importance to long term morbidity after critical illness and yet very difficult to objectively quantify in the individual patient. Different disease severity scoring strategies or diagnostic labels, while useful, give us little insight into the true extent or severity of end organ damage and resultant baseline end organ reserve. Given that critical illness is a severe and generalized monophasic event, it is likely that there will be evidence of compromised reserve in all end organs if one looks hard enough. It remains challenging but important to devise new strategies to quantify the extent to which critical illness imparts a worsening of end organ reserve so that we can better understand what is truly ICU-acquired organ dysfunction. Furthermore, it is crucial to understand which end organs are the most vulnerable to this insult and in which organ systems this incremental disability is of the most functional consequence.

Physical resilience is defined as an individual's intrinsic capacity to rehabilitate from severe physical disability. This is included as a discrete predictor of morbidity because it defines the innate and dynamic aspect of an individual patient's ability to recover. The ability to predict physical recovery is more complex than simply defining the extent of residual organ reserve. Rather, we need to identify those traits that enable some patients to achieve remarkable outcomes from a severely compromised state. This process is modified by intrinsic host factors such as personality traits, intellectual ability (level of education as a surrogate measure), and access to monetary resources expressed as socioeconomic status.

Emotional and cognitive resilience is defined as an individual's intrinsic capacity to regain neuropsychological health after an episode of critical illness. There is tremendous individual heterogeneity in this recovery response and the process, like physical resilience, is intimately linked to personal and economic resources (modifiers). There is an important emerging literature evaluating the emotional and cognitive sequelae of the acute respiratory distress syndrome (ARDS). It is possible that early intervention by a neuropsychologist or psychiatrist may ameliorate some of this disability.

The stability of an individual's friendship and family network may be an important predictor of morbid outcome. With constrained health care resources, family members now assume a greater caregiver role and actively participate in nursing and rehabilitation of the patient within the home. In the early stages of physical recovery, intact family/friend support may be an important asset for advocacy with health care professionals such that specific obstacles to rehabilitation are identified and dealt with expeditiously. This may impact both on the rate and the extent of recovery that the patient ultimately achieves. An additional physician driven support network in the form of a post-ICU ambulatory follow-up clinic may prove to be another valuable resource. A formal follow-up process may facilitate early identification of morbid issues and referral to other subspecialists and health care professionals. As with the other two predictors, support systems would also be modified by individual and economic factors.

ICU care is another important and equally complex predictor of morbidity. It may be very difficult to ascertain the isolated impact of specific ICU process and care issues on individual patient outcome because there is so much heterogeneity in practice patterns and environmental factors both within and across different units. In addition, practice patterns are modified both by premorbid health status and extrinsic factors such as the advocacy of a vigilant friend/family network. Furthermore, the impact of ICU interventions may manifest differently according to baseline health status and organ reserve.

This chapter will evaluate the current understanding of morbidity and functional limitation in survivors of ARDS. Within the proposed model of morbidity in Figure 1, it will specifically outline the end-organ damage – both pulmonary and extrapulmonary – that may be responsible for the compromised physical function reported in these patients. The relative contribution of premorbid health status, physical resilience, physician support network in the form of a post-ICU ambulatory follow-up clinic and ICU care – four of the predictors of morbidity from the proposed model – will be discussed as they relate to this pulmonary and extrapulmonary morbidity. The ARDS population was chosen to highlight the complexity of factors influencing long-term morbidity. These include the sequelae of severe multiple organ dysfunction, the heterogeneity of intra-ICU management of respiratory and organ failure and the variable degree of emotional, cognitive and physical resilience in those who survive.

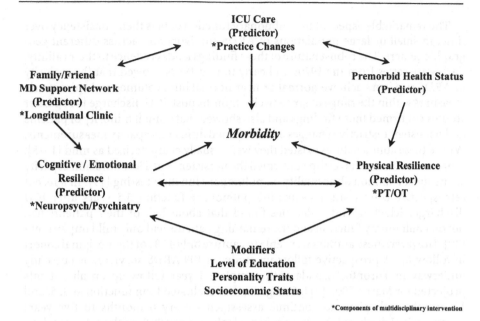

ICU Care
(Predictor)
*Practice Changes

Family/Friend
MD Support Network
(Predictor)
*Longitudinal Clinic

Premorbid Health Status
(Predictor)

Morbidity

Cognitive / Emotional
Resilience
(Predictor)
*Neuropsych/Psychiatry

Physical Resilience
(Predictor)
*PT/OT

Modifiers
Level of Education
Personality Traits
Socioeconomic Status

*Components of multidisciplinary intervention

Fig. 1. Model of predictors and modifiers of morbidity in survivors of critical illness

Pulmonary Morbidity

Evaluation of pulmonary function in survivors of ARDS has been the dominant theme in the outcomes literature since the first description of the syndrome in 1967 [1]. For the purposes of this review, pulmonary morbidity will be evaluated under the following headings: i) pulmonary function testing; ii) gas exchange at rest and with exercise; iii) chest radiology.

Pulmonary Function Testing

Until recently, studies of pulmonary function in ARDS survivors have suffered from the following limitations:
1) lack of consecutive patient selection and loss to follow-up resulting in compromised study validity because of selection bias;
2) limited sample size;
3) follow-up limited to a one year period, and
4) study of pulmonary function in isolation without simultaneous measurement of other relevant health and quality of life outcomes.

Perhaps the latter point has been the most limiting in ascertaining the true contribution of pulmonary dysfunction to overall functional and quality of life impairment in ARDS survivors.

The remarkable aspect of the pulmonary function data is their consistency over time, in small or large populations of ARDS survivors and across different geographic centers. The robust nature of these findings lends credence to their validity. Early case series from the 1970s and early to mid 1980s showed that the majority of ARDS survivors achieve normal or near normal lung volumes and spirometric measures within the range of six to twelve months post-ICU discharge [214]. Later studies confirmed these findings and also showed that a small minority of patients had persistent restrictive changes and abnormal diffusion capacity measurements. Where these abnormalities existed they were usually characterized as mild [1518]. More recent studies have also confirmed the persistence of a low diffusion capacity as the most common abnormality on pulmonary function testing [19]. In a recent retrospective cohort study evaluating pulmonary function 5.5 years after ICU discharge, Schelling and colleagues found that about half of their patients had normal pulmonary function and the remaining patients had only mild impairment [20]. However, these authors were able to capture only 42 % of their original cohort in follow-up. A prospective follow-up study on 109 ARDS survivors is currently underway in Toronto, Canada with complete 1-year follow-up on all patients projected for March 2002 [21]. Our group has evaluated lung function at 3, 6, and 12 months with plans to continue assessments every 6 months to five years following ICU discharge. We have achieved follow-up of 89 % of the cohort to date. Findings are similar to those outlined above in that volumetric and spirometric measures are normal or near normal by 6 to 12 months post-ICU discharge. Diffusion capacity is normal or near normal in most cases by 1 year. Where abnormalities persist beyond 1 year, they are mild.

Gas Exchange at Rest and on Exercise

Fewer studies have evaluated gas exchange at rest or on exertion in the ARDS population. One can imagine how important an adjunct these data may be in determining the pulmonary contribution to reported physical disability. In an early review of outcomes in ARDS patients, Alberts and colleagues qualitatively pooled data from 21 publications that evaluated varied outcome measures in ARDS survivors [13]. They found that resting arterial blood gas levels were measured at least once during follow-up in 91 ARDS patients. The levels were normal in 74 % of patients and there was some mild degree of hypoxia in the remainder. Of the 65 patients who were exercised, 48 % had a decline in their PaO_2. Three percent of patients developed hypercapnia with exercise. Qs/Qt calculations were reported in 38 patients and were normal in 90 % of this group. In their case series of 16 patients, Luhr and colleagues reported normal blood gas data in 15 of their patients [19]. Recent results from Schelling and co-workers reported PO_2 in the normal range at rest in all patients and only 6 % showed a mild degree of hypoxia during exercise, defined as below 80 % of predicted [20]. The Toronto ARDS follow-up group evaluated oxygen saturation at rest and on exercise in the context of a structured 6 minute walk test at 3, 6, 12 months and then every 6 months to five years. The data are consistent with those presented above. No ARDS survivor in this cohort has required home oxygen on an ongoing basis at one year post ICU discharge [21].

Chest Radiology

Several authors have looked at chest x-ray data in ARDS survivors. Without exception, the vast majority of ARDS survivors (>80 %) have normal chest radiographs with the average time to clearance of the lung fields measured in months [13, 19, 21]. A small minority has changes of hyperinflation (7 %) and interstitial infiltrates (11 %) [13].

When more detailed imaging is carried out, there is greater evidence of the sequelae of the episode of severe lung injury. Desai and colleagues [22] found that a reticular pattern with an anterior distribution was the most prevalent and extensive abnormality on computed tomography (CT) scanning in ARDS survivors. They determined a relationship between the extent of these reticular changes and total duration of mechanical ventilation and specifically to duration of pressure-controlled inverse-ratio ventilation. Nobauer-Huhmann recently published similar findings to the Desai paper [23]. They found fibrotic changes in 87 % of their patients and these were most pronounced in the ventral distribution. These authors found a correlation with duration of mechanical ventilation, high peak inspiratory pressures and exposure to high inspired oxygen fractions (FiO_2, >70 %).

It seems clear that virtually all ARDS survivors have some pulmonary sequelae of their severe episode of lung injury. The CT studies illustrate the fact that if you look hard enough you will be able to document some physical damage. However, the more relevant question is: What is the functional consequence of this injury? Based on the physiologic data presented, the overwhelming message is that functional pulmonary impairment is modest in most cases and when it does exist is generally mild. There are certainly outliers who have a greater degree of pulmonary dysfunction, but as a whole this group is not impressively disabled from a lung standpoint.

Who are the patients with poor long-term pulmonary function and what can we learn from them? If we return to our morbidity construct in Figure 1, we may gain some insight into this and future interventions that might minimize pulmonary dysfunction. It is possible that premorbid health status may play an important role here. This population of patients may have had significant but relatively asymptomatic intrinsic lung disease prior to their episode of acute lung injury. Even a modest loss of pulmonary function following ARDS may be enough to compromise reserve such that the patient is now quite compromised.

Heterogeneity in ICU practice may be an important determinant of pulmonary outcome as well. There may be differences in the degree to which patients were managed with lung protective strategies during their episode of ARDS or differences in the surveillance and management of ventilator associated pneumonias or other nosocomial pulmonary complications. Clearly, there are a myriad of possible interventions within the ICU that may have some beneficial impact on long-term pulmonary dysfunction in the susceptible host. The challenge will be to determine which of these interventions results in the greatest pulmonary benefit to the patient. Gaining a better understanding of intrinsic host factors that determine recovery from diffuse alveolar damage may also yield valuable insights into how to better manage this susceptible group of patients. Knowledge of the cellular/genetic basis of physical resilience may enable us to optimize pulmonary outcomes in our most vulnerable patients.

Finally, there may simply be too much heterogeneity in the population to be able to ascertain the natural history of the disease under study. The Toronto ARDS Outcomes group has found a 5 % incidence of bronchiolitis obliterans organizing pneumonia (BOOP) and bronchiolitis obliterans (BO) in those recruited as ARDS patients because they fulfill ARDS criteria [21]. The natural history of untreated BOOP/BO is very different from that of diffuse alveolar damage and it is possible that this heterogeneity is one explanation for the differences in observed pulmonary outcome. Through a long-term follow-up clinic, ARDS patients might be screened to determine if they may fall into this subset. Early identification and treatment of this group with steroids may offer better long-term pulmonary outcomes.

Extrapulmonary Morbidity

In 1994, McHugh and her colleagues from Seattle addressed some of the limitations of the previous ARDS follow-up studies [18]. Specifically, they set out to simultaneously measure pulmonary function at defined time intervals and combine this with a generic quality of life assessment to determine the relationship between any observed pulmonary dysfunction and self-report functional disability. The Sickness Impact Profile (SIP) measures the subject's self-perceived physical and psychological condition [24, 25]. The psychosocial aspect of the score measures emotional behavior, communication, and social interaction. The physical aspect evaluates patient's perceptions of mobility, ambulation, and self care. These authors found that the SIP scores were very low at the time of extubation, rose substantially in the first 3 months and then exhibited only slight improvement to 1 year. When combined with an additional lung score, patients perceived that only a modest proportion of their overall dysfunction was due to their lungs.

Weinert and colleagues also identified important functional impairment in a cohort of survivors from acute lung injury [26]. They administered a different generic quality of life measure, the Medical Outcomes Study 36-item short-form health survey (SF-36), to their patients. This health profile provides scores in eight domains including physical and social functioning, role limitations because of emotional or physical problems, mental health, vitality, bodily pain, and general health perceptions [27]. While all domains of the SF-36 were reduced in their ARDS survivors, the largest decrement was in the role functioning physical domain. This domain is defined as the extent to which physical health interferes with work or other daily activities, including accomplishing less than wanted, limitations in the kind of activities, or difficulty in performing activities. While some of this dysfunction was attributed to pulmonary specific issues, many patients reported a more global and generalized disability. The following is a quotation from one of the ARDS survivors who participated in their focus group: "One thing I find somewhat alarming is that when they measure my lung capacity it measures 80 % which they consider normal so in a sense they're telling me I'm fine now and there is nothing wrong with me. And yet I can't do any of the things that I took for granted."

Schelling and coworkers have administered the SF-36 to their ARDS survivors in two separate studies and in both studies noted that the largest decrements in each case occurred in the role-physical domain [20, 28]. These authors inferred that this physical disability was on a pulmonary basis but did not provide any corroborative data to support this contention.

Davidson and colleagues designed a study to determine if there were differences in the health-related quality of life in ARDS survivors and comparably ill controls [29]. They used both a generic quality of life measure (SF-36) and a pulmonary disease specific questionnaire (St. Georges Respiratory Questionnaire [SGRQ]) to ascertain the degree to which perceived disability in ARDS survivors was related to pulmonary dysfunction. Similar to previously published quality of life reports, these authors found that all domains of the SF-36 were reduced and that the largest decrement was in the role-physical domain (Table 1).

The SGRQ is a 76-item pulmonary disease-specific questionnaire comprised of three domains: symptoms, activity, and impacts [30]. This questionnaire has only been validated in patients with intrinsic lung disease. The ARDS survivors had significantly worse scores on the SGRQ than similarly ill critical care controls. These authors concluded that there was a significant and ARDS specific, pulmonary component to this reported functional disability (Table 1).

The Toronto ARDS Outcomes group also administered both the SF-36 and SGRQ to their ARDS survivors [21, 31]. However, in contrast to the Davidson study where the questionnaire was administered once at a median of 23 months from time of hospital admission, the questionnaires were simultaneously administered at each follow-up time interval. Similar to the other studies, the Toronto data demonstrate that all domains of the SF-36 are reduced with the largest reductions in the physical functioning and role-physical domains. The Toronto SGRQ data are also abnormal but the reader will note in Table 2 that the most dynamic domain in the scoring system is that of activity. Activity score improves over time and is the main determinant of the abnormality reported in the total score [31]. In our dataset, the improvement in the SGRQ score coincides with the improvement in the role-physical and physical functioning domains of the SF-36. It may be inferred from these data that the disability represented by an increased score in the SGRQ activity domain may not be specific to intrinsic pulmonary dysfunction – and we have already seen that pulmonary dysfunction in ARDS survivors is modest – but rather reflects any cause of impaired physical functioning. Furthermore, symptoms such as dyspnea thought to be lung specific – may also be reported in the context of any physical dysfunction that results in an increased perceived work of breathing. Extrapulmonary factors such as muscle loss/weakness or neuromuscular disease may similarly be reflected as abnormal SGRQ symptom scores.

The quality of life data from most studies are consistent and underscore the functional limitation experienced by ARDS survivors. In the context of all of the previously presented pulmonary morbidity data, which supports mostly mild intrinsic pulmonary dysfunction, there must be other important determinants of this reported disability.

Table 1. Domains of the SF-36 and the St. George's Respiratory Questionnaire (expressed as mean SD) in ARDS cases reported a median of 23 months following hospital admission. From [29] with permission

	Matched Controls (n=73)	All ARDS Cases (n=77)
Short Form 36*		
Physical Functioning	84±17	61±25
Role-physical	58±32	33±33
Bodily Pain	68±20	53±25
General Health	65±19	49±21
Vitality	64±14	49±20
Social Functioning	78±18	60±27
Role-emotional	72±36	64±41
Mental Health	75±15	64±18
St. George's Respiratory Questionnaire**		
Symptoms	26±21	45±22
Activity	18±17	39±23
Impacts	6± 9	15±16
Total	13±11	27±17

* higher score denotes better quality of life
** lower score denotes better quality of life

Table 2. Changes in the domains of the St. Georges Respiratory Questionnaire (expressed as mean SD) from 3 to 12 months after ICU discharge in ARDS survivors. From [31] with permission

	3 Months	6 Months	12 Months	p value
St. Georges Respiratory Questionnaire*				
Symptoms	23±20	25±17	21±20	0.85
Activity	**53±26**	**45±28**	**30±26**	**0.05**
Impacts	23±18	21±23	15±17	0.56
Total	33±18	28±20	21±18	0.19

* lower score denotes better quality of life

Objective Measures of Function

One of the great deficiencies in the ARDS morbidity literature has been the absence of any data that could objectively quantify functional disability. In the context of an ARDS follow-up study seeking to determine if a ventilation strategy to prevent barotrauma changed long term outcome, Cooper and his colleagues [32] were among the first to combine a simple measure of exercise distance walked in 6 minutes – with pulmonary function and quality of life. They were able to evaluate only a limited subset of the survivors from their randomized controlled trial approximately 1 to 2 years after ICU admission, but their qualitative results were informative. Their survivors also reported a functional limitation and this was in the context of very modest pulmonary dysfunction and normal arterial blood gases at rest. The patients were only able to walk on average 373 meters during the 6-minute exercise test and this exercise capacity was comparable to patients with chronic respiratory disease.

The Toronto ARDS follow-up group [21] combined a 6-minute walk distance with the other outcome measures that have been discussed previously. We found that distance walked in 6-minutes, although it improved substantially from the 3 month to 12 month visits, remained below that predicted for age and gender matched controls.

Neuromuscular and Skeletal Dysfunction

Following ICU discharge, all ARDS survivors are cachectic, deconditioned, and have lost approximately 20 % of their baseline weight [21]. Many patients have to learn how to weight bear and walk again. Virtually all patients have some important proximal muscle weakness such that they cannot fully abduct their arms nor can they get out of chairs or climb stairs. They attribute their inability to perform activities of daily living to profound generalized weakness secondary to loss of muscle mass and deconditioning [21]. These patients report exertional dyspnea and perceive it to be on an extrapulmonary basis. Other important neuromuscular and skeletal sequelae that may contribute to functional impairment are outlined under the following headings: a) critical illness polyneuropathy; b) entrapment neuropathies; c) ICU acquired myopathy; d) heterotopic ossification.

Critical Illness Polyneuropathy: In the 1980s, an acute polyneuropathy was described in multiple organ dysfunction and sepsis. Termed critical illness polyneuropathy, this condition is characterized both electrophysiologically and morphologically by a primary axonal degeneration of motor and sensory fibers [33–36]. Critical illness polyneuropathy has a reported prevalence of 70 % [36] and has been found in populations of patients with sepsis/multiple organ dysfunction and ARDS [37]. While the precise etiology of this condition remains unknown, there is increasing evidence that critical illness polyneuropathy may be due to ischemia secondary to a disturbance in the microcirculation. The severity of critical illness polyneuropathy is associated with the severity of multiple organ dysfunction [38] and not the concurrent administration of neuromuscular blocking agents or steroids [39]. This lends support for the argument that this polyneuropathy should be regarded as another vulnerable end organ system in the multiple organ failure syndrome. This entity is likely under diagnosed and may contribute significantly to functional limitation in ARDS survivors. Consistent with the functional outcome data previously presented, recovery was complete or near complete in those who had mild or moderately severe involvement. No patients who had severe involvement were able to survive their ICU stay [36].

Entrapment Neuropathies: The Toronto ARDS Outcomes study evaluated the incidence of entrapment neuropathies in our population of ARDS survivors. The incidence of peroneal nerve palsy with resultant foot drop was approximately 5 % [21]. Although only a small proportion of our patients suffered from this, it was a very morbid event and had a profound impact on their rehabilitation and in one case precluded return to original work. Others have also noted that compression neuropathies may cause permanent sequelae [40].

ICU-acquired Myopathy: The incidence of an ICU-acquired myopathy and its impact on disability and prolonged rehabilitation in the post-ICU period remains uncertain. There are several reports of ICU-acquired muscle lesions but these are often described as heterogeneous ranging from non-specific myopathic changes to discrete type II fiber atrophy [39]. Myopathic changes have been postulated to be on a catabolic basis [34] and have been documented in the absence of corticosteroid or neuromuscular blocker use [41]. Several patients from the Toronto ARDS cohort who had persistent complaints of muscle weakness underwent open muscle biopsy [21]. All of these patients had evidence of a myopathic process secondary to a monophasic illness. Several had significant type II fiber drop-out, the sort of muscle injury observed in prolonged immobilization and disuse. This lesion is very responsive to rehabilitation. These observations may again underscore the importance of detailed characterization of end organ morbidity because they have implications for rehabilitation and amelioration of ultimate functional disability.

Heterotopic Ossification

Heterotopic ossification is the deposition of para-articular ectopic bone and is associated with polytrauma, burns, pancreatitis, and ARDS [43, 44]. It is known to follow paralysis from traumatic and atraumatic neurologic insults. It follows that our critically ill patients, often paralyzed and usually sedated, would be at risk for this condition. In the Toronto ARDS Outcomes cohort [21], the incidence of heterotopic ossification was 3 %. This is low, but in each case a large joint was completely immobilized by this para-articular bony deposition. Patients could not walk and in one case had no functional use of a dominant arm/hand. This entity is important to identify because it requires surgical debridement of the bony deposition to achieve a good functional outcome at the affected joint site.

If we again consider the construct of morbidity outlined in Figure 1, it might assist us in considering the important predictors of extrapulmonary outcomes and how to design interventions to minimize this morbidity. For this discussion, we will focus on the potential impact of ICU care and a post ICU follow-up clinic on these outcomes.

While there does appear to be evidence to support individual susceptibility to extrapulmonary morbid events, the nature of ICU care is clearly an important determinant of these outcomes. Entrapment neuropathies should be a wholly preventable morbid outcome if we are rigorous about patient positioning during ICU care. In the context of a patient who has a high acuity of illness and is difficult to oxygenate, mundane issues such as positioning are frequently overlooked. However, if that patient survives and has foot drop, that may be the most morbid event of their critical illness and ICU stay.

It may be more difficult to minimize critical illness myopathies and heterotopic ossification. Given that the literature supports a significant degree of type II muscle cell drop out in survivors of ARDS and critical illness, one might postulate that minimal use of sedation and paralytics and early mobilization/rehabilitation within the ICU might be important in minimizing some of this morbidity. This same argument might follow for those at risk of heterotopic ossification since the literature indicates that immobility is a major predisposing factor.

Early identification and intervention of these extrapulmonary sequelae may be facilitated through a post ICU follow-up clinic and may help minimize some of this disability. Those patients with type II muscle cell myopathy and critical illness polyneuropathy need intensive rehabilitation therapy and a follow-up clinic will not only help identify those who are most profoundly affected but may also serve to facilitate rehabilitation referrals. Those with heterotopic ossification need to have surgical debridement of the para-articular bone deposits or they will not regain good function of the involved joint. A post ICU follow-up clinic will identify these patients and make appropriate referral to an orthopedic surgeon skilled in treating this complication.

Conclusion

This chapter has proposed a new construct for considering the complexity of morbidity in patients who survive an episode of critical illness. This author suggests that we need to fully characterize the morbidity of critical illness across all organ systems to better understand the predictors and modifiers of disability. In addition, we need to determine which organ system impairments are the most consequential in terms of functional outcome and make these the focus for future intervention.

ARDS survivors were used to illustrate the complexity of the determinants of functional outcome. The current literature would suggest that the disability in these patients is multifactorial. There appears to be only mild pulmonary dysfunction in ARDS survivors. Most patients attribute their functional disability to profound loss of muscle mass and resultant generalized weakness. In some patients there may be additional mobility problems related to discrete neuromuscular diagnoses or heterotopic ossification.

References

1. Ashbaugh DG, Bigelow DB, Petty TL (1967) Acute respiratory distress in adults. Lancet 2:319–323
2. Downs JB, Olsen GN (1974) Pulmonary function following adult respiratory distress syndrome. Chest 65:92–93
3. Yernault JC, Englert M, Sergysels R, et al (1975) Pulmonary mechanics and diffusion after "shock lung" Thorax 30:252–257
4. Lakshminarayan S, Stanford RE, Petty TL (1976) Prognosis after recovery from adult respiratory distress syndrome. Am Rev Respir Dis 113:716
5. Klein JJ, van Haeringen JR, Sluiter HJ, et al (1976) Pulmonary function after recovery from the adult respiratory distrss syndrome. Chest 69:350–355
6. Richardson JV, Light RW, Baskin TW, et al (1976) Late pulmonary function in survivors of adult respiratory distress syndrome. South Med J 69:737–740
7. Rotman HH, Lavelle TF, Dimcheff DG, et al (1977) Longterm physiologic consequences of the adult respiratory distress syndrome. Chest 72:190–192
8. Simpson DL, Goodman M, Spector SL, et al (1978) Long-term follow-up and bronchial reactivity testing in survivors of the adult respiratory distress syndrome. Am Rev Respir Dis 117:449–454
9. Yahav J, Lieberman P, Molho M (1978) Pulmonary function following the adult respiratory distress syndrome. Chest 74:247–250
10. Lakshminarayam S, Hudson LD (1978) Pulmonary function following the adult respiratory distress syndrome. 74: 489–490
11. Shaw RA, Whitcomb ME, Schonfeld SA (1981) Pulmonary function after adult respiratory distress syndrome associated with Legionnaires disease pneumonia. Arch Intern Med 141:741–742
12. Elliott CG, Morris AH, Cengiz M (1981) Pulmonary function and exercise gas exchange in survivors of the adult respiratory distress syndrome. Am Rev Respir Dis 123: 492–495
13. Alberts WM, Priest GR, Moser KM (1983) The outlook for survivors of ARDS. Chest 84:272–274
14. Halevy A, Sirik Z, Adam YG, et al (1984) Long-term evaluation of patients following the adult respiratory distress syndrome. Respir Care 29:132–137
15. Elliott CG, Rasmusson BY, Crapo RO, et al (1987) Prediction of pulmonary function abnormalities after adult respiratory distress syndrome (ARDS). Am Rev Respir Dis 135:634–638
16. Ghio AJ, Elliott CG, Crapo RO (1989) Impairment after adult respiratory distress syndrome: an evaluation based on American Thoracic Society recommendations. Am Rev Respir Dis 139:1158–1162
17. Peters JI, Bell RC, Prihoda TJ, et al (1989) Clinical determinants of abnormalities in pulmonary functions in survivors of the adult respiratory distress syndrome. Am Rev Respir Dis 139:1163–1168
18. McHugh LG, Milberg JA, Whitcomb ME, Schoene RB, Maunder RJ, Hudson LD (1994). Recovery of function in survivors of the acute respiratory distress syndrome. Am J Respir Crit Care Med 150:90–94
19. Luhr O, Aardal S, Nathorst-Westfelt U, et al (1998) Pulmonary function in adult survivors of severe acute lung injury treated with inhaled nitric oxide. Acta Anaesthesiol Scand 42:391–398
20. Schelling G, Stoll C, Vogelmeier C, et al (2000) Pulmonary function and health-related quality of life in a sample of long-term survivors of the acute respiratory distress syndrome. Intensive Care Med 26:1304–1311
21. Herridge MS, Cheung AM, Tansey CM, et al (2001) Long term outcomes in survivors of ARDS. Am J Respir Crit Care Med:A253 (abst)
22. Desai SR, Wells AU, Rubens MB, Evans TW, Hansell DM (1999) Acute respiratory distress syndrome: CT abnormalities at long term follow-up. Radiology 21:29–35

23. Nobauer-Huhmann IM, Eibenberger KR, Schaefer-Prokop CR, et al (2001) Changes in lung parenchyma after acute respiratory distress syndrome (ARDS): assessment with high-resolution computed tomography. Eur Radiol 11:2436–2443

24. Gilson BS, Gilson JS, Bergner M, et al (1975) The sickness impact profile: development of an outcome measure of health care. Am J Public Health 65:1304–1307

25. Bergner M, Bobbit RA, Carter WC, et al (1981) The sickness impact profile:development and final revision of a health status measure. Med Care 19:787–805

26. Weinert CR, Gross CR, Kangas JR, Bury CL, Marinelli WA (1997) Health-related quality of life after acute lung injury. Am J Respir Crit Care Med 156:1120–1128

27. Ware JE, Sherbourne CD (1992) The MOS 36-item ahort form health survey (SF-36). I. Conceptual framework and item selection. Med Care 30:473–483

28. Schelling G, Stoll C, Haller M, et al (1998) Health-related quality of life and posttraumatic stress disorder in survivors of the acute respiratory distress syndrome. Crit Care Med 26: 651–659

29. Davidson TA, Caldwell ES, Curtis JR, Hudson LD, Steinberg KP (1999) Reduced quality of life in survivors of acute respiratory distress syndrome compared with critically ill control patients. JAMA 281:354–360

30. Jones PW, Quirk FH, Baveystock CM (1991) The St. Georges respiratory questionnaire. Respir Med 85:25–31

31. Tansey C, Cheung AM, Matte-Martyn A, et al (2002) Serial St. Georges Respiratory Questionnaire (SGRQ): Measures in ARDS survivors. Am J Respir Crit Care Med (abst, in press)

32. Cooper AB, Ferguson ND, Hanly PJ, et al (1999) Long-term follow-up of survivors of acute lung injury: Lack of effect of a ventilation strategy to prevent barotrauma. Crit Care Med 27:2616–2621

33. Bolton CF, Gilbert JJ, Hahn AF, Sibbald WJ (1984) Polyneuropathy in critically ill patients. J Neurol Neurosurg Psychiatry 47:1223–1231

34. Zochodne DW, Bolton CF, Wells GA, et al (1987) Critical illness polyneuropathy: a complication of sepsis and multiple organ failure. Brain 110: 819–842

35. Bolton CF, Laverty DA, Brown JD, Witt NJ, Hahn AF, Sibbald WJ (1986) Critically ill polyneuropathy: electrophysiological studies and differentiation from Guillain-Barre syndrome. J Neurol Neurosurg Psychiatry 49:563–573

36. Witt NJ, Ochodne DW, Bolton CF, et al (1991) Peripheral nerve function in sepsis and multiple organ failure. Chest 99:176–184

37. Lopez Messa JB, Garcia A (1990) Acute polyneuropathy in critically ill patients Intensive Care Med 16:159–162

38. Leijten FSS, DeWeerd AW, Poortvliet DCJ, et al (1996) Critical Illness polyneuropathy in multiple organ dysfunction syndrome and weaning from the ventilator. Intensive Care Med 22:856–861

39. Zifko UA, Zipko HT, Bolton CF (1998) Clinical and electrophysiological findings in critical illness polyneuropathy. J Neurol Sci 14:186–193

40. Wijdicks EF, Litchy WJ, Harrison BA, Gracey DR (1995) The clinical spectrum of critical illness polyneuropathy. Mayo Clin Proc 70:198–200

41. Deconinck N, Van Parijs V, Beckers-Bleukx G, Van den Bergh P (1998) Critical illness myopathy unrelated to corticosteroids or neuromuscular blocking agents. Neuromuscul Disord 8:186–192

42. Clements NC, Camilli AE (1993) Heterotopic ossification complicating critical illness. Chest 104:1526–1528

43. Jacobs JW, De Sonnaville PB, Hulsmans HM, van Rinsum AC, Bijlsma JW (1999) Polyarticular heterotopic ossification complicating critical illness. Rheumatology 38:1145–1149

Health-related Quality of Life

K. M. Rowan, C. Jenkinson, and N. Black

Introduction

The primary aims of health care are the reduction of mortality and morbidity, and the maintenance or improvement of functional capacity and quality of life. Traditionally, the assessment of critical care has focused largely on mortality and assessment of the health of survivors in terms of physiological, radiological, and biochemical measurements of impairment. This is now changing. Recently, there has been a move away from these objective measures towards subjective measures of functional status and health-related quality of life (HRQL), with data collected directly from patients [1]. Interest in patients' perspectives in the evaluation of health care has led to the development of numerous subjective measures.

The ideal outcome of health care is for the patient to return to their pre-existing state or that expected for a person of the same age and medical condition [2, 3]. Whether objective or subjective measures are used, they must provide information that is valid, reliable and responsive (Table 1).

Outcome measures can be divided into measures of impairment, functional status (also known as health status or disability) and HRQL (also known as handicap or well-being). Impairment refers to objective measures of anatomical, physiological or biochemical aspects such as hemoglobin concentration or respiratory rate. These are the underlying features of ill-health that can be assessed or measured by another person, rather than the symptoms or problems that patients report.

Impairment may, or may not, affect a person's functional status by giving rise to symptoms or limitations in their ability to function. For example, low hemoglobin (impairment) may be associated with breathlessness (disability), which may be associated with an inability to go for a walk in the country (quality of life). As Table 2 illustrates, measures of impairment, functional status and HRQL may either be generic or specific to a particular condition.

As patients admitted to critical care are a heterogeneous group, there is a need for generic outcome measures, which can be used across a wide range of medical and surgical conditions, as well as condition-specific ones.

Most of the measures that are available to be used in critical care are multi-item scales; that is, they are made up of several (or many) questions/items. Some multi-item scales not only provide a total score indicating the overall aspect being

Table 1. Validity, reliability and responsiveness (based on [4])

Validity

A valid assessment is one that measures what it claims to measure. The evaluation of the validity of a measure usually involves comparison with some standardized criterion or criteria. This is no easy thing in the social sciences as there are rarely 'gold standards' against which measures can be compared. However, a number of standard criteria for validity are usually assessed for any properly constructed questionnaire.

Face validity refers to whether items on a questionnaire appear both appropriate to the phenomenon being measured and to make sense, as well as being easily understood.

Content validity refers to choice of, and relative importance given to, items on a questionnaire. It is important that items appropriate to the phenomenon under investigation are chosen and if they are weighted in some way, that the weights reflect the perceived level of difficulty or health problem.

Construct validity is an important aspect of validity, especially where the variable being measured cannot be observed directly. It refers to where hypotheses are generated and a questionnaire is tested to determine if it actually reflects these prior hypotheses. For example, the construct validity of a measure can be checked to ensure that certain groups (e.g., older, lower social classes, those with illnesses) would gain worse scores than other groups (e.g., younger, higher social classes, those without illnesses).

Criterion validity refers to the ability of an instrument to correspond with other measures held up as 'gold standards'. In practice, few studies can truly claim to have evaluated criterion validity, as 'gold standards' are hard to find in this area of research.

Reliability

As with validity, there are a number of methods of assessing reliability. The most commonly used method is referred to as **internal reliability** or internal consistency and is measured using Cronbach's α statistic (for items with more than two response categories, such as: "Never"; "Sometimes"; "Always").

In **test-retest reliability** the questionnaire is administered on two occasions separated by a few days. Ideally respondents should not have changed in any way between the two administrations of the questionnaire and consequently the two administrations should produce almost identical results.

Responsiveness

It is essential that evaluative instruments are able to detect change and the level of this change is interpretable in some way. The sensitivity to change or responsiveness of an instrument is a very important criterion to consider when selecting measures.

The effect size statistic is the most commonly cited interpretation of change scores. This is usually calculated by subtracting the mean value before treatment with that gained after treatment, then dividing the result with the baseline standard deviation.

Table 2. Outcome measures – example for osteoarthritis of the hip

	Impairment	Functional status	Health-related quality of life
Disease specific	X-ray changes	Pain in hip Poor mobility	Unable to garden
Generic		Activities of Daily Living scale	Perceived Quality of Life scale

measured, for example, physical functional status, but also generate sub-scales, which provide information on particular aspects, for example, mobility. However, not all measures are multi-item. Some single item measures exist which generally consist of a global question that attempts to encompass the person's overall state of health.

This chapter provides a methodological review of the existing literature on outcome measures of HRQL that have been used with adults following discharge from critical care (intensive care and high dependency care) and identifies the key gaps for further research. It is based on a comprehensive review of the literature on outcome measures of impairment, functional status and HRQL used in critical care funded by the National Health Service Health Technology Assessment Program [5]. The review encompassed a comprehensive search for relevant methodological studies. Searching included: electronic databases; manual searching of both journals and conference proceedings not indexed by the electronic databases; cross-referencing with reference lists of other reviews; snowballing from the reference lists of retrieved, relevant studies; and contact with experts in the field.

The objectives of this chapter are to:
- describe the main measures of HRQL that have been used in adult survivors of critical care;
- review the validity, reliability and responsiveness of HRQL that have been used in adult survivors of critical care;
- review what is currently known about the HRQL of adult survivors of critical care
- conclude, making recommendations for further research.

We have confined ourselves to survivors of adult (16 years and over) critical care, and exclude survivors of units that fulfil a specialized function such as coronary care, burns and post-anesthesia care but includes intensive care units (ICUs) that restrict admission to certain groups, such as post-surgical. We exclude studies where the sample size was less than twenty patients. Some degree of overlap exists within some measures. If a measure included functional status in addition to HRQL, it was included. Both multi-item and single item, generic and disease-specific measures are included. For inclusion, a measure had to have been used in at least two studies. In addressing the third objective, we include only those measures that have been used in at least ten studies – to enhance the external validity of the conclusions.

Main Measures of HRQL that have been Used in Adult Survivors of Critical Care

Nine measures of HRQL had been used in studies of critical care survivors (Table 3). A brief description of each is found below. A more detailed description can be found elsewhere [6].

Sickness Impact Profile (SIP)

The SIP was developed by Bergner and colleagues as a measure of perceived health status across a wide number of health problems and diseases [7, 8]. The SIP focuses on the resultant impact that sickness has on functional status and quality of life. It assesses: work, recreation, emotion, affect, home life, sleep, rest, eating, ambulation, mobility, communication, and social functioning. Scores can be obtained for the twelve dimensions as well as summary physical and psychosocial scores and a global aggregated score (all measured on the range 0–100 with a lower score representing good health). In the UK, modifications to the SIP have resulted in the Functional Limitations Profile (FLP) [9].

Perceived Quality of Life Scale (PQOL)

The PQOL was developed as a cognitive measure of quality of life and satisfaction for medical patients in critical care [10]. It comprises eleven items: health, thinking,

Table 3. Main generic and disease-specific measures of health-related quality of life that have been used in adult survivors of critical care

Sickness Impact/Functional Limitation Profile (SIP/FLP)

Perceived Quality of Life Scale (PQOL)

Nottingham Health Profile (NHP)

Short Form-36 (SF-36)

Rosser Disability and Distress Categories

Spitzer Quality of Life Index

Psychological General Well-Being Schedule (PGWB)

Fernandez questionnaire

Whiston Hospital questionnaire

happiness, family, help, community, leisure, income, respect, meaning, and work (all measured on the range 0–100 with a higher score representing good health). The average of the question scores provides a summated rating score.

Nottingham Health Profile (NHP)

The NHP was developed in the UK and is based on lay perceptions of functional status and quality of life [11]. The NHP was designed to measure the experience of ill health, and comprises two parts. Part I measures perceived or subjective functional status by requiring a yes or no answer to 38 statements associated with six dimensions: physical mobility, pain, sleep, energy, emotional reactions, and social isolation (all measured on the range 0–100 with a lower score representing good health). Part II of the questionnaire focuses on quality of life and asks the subjects about the effects of their functional health status on seven areas of daily life: work, looking after the home, social life, home life, sex life, interests/hobbies, and holidays.

Short Form 36 (SF-36)

The Short Form 36 (SF-36) is the product of two large studies conducted in the USA: the Health Insurance Experiment and the Medical Outcomes Study [2]. The SF-36 comprises eight dimensions: physical functioning, social functioning, role limitations due to physical problems, role limitations due to emotional problems, general mental health, energy/vitality, bodily pain, and general health perceptions. Item scores for each of these dimensions are summated and transformed using a scoring algorithm (all measured on the range 0–100% with a higher score representing good health).

Rosser Disability and Distress Categories

Rosser Disability and Distress Categories measure the degree of disability and distress experienced. The measure is composed of four dimensions: general mobility, usual activity, self-care, and social and personal relationships [12]. General mobility and usual activity are scored from 1 to 6 and from 1 to 4, respectively. The other two dimensions are scored from 0–4. The maximum score is 18 (with a lower score representing good health). An allocation method then enables the scores to be categorized from I to VII, where I is least disabled and VII is most disabled.

Spitzer Quality of Life Index

This Index was developed by Spitzer and colleagues to be used by clinicians in assessing chronically ill patients and those suffering from cancer [13]. The Quality of Life Index comprises the following dimensions: activity, performance of activities of daily living, perception of health, support from family and friends, and outlook on life. Respondents select items in terms of the applicability of statements to them. The Index also includes a visual-analog scale (uniscale), which requests the respondent and the interviewer to mark an X on a line, which rates quality of life from 'lowest quality of life to highest quality of life'. The scale can be summed to give an overall single score or each item in the Index can be presented separately.

Psychological General Well-being Schedule (PGWB)

The PGWB was designed to measure feelings of well-being and distress rather than a broader concept of quality of life [14, 15]. The domains include: anxiety, depression, positive well-being, self-control, general health, and vitality. The Schedule consists of eighteen questions and utilizes a six-point response scale for intensity or frequency (for 14 items) and a 0–10 rating scale defined by adjectives at each end (for 4 items). Total scores from 0–60 reflect severe psychological distress, 61–72 represent moderate psychological distress, and 73–110 represent positive psychological well-being.

Fernandez Questionnaire

Fernandez and colleagues developed a questionnaire based in part on the Activities of Daily Living Scale, which comprised fifteen items grouped into three subscales assessing: physiological activities, normal daily activities, and emotional state [16]. Scores range from 0–29 (with a lower score representing good quality of life).

Whiston Hospital Questionnaire

The Whiston Hospital Questionnaire was developed by Jones and colleagues [17]. It comprises a pre-morbid health questionnaire and a reworded follow-up questionnaire, which is loosely based on the FLP. The information collected includes: previous/current health, mobility, work, leisure, and contact with friends or relatives (all measured on the range 0–3 with a lower score representing good health). The maximum possible total score is 25.

Validity, Reliability and Responsiveness of HRQL Measures that have been Used in Adult Survivors of Critical Care

Information on three measurement properties (validity, reliability and responsiveness – see: Table 1 for definitions) in adult critical care were sought for each of the nine measures considered. If the measurement properties were not reported explicitly, an attempt to infer some information from the data presented, was made.

Table 4. Evidence for the validity, reliability and responsiveness of the nine main measures of health-related quality of life

	Construct validity	Criterion validity	Internal reliability	Test- retest reliability	Responsiveness
SIP	[18, 19, 20, 21, 22, 23]	[17, 23, 24, 25]	[23]	[17]	[21]
PQOL	–	[10, 17, 26, 27]	[10]	–	[28, 29]
NHP	[27, 30, 31]	[27, 30, 32, 33]	–	–	–
SF-36	[34, 35, 36, 37]	[36]	[36, 37, 38]	–	[34]
Rosser	–	–	–	–	[29]
Spitzer	[39]	–	–	–	[39, 40]
PGWB	–	[10]	–	–	–
Fernandez	[41, 42]	[16]	[16, 41]	[16, 41]	[41, 42]
Whiston	[17, 26]	[17, 26]	–	–	–

The studies providing evidence for the measurement properties of the nine main measures are summarized in Table 4.

SIP

Construct validity was assessed using the variable age. Weak associations were found between age and several dimensions of SIP [18, 19] and with the total SIP score [20]. One study did not find an association with age [21]. Direct and proxy measures of severity (Therapeutic Intervention Scoring System [TISS], Acute Physiology And Chronic Health Evaluation II [APACHE II], Injury Severity Score [ISS], length of stay) were either weakly or not associated with SIP scores [20, 21, 22]. One study considered pre-admission employment status, income and educational level and demonstrated only weak association [23].

Criterion validity was assessed using a variety of measures. SIP scores were significantly associated with one measure of impairment (electroencephalography) [24] but not with another (DLCO) [25]. There was also no association with the level of social networks a subject had, but SIP scores were associated with their employment status [23]. There was also evidence of the criterion validity of the SIP in the observed associations with the PQOL and the Whiston Hospital Questionnaire [17].

Table 5. Detail of studies using the SIP or FLP

Study	N	N available for follow-up	N (%) followed up	Type of critical care patients	Mean age in years ± SD or (range)	Male (%)	Severity, mean ± SD [median] (range)	Mean follow up period in months [median] or (range)	Mode
[18]	472	N/A	424 (N/A)	CPR	N/A	N/A	N/A	6	I
[19]	337	254	140 (55)	General	58.4	50	APACHE II 13.3 TISS 104	(15-20)	Q (mail/tel)
[43]	156	119	59 (50)	General	74.5	50	N/A	18 (16-20)	Q (mail/tel)
[44]	193	110	69 (63)	Medical/respiratory	68.9 ± 8.4	52	APACHE II 13.0 ± 7	N/A	I (face)
[10]	160	90	69 (77)	Medical/respiratory	69 ± 8.0	52	APACHE II 13.0 ± 6	[19]	I (face)
[45]	1345	1261	887 (70)	General	59 ± 18.2	57	N/A	6	Q (mail)
[46]	131	131	131(100)	Mild head injury Moderate head injury Severe head injury	36 ± 14.1 43 ± 18.2 39.5 ± 17.1	80	GCS 6.2 ± 1.97 GCS 13.3 ± 2.0 GCS 13.2 ± 2.6	(4-98)	I
[47]	1308	N/A	N/A	General	N/A	N/A	N/A	(12 - 60)	Q (mail)
[22]	330	256	157 (61)	General	47 ± 23.5 (1 - 92)	63	N/A	N/A	I (face)
[24]	112	N/A	17 (N/A)	Liver and heart transplant	45.8 ± 12.1	67	N/A	3 6 12	I (face)
[17]	216	147	49 (33)	General	N/A	58	APACHE II [12] (2 - 21)	6	Q (mail)
[26]	N/A	N/A	60 (N/A) 44 (N/A)	General	N/A	N/A	N/A	6 12	Q (mail)

Table 5. *(Continued)*

Study	N	N available for follow-up	N (%) followed up	Type of critical care patients	Mean age in years ± SD or (range)	Male (%)	Severity. mean ± SD [median] (range)	Mean follow up period in months [median] or (range)	Mode
[21]	477	164	69 (42) 12 (7)	CPR	64 ± 19	64	APACHE II 20.1 ± 8.6 TISS 29.3 ± 11.9	6 24	Q (mail) I (face)
[25]	216	82	20 (24)	Acute respiratory distress syndrome	41 (19 – 73)	62	N/A	3 6 12	I (face/tel)
[20]	6424	N/A	3655 (N/A)	General	60.1 ± 15	N/A	APACHE II 9.7± 5.2	12	Q (mail)
[48]	100	71	57 (80)	General	(0.3 94)	50	N/A	6	I (face)
[49]	3619	2313	1746 (75)	General	62.1	55	N/A	2	
[50]	58	29	6 (21)	General	61.4 ± 19.9	53	APACHE III 66.5 ± 25.3	6	N/A
[51]	269	N/A	219 (N/A)	Heart transplant	53 ± 9 (24 – 71)	80	N/A	6	Q (mail)
[23]	228	N/A	109(N/A)	Trauma	37.4 ± 16.8	68	ISS 15.5 ± 9.9 (1-51)	3	I (tel)

N/A: not available; N: Number; CPR: Cardiopulmonary resuscitation; GCS: Glasgow Coma Score; TISS: Therapeutic Intervention Scoring System; ISS: Injury Severity Score; Q: Questionnaire; I: Interview; tel: telephone

Cronbach's α as a measure of internal reliability was cited as 0.94 (it is assumed that this figure related to the overall SIP score, though this was not made explicit) [23]. Test-retest (inter-rater) reliability of 0.85 (p < 0.0001) was reported between patients and relatives responses to the SIP [17].

In terms of responsiveness, Miranda reported no significant differences in the SIP scores administered at two different time points [21]. Significant differences were found between pre-admission and follow-up SIP scores, using Chi squared analyses for housework, leisure activity, and social contact (p < 0.01).

PQOL

There was no evidence for the construct validity of the PQOL in critical care. Criterion validity was assessed. Patrick and colleagues demonstrated correlation between the PQOL and the SIP (r^2=0.24, p = 0.0001) and the PGWB (r^2=0.29, p = 0.001) [10]. Jones and colleagues obtained r^2=0.46 (p < 0.0001) with the Whiston Hospital Questionnaire and the POMS (r^2=0.46, p = 0.01) [17, 26]. Another study compared the PQOL with the NHP and obtained a z score of 9.853 (p = 0.0001) [27].

The internal reliability for the PQOL has been reported (Cronbach's α = 0.88) [10]. Apart from that, there was no evidence for the reliability of the PQOL. With regard to responsiveness, although one study assessed PQOL at more than one time point, it did not address responsiveness over time [28]. Ridley and colleagues reported no significant changes in PQOL scores between those obtained on admission to ICU and follow-up [29].

NHP

With regard to construct validity, two studies found no association with age [30, 31] and two studies found no association with patient gender [27, 30]. Criterion validity was also assessed. One study used a global quality of life question and the Hospital Anxiety and Depression (HAD) scale [30], others used the PQOL [27, 32] and one used a satisfaction scale [33]. There was no evidence for the reliability or responsiveness of the NHP.

SF-36

Ridley and colleagues reported on the construct validity of the SF-36 when used in critical care using the variable of pre-morbid employment status (p < 0.001) [34]. Another study used a linear regression model and reported no significant effects of age, acute severity or comorbid disease [35]. One study reported a significant correlation between age and the physical component of the SF-36 (r^2= 0.14) [36]. Another study used a general linear model to identify a significant difference in score distribution due to age (F = 6.3, p < 0.001) and sex (F = 9.2, p < 0.001) [37]. Criterion validity was explored by Weinert and colleagues who reported significant correlation between the Karnofsky Index and the physical component (r^2= 0.56) and the mental component of the SF-36 (r^2= 0.37) [36].

Three studies assessed reliability of the SF-36 in the context of critical care. One reported Cronbach's α of 0.87 for social function, 0.77 for mental health and 0.93 for physical functioning [37], another reported Cronbach's α of 0.70 for vitality to 0.98 for emotional and role function. Most multi-item scales had Cronbach's αvalues ranging between 0.93 and 0.98 indicating good reliability [38]. The third study reported Cronbach's α ranging from 0.85 to 0.93 [36]. There was no evidence for test-retest reliability.

With regard to responsiveness, Ridley and colleagues obtained data at two time points and reported differences in specific dimensions of the SF-36. They presented data for the mean change over time from ICU discharge to 6 month follow up with 95% CI. Significant increases were reported in mental health, vitality, social functioning and reduction in bodily pain scores although no values were provided [34].

Rosser Disability and Distress Categories

There was no evidence for the validity or reliability of the Rosser Disability and Distress Categories in the follow-up of critical care survivors. However, with regard to responsiveness, one study found no change in responses in 61% of their sample between critical care admission and follow-up [29].

Spitzer Quality of Life Index

One study examined construct validity with the variable age, although not explicitly [39]. There was no evidence for criterion validity or reliability. With regard to responsiveness, the same study reported a significant decrease in levels of activity between baseline and follow-up at twelve months (p < 0.001) and yet perceived health was reported to have improved at follow up (p < 0.05) [39]. One further study assessed pre-admission quality of life with respect to one month before admission (retrospectively obtained at follow-up) and also reviewed quality of life one month after discharge (p < 0.001) [40].

PGWB

There was no evidence for construct validity but one study examined criterion validity – it reported a modest correlation (r^2= 0.29, p = 0.001) between the PGWB and the PQOL scale [10]. There was no evidence for the reliability or responsiveness of the PGWB.

Fernandez questionnaire

Two studies reported on construct validity [41, 42]. Both found a moderate correlation with age, APACHE II scores and, in one of the studies, with the ISS. There was also some evidence of criterion validity in a further study that reported a significant correlation with the Glasgow Outcome Scale (GOS) [16]. Quality of life as measured by their scale and the GOS decreased six months after discharge from the ICU. The magnitude of the differences between the two scales was compared and a weighted kappa index of 0.56 (p < 0.001) was reported.

Internal consistency for the global quality of life scale (Cronbach's $\alpha = 0.85$) and for the physiological activities (Cronbach's $\alpha = 0.66$), physical capacities (Cronbach's $\alpha = 0.81$) and emotion (Cronbach's $\alpha = 0.82$) subscales, was reported. Cronbach's α ranged between 0.82 and 0.85 when each item in turn was removed from the scale [16]. Vazquez Mata and colleagues reported the internal consistency as α 0.67 [41].

This same study also reported on test-retest (inter-observer) reliability as >0.9 for the global scale and the physical capacities subscale, 0.77 for the emotional subscale and 0.61 for the basic physiological activities subscale and test-retest (intra-observer) reliability as >0.9 for the global scale and the physical capacities subscale, 0.84 for the emotion subscale and 0.93 for the basic physiological activities subscale [41]. Another study also examined test-retest (inter-observer) reliability between the responses of patients and those of close relatives and they reported correlation coefficients of >0.9 for the global scale and the physical capacities subscale and 0.82 and 0.76 for the emotion and the basic physiological activities subscales, respectively. Correlation coefficients of >0.95 for the global scale and the physical capacities subscale and 0.81 and 0.86 for the emotion and the basic physiological activities subscales, respectively, were also reported for the reliability between direct and telephone interviews [16].

With regard to responsiveness, one study reported a deterioration in quality of life between the first and second administration of the questionnaire (p < 0.01) [41]. Another study reported significant correlations between quality of life scores at one and two years ($r^2 = 0.908$, p < 0.0001). There was a weak correlation between baseline and one year ($r^2 = 0.167$, p < 0.0001) and admission and two years ($r^2 = 0.198$, p < 0.0001) [42].

Whiston Hospital Questionnaire

Two studies provided some information on construct and criterion validity [17, 26]. There was no significant correlation between the score and the APACHE II score on admission [17]. Reasonably high correlation with the FLP and PQOL suggested criterion validity existed (though the former association is not surprising given the origins of the questionnaire) [17] and the other study found no significant association with the Profile Of Mood States [26]. There was no evidence for the reliability or responsiveness of the Whiston Hospital Questionnaire.

What is Currently Known about the HRQL of Adult Survivors of Critical Care

There are considerable difficulties in summarizing the HRQL of adult survivors of critical care. Even for those measures that have been used in at least ten studies (selected in an attempt to enhance the external validity of any results), reported results vary considerably depending on the sample size (original and at follow-up), the case mix and the follow-up period for the population studied. Mode of administration of the measure also varies from study to study. In addition, the actual results presented for the same measure differ from study to study making comparison difficult. A further methodological difficulty is relating results from studies using one measure to those using another HRQL measure.

The majority of these methodological difficulties can best be demonstrated when reviewing the studies that have used the SIP, the HRQL measure in this review with the greatest evidence for validity, reliability, and responsiveness in adult survivors of critical care.

Twenty studies used either the SIP or, the anglicized version, the FLP (Table 4). Where reported, the number of subjects eligible for follow-up ranged from 29 to 2313 and the percentage of available subjects who were followed-up ranged from 21 to 100 %. Only eleven studies were based on general critical care patients. The mean age of the subjects ranged from 36 to 75 years and the percentage of males ranged from 50–80 %. Acute severity scores were only reported for 9 studies and, for APACHE II mean scores ranged from 10–20. Follow-up periods across studies ranged from two to eighteen months. In some studies, the follow-up period within a study ranged from four to ninety-eight months or twelve to sixty months.

Of the 20 studies, 10 administered the SIP in an interview, nine as a questionnaire by mail (some followed by a telephone follow-up/interview) and in one study it was unclear. Results were also presented in different ways: some studies did not present results for the SIP, some presented solely a mean global aggregated SIP score with standard deviation or 95 % confidence interval, some presented solely scores for the twelve dimensions, and some studies presented the results, as expected, with mean global aggregated SIP scores and mean physical and psychosocial summary scores.

Despite these methodological differences, consistent findings were that the five dimensions which had the highest scores (poorest quality of life) at follow-up were work, home life, recreation, sleep, and rest.

Conclusion

To date, selection of HRQL measures has been somewhat *ad hoc* and unsupported by evidence for their validity, reliability and responsiveness. Some evidence for validity exists but rather little as to reliability or responsiveness.

Those studies providing evidence for the validity, reliability and responsiveness of HRQL measures frequently reported on associations between the measure and patient characteristics, such as age and severity of illness. However, an explicit hypothesis was rarely provided as to whether or not any association was expected so it was difficult to use such evidence to throw light on the construct validity of the measure in question. Similarly, in those studies reporting serial values for some measures over time, again, it was impossible to judge whether stability or change over time indicated responsiveness of the measure or not.

The current poor state of evidence for the measurement properties of appropriate HRQL measures for adult survivors of critical care means that it is difficult to make clear recommendations as to which particular measures should be used.

A first recommendation is for the critical care community is to agree on a limited list of HRQL measures to be used. This would enable a considerable body of experience and knowledge to be built up around a few measures. In addition, it would allow investigators to make comparisons between studies and facilitate overviews based on secondary research of published results.

A second recommendation is for the critical care community to respond to the need for rigorous assessment of the measurement properties of the agreed measures. All studies assessing the HRQL of adult survivors of critical care could include an explicit hypothesis to explore at least one methodological characteristic of the measure being used.

A third recommendation is for better design and reporting of results. Given the current methodological limitations, it is almost impossible to arrive at an accurate and generalizable overview of the HRQL of adult survivors of critical care. It is apparent from the literature that differences in HRQL exist between studies. However, due to issues such as: the different measures used, the number and variation in subjects studied, the failure to follow-up all survivors, the time differences in follow-up, and the non-standard presentation of results, combining results cannot be justified and would be difficult to interpret.

References

1. Geigle R, Jones SB (1990) Outcomes measurement: A report from the front. Inquiry 27:7–13
2. Ware JE, Snow KK, Kosinski M, Gandek B (1993) SF-36 Health survey: Manual and Interpretation Guide. The Health Institute, Boston
3. Silver GA. Paul Anthony Lembke (1990) A pioneer in medical care evaluation. Am J Psychol 80:342–348
4. Jenkinson C, McGee H (1998) Health Status Measurement. Radcliffe Medical Press, Abingdon
5. Hayes JA, Black NA, Jenkinson C, et al (2000) Outcome measures for adult critical care: a systematic review. Health Technology Assessment 4. Dept of Health, London
6. Bowling A (1995) Measuring Disease. Open University Press, Buckingham
7. Bergner M, Bobbitt RA, Kressel S, Pollard WE, Gilson BS, Morris J (1976) The Sickness Impact Profile: conceptual formulation and methodology for the development of a health status measure. Int J Health Serv 6:393–415
8. Bergner M, Bobbitt RA, Pollard WE, et al (1976) The Sickness Impact Profile: validation of a health status measure. Med Care 14:57–67
9. Patrick D (1981) Standardization of Comparative Health Status Measures: Using Scales Developed in America in an English Speaking Country. Health Survey Research Methods, 3rd Biennial Conference. DHEW Publications, Washington
10. Patrick DL, Danis M, Southerland LI, Hong G (1988) Quality of life following intensive care. J Gen Intern Med 3:218–223

11. Hunt SM (1984) Nottingham Health Profile. In: NK Wenger, ME Mattson CD Furberg, et al (eds) Assessment of Quality of Life in Clinical Trials of Cardiovascular Therapies. Le Jacq, New York

12. Kind P, Rosser RM, Williams A (1982) Valuation of quality of life: some psychometric evidence. In: MW Jones-Lee (ed) The Value of Life and Safety. North Holland Publishing Company, Amsterdam, pp 159–170

13. Spitzer WO, Dobson AJ, Hall J, et al (1981) Measuring quality of life of cancer patients: A concise QL-Index for use by physicians. J Chronic Dis 34:585–597

14. Dupuy HJ (1974) Report of the national conference on evaluation in alcohol, drug abuse and mental health programs: Utility of the national center for health statistics General Well-Being Schedule in the assessment of self representations of subjective well-being and distress. ADA MHA, Washington

15. Dupuy HJ (1978) Self representations of general psychological well-being of American adults. Paper presented at American Public Health Association Meeting, Los Angeles, October, 1978

16. Fernandez RR, Sanchez Cruz JJ, Vazquez Mata GV (1996) Validation of a quality of life questionnaire for critically ill patients. Intensive Care Med 22:1034–1042

17. Jones C, Hussey R, Griffiths RD (1993) A tool to measure the change in health status of selected adult patients before and after intensive care. Clin Intensive Care 4:160–165

18. Bergner L, Bergner M, Hallstrom AP, Eisenberg M, Cobb LA (1984) Health status of survivors of out-of-hospital cardiac arrest six months later. Am J Public Health 74:508–510

19. Sage WM, Rosenthal MH, Silverman JF (1986) Is intensive care worth it? An assessment of input and outcome for the critically ill. Crit Care Med 14:777–782

20. Tian ZM, Miranda DR (1995) Quality of life after intensive care with the sickness impact profile. Intensive Care Med 21:422–428

21. Miranda DR (1994) Quality of life after cardiopulmonary resuscitation. Chest 106:524–530

22. Hulsebos RG, Beltman FW, Reis Miranda D, Spangenberg JFA (1991) Measuring quality of life with the Sickness Impact Profile: a pilot study. Intensive Care Med 17:285–288

23. Richmond TS, Kauder D, Schwab CW (1998) A prospective study of predictors of disability at 3 months after non-central nervous system trauma. J Trauma 44:635–643

24. Riether AM, Smith SL, Lewison BJ, Cotsonis GA, Epstein CM (1992) Quality-of-life changes and psychiatric and neurocognitive outcome after heart and liver transplantation. Transplantation 54:444–450

25. McHugh GJ, Havill JH, Armistead SH, Ullal RR, Fayers TM (1997) Follow up of elderly patients after cardiac surgery and intensive care unit admission, 1991 to 1995. N Z Med J 110:432–435

26. Jones C, Griffiths RD, Macmillan R, Palmer TEA (1994) Psychological problems occurring after intensive care. Br J Intensive Care 4:46–53

27. Hurel D, Loirat P, Saulnier F, Nicolas F, Brivat F (1997) Quality of life 6 months after intensive care: results of a prospective multicentre study using a generic health status scale and a satisfaction scale. Intensive Care Med 23:331–337

28. Chelluri L, Pinsky MR, Donahoe MP, Grenvik A (1993) Long-term outcome of critically ill elderly patients requiring intensive care. JAMA 269:3119–3123

29. Ridley SA, Biggam M, Stone P (1994) A cost-utility analysis of intensive therapy II: Quality of life in survivors. Anaesthesia 49:192–196

30. Rowan KM (1992) Outcome comparisons of intensive care units in Great Britain and Ireland using APACHE II method [D.Phil thesis]. University of Oxford, Oxford

31. Munn J, Willatts SM, Tooley MA (1995) Health and activity after intensive care. Anaesthesia 50:1017–1021

32. Thiagarajan J, Taylor P, Hogbin E, Ridley S (1994) Quality of life after multiple trauma requiring intensive care. Anaesthesia 49:211–218

33. Dixon JJ, Manara AR, Willats SM (1997) Patient and relative satisfaction with intensive care. Importance of duration and quality of life. Clin Intensive Care 8:63–68

34. Ridley SA, Chrispin PS, Scotton H, Rogers J, Lloyd D (1997) Changes in quality of life after intensive care: comparison with normal data. Anaesthesia 52:195–202

35. Davidson TA, Caldwell ES, Curtis JR, Hudson LD, Steinberg KP (1999) Reduced quality of life in survivors of acute respiratory distress syndrome compared with critically ill control patients. JAMA 281:354–360
36. Weinert CR, Gross CR, Kangas JR, Bury CL, Marinelli WA (1997) Health related quality of life after acute lung injury. Am J Respir Crit Care Med 156:1120–1128
37. Chrispin PS, Scotton H, Rogers J, Lloyd D, Ridley SA (1997) Short Form 36 in the intensive care unit: assessment of acceptability, reliability and validity of the questionnaire. Anaesthesia 52:15–23
38. Schelling G, Stoll C, Haller M, et al (1998) Health-related quality of life and posttraumatic stress disorder in survivors of the acute respiratory distress syndrome. Crit Care Med 26:651–659
39. Konopad E, Noseworthy TW, Johnston R, Shustack A, Grace M (1995) Quality of life measures before and one year after admission to an intensive care unit. Crit Care Med 23:1653–1659
40. Slatyer MA, James OF, Moore PG, Leeder SR (1986) Costs, severity of illness and outcome in intensive care. Anaesth Intensive Care 14:381–389
41. Vasquez Mata G, Riviera Fernandez R, Gonzalez Carmona A, et al (1992) Factors related to quality of life 12 months after discharge from an intensive care unit. Crit Care Med 20:1257–1262
42. Vasquez Mata G, Riviera Fernandez R, Perez Aragon A, Gonzalez Carmona A, Fernandez Mondejar E, Navarrete Navarro P (1996) Analysis of quality of life in polytraumatised patients two years after discharge from an intensive care unit. J Trauma 41:326–332
43. Sage WM, Hurst CR, Silverman JF, Bortz II WM (1987) Intensive care for the elderly: outcome of elective and nonelective admissions. J Am Geriatr Soc 35:312–318
44. Danis M, Patrick DL, Southerland LI, Green ML (1988) Patients' and families' preferences for medical intensive care. JAMA 260:797–802
45. Mundt DJ, Gage RW, Lemeshow S, Pastides H, Teres D, Avrunin JS (1989) Intensive Care Unit Patient follow-up. Mortality, functional status, and return to work at six months. Arch Intern Med 149:68–72
46. Stambrook M, Moore AD, Peters LC, Deviaene C, Hawryluk GA (1990) Effects of mild, moderate and severe closed head injury on long-term vocational status. Brain Injury 4:183–190
47. Schuster HP (1991) Intensive care in old age. Med Klin 86:473–481
48. Sawdon V, Woods I, Proctor M (1995) Post-intensive care interviews: implications for future practice. Intensive Crit Care Nurs 11:329–332
49. Wu AW, Damiano AM, Lynn J, et al (1995) Predicting future functional status for seriously ill hospitalized adults: the SUPPORT prognostic model. Ann Intern Med 122:149–150
50. Douglas SL, Daly BJ, Brennan PF, Harris S, Nochomovitz M, Dyer MA (1997) Outcomes of long term ventilator patients: a descriptive study. Am J Crit Care 6:99–105
51. Grady KL, Jalowiec A, White-Williams C (1998) Quality of life 6 months after heart transplantation compared with indicators of illness severity before transplantation. Am J Crit Care 7:106–116

The Neuropsychological Consequences of Intensive Care

K. T. Sukantarat and S. Brett

Introduction

Understanding the complex series of factors that contribute to a patient's recovery from an episode of critical illness is not simple. Defining 'recovery' implies that we understand what the patient regards as an acceptable outcome, and of course patients may have very different expectations. For example an elderly patient having surgery for aortic valve disease may be satisfied with relief of dyspnea and chest pain, whereas a young person recovering from severe trauma wishes to return to the same functional status that he or she had prior to their accident. In addition, the patient may wish to return to a physically and mentally active occupation to provide for their family; any deficit perceived in one area is likely to have a negative impact on another. Thus from the patient's perspective there may be a number of possible definitions of 'recovery'. The sorts of factors that may impair an individual's recovery are outlined in the Venn diagram in Figure 1. The zones do not overlap because the relative importance and interaction of these zones is highly individual. The complexity of these interactions is exemplified by cardiac surgical patients, many of whom have cognitive deficits measurable during recovery, but whose quality of life is increased because the overwhelming factor is an improvement in physical symptoms after surgery [1, 2]. Because intensive care follow-up is a relatively novel phenomenon, this area has been inadequately studied, but some important research is now underway and some published studies are beginning to alert people to these problems. The purpose of this review is to define the current status of this research and place this in the context of 'recovery' in its broadest sense.

Neuropsychology

This is defined as: "The study of the relationship between behavior and brain function" [3].

Although our understanding of the impact of critical illness on the brain is rudimentary at best, it may be possible to provide some illumination by studying aspects of brain dysfunction in the recovery period. A bewildering variety of potential aspects of normal brain functioning are possible targets, but a few obvious candidates likely to have a major impact on recovery include: memory, ability to

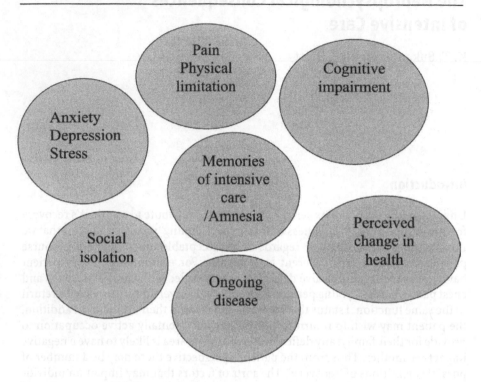

Fig. 1. Factors contributing to quality of recovery

concentrate, cognitive function and 'executive' function. In addition, a number of manifestations of psychological dysfunction, such as depression, anxiety, post-traumatic stress disorder and memories of delusions are of obvious importance.

Unfortunately these tests take time to perform, and in many cases the patients remain very frail at their follow-up appointments. Presenting a patient with many complex and mentally tiring tests is a flawed strategy; motivational factors, in a patient who may have elements of depression or anxiety, will impair test performance. Thus, studies must have realistic ambitions. Some tools have been well validated in the non-intensive care unit (ICU) population but they may be less applicable to those recovering from critical illness. The tests themselves do not necessarily measure only one isolated aspect of dysfunction. Thus, anxiety or increased alertness is a component of post-traumatic stress disorder, and studies using conventional measures of anxiety may miss-label patients whose anxiety is part of a post-traumatic stress disorder complex.

A further complicating factor is the variable impact of precipitating illness. Clearly primary head injury has a major and obvious impact, and cardiopulmonary bypass has an effect that has been studied. Less well characterized are the general effects of critical illness of all types. Septic encephalopathy is a well-recognized entity [4], but only recently have practical tools been developed that will allow the identification, and to some extent quantification of delirium in large groups of intensive care patients [5].

Baseline Data

The extreme scarcity of baseline data presents a considerable challenge to investigators working in this area. With the exception of defined populations undergoing elective surgery, a predictable proportion of whom will sustain critical illness, baseline data do not exist. Thus, comparisons must be made with population derived 'normative' data. Such data must be used with extreme caution, given that the development data sets may have come from populations with obvious or occult peculiarities, not the least being that they were prepared to spend their time being control subjects. This can be somewhat improved by studying patients at various time-points and examining recovery towards population normal. The obvious difficulty here is estimating the effects of learning on repeat testing; for some instruments this has been studied in population normal data sets. Additionally the patient group tends to undergo attrition as time passes and patients die or loose motivation to continue with the study.

Assessing Quality of Life

A multiplicity of factors contributes to perceived quality of life; a similar diagram to Figure 1 could be designed with equal limitations. The Sickness Impact Profile (SIP) [6] attempts to describe these interactions but has now probably been superseded, given that it was designed several decades ago and expectations of health have changed. The Medical Outcomes Study 36-Item Short Form Health Survey Standard Form (SF-36) [7] has been used in a number of insightful studies of critical care survivors [e.g., 8–10]. Eight domains of existence (Table 1) are examined with a questionnaire that can be self-administered. This tool has been shown to be reliable and valid in a wide variety of acute and chronic disease [11], and specifically in survivors of critical illness [12]. The SF-36 takes a broad overview of health status, including physical and "mental" domains. It is limited in that, in order to have a practical tool and data output, the individual domains are not explored in real depth. Having said this, robust population norms exist and thought provoking data have been produced, especially in studies which have included detailed disease-specific tools such as the St. George's Respiratory Questionnaire [12].

Anxiety and Depression

Not surprisingly, anxiety and depression are seen in survivors of critical illness, although formal reporting of this in the literature is scarce. How much is pure reactive affective disorder consequent upon direct effects on the brain and how much is due to factors such as post-traumatic stress disorder, fear about health

Table 1. The Short Form-36 Domains [7]

General health perception

Physical functioning

Role physical - restriction of activity by physical symptoms

Role emotional - restriction of activity by emotional symptoms

Social functioning

Bodily pain

Energy and vitality

Mental health

status or post-discharge social isolation, etc., is impossible to say. Scragg and colleagues [13] used a postal self-administered Hospital Anxiety and Depression Scale (HAD) as part of a study assessing contributors to post-traumatic stress disorder. Almost half of their sample (80 fully completed questionnaires from an original discharge cohort of 222 patients) reported significant anxiety and/or depression scores. Subsequent multivariate regression analysis did not take their analysis further, but this level of affective disorder is substantially greater than that reported in a large cohort of patients with chronic medical disease [14]. Unlike conventional psychiatric practice, in which patients often present a predominantly anxious or depressive affective disorder, ICU survivors seem to score simultaneously on both anxiety and depression scales (Figure 2). It is possible that the HAD has discriminatory limitations in the post-ICU setting. The HAD scale is in fact designed as a screening tool and clinical diagnosis of an affective disorder requires a face to face consultation, clearly impractical in large scale follow up studies.

Assessing affective disorders during critical illness is an almost insuperable challenge. Psychiatrists are generally not interested until the patient can talk. However, intensivists recognize patients whose level of anxiety seems greater than anticipated, or alternatively seem withdrawn and de-motivated. Such clinical pictures often become apparent during prolonged weaning episodes, and little is published about this scenario. Pochard and colleagues [15] bravely attempted this in a difficult, questionnaire-based study, which could only include 32 of a potential 54 ventilated patients. Their results suggested overall psychological status was poor. Does it matter? Intuitively it does; we all recognize patients who are determined to recover, and those who appear to have given up. The SUPPORT investigators studied a large cohort of seriously (although not necessarily critically) ill patients who could complete a Profile of Mood States Depression sub-scale [16]. Depressed mood was associated with worse level of physical functioning, greater severity of illness and decreased survival time (hazard ratio 1.134, confidence interval 1.07–1.2, p</=0.001). There are no trials of interventions for depression in

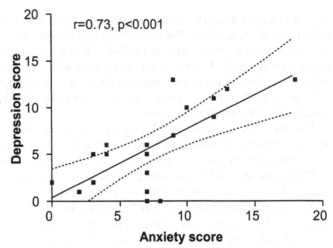

Fig. 2. Preliminary data from a study of neuropsychological consequences of critical illness. Patients studied at 3 months post ICU discharge. Clear relationship between anxiety and depression scores is demonstrated.

this group, but the use of selective serotonin re-uptake inhibitors appears to be becoming more widespread.

Post-traumatic Stress Disorder

More commonly associated with the after effects of conflict, trauma, assault, etc., post-traumatic stress disorder is now increasingly recognized as a possible consequence of critical illness. It consists of a triad of symptom complexes: intrusive unpleasant and unsettling flashbacks associated with emotional upset; subsequent avoidance of situations that tend to trigger these flashbacks; and finally an increased level of alertness or chronic anxiety state. A variety of questionnaire-based screening tools are available and studies have been performed in ICU survivors. Schelling and colleagues [17] studied 80 survivors of acute respiratory distress syndrome (ARDS) using a postal questionnaire that included a Post-Traumatic Stress Syndrome 10-Question Inventory (PTSS-10). Unusually this study included several "control" groups, one of which was a group of soldiers who had seen active service, and another, routine major surgical patients. The mean age of patients was 36 years, and the mean follow-up interval was 4 years. Using the PTSS-10, 27.3% of ARDS survivors exhibited symptoms of post-traumatic stress disorder, a greater incidence than for the other two groups. In addition, the individuals with high PTSS-10 scores also exhibited lower quality of life scores on the SF-36, and had more memories of unpleasant events. Only 61.3% of the ARDS group was employed in any capacity.

However, concerns exist that tools designed specifically for the intensive care setting are required, and a number have been developed. Scragg and colleagues [13] developed the Experience After Treatment in Intensive Care-7 (ETIC-7) scale. This was compared with the Trauma Symptom Checklist-33 (TSC-33) that measures symptoms found in psychologically traumatized individuals [18], and the

Impact of Events Scale (IES) that measures intrusion and avoidance as markers of post traumatic stress [19]. The ETIC-7 was highly correlated with the IES, TSC-33 and HAD scale; 38 % of patients studied exhibited symptoms of post-traumatic stress disorder, and 15 % had scores consistent with a diagnosis of full post-traumatic stress disorder. Younger age and time since discharge were factors apparently associated with worse outcome, perhaps reflecting that younger patients' admissions were often post trauma.

The impact of memories of ICU stay on subsequent morbidity has been studied recently. Jones and colleagues were interested in the interaction of factual and delusional memory and development of morbidity [20]. To this end they developed an "ICU memory tool" which was first validated and then used prospectively on a cohort of recovering patients who were also assessed with the IES, Fear Index and HAD scale; patients were studied at 2 and 8 weeks post-ICU discharge. At 2 weeks patients without factual memories, but with delusional memories scored highly on the HAD scale. At 8 weeks this group scored highly on the IES. Those patients with factual memories seemed less likely to develop post-traumatic stress disorder-type symptoms. Pre-morbid anxiety-prone personality type was correlated with subsequent post-traumatic stress disorder symptoms and scores on the Fear Index. Interestingly at 2 weeks 16 % of patients failed to recall any factual events, but by 8 weeks this figure had risen to 37 %; by contrast patients describing delusions at 2 weeks remembered them at 8 weeks. This small but fascinating study raises a number of important issues:

1. Memories of factual events may protect against subsequent post-traumatic stress disorder symptoms.
2. Memories of delusions and hallucinations may be laid down with a 'firmer' trace, possibly because their occurrence is associated with more anxiety.
3. If 1 and 2 are confirmed we may need to review our concepts of optimal sedation and to evolve strategies to reinforce and help retain factual memories.

Our understanding of the causation of delusions and its relationship to delirium are limited, and the assessment of delirium in the ICU is non-trivial. Recently an excellent and practical tool has been developed to allow the quantification of delirium by ICU nursing and house staff [5]. This is likely to prove very valuable.

Why should the studies by Schelling et al. [17] and Jones et al. [20] have produced conflicting results? There are substantial differences between the studies: Jones looked at patients face to face very soon after illness, whereas Schelling used a postal questionnaire 4 years after illness; Schelling's patients were younger and thus, according to Scragg's data [13], may have been more likely to score highly for post-traumatic stress disorder. Whatever the reasons, both are important contributions. The real incidence of post-traumatic stress disorder (and indeed the natural history) remains unknown given that the tools described are essentially for screening and proper diagnosis requires a specialist psychiatry consultation. However, screening tools are being validated in the ICU setting [21]. What we can say is that for a substantial group of patients post-traumatic stress disorder is likely to be important, and that we do not know enough about its causation and natural history, or how to reduce the likelihood of occurrence.

Cognitive Dysfunction

The term 'cognitive function' has come to be regarded as a generic term to encompass various aspects of intellectual function including: memory; attention, and ability to concentrate; linguistic and numerical skills; and executive function, which describes our ability to assimilate information and respond. This area has not been well explored. By contrast the impact of cardiac surgery has been studied extensively using a bewildering variety of tests. Clearly cardiac surgery is associated with a number of direct insults to the brain, and substantial efforts have been directed at reducing post-operative morbidity; a recent study identifying deficits in 53 % of patients at discharge [22]. These data have only limited applicability to critical care but some interesting points are illustrated. Kilminster and colleagues [1] were able to examine 130 patients pre- and 6–8 weeks post-cardiac surgery using a battery of neuropsychological tests. Overall, 10 tests improved, including the HAD scale and a general health questionnaire. Three tests were worse, generally tests of memory function, and 12 tests remained the same. Physical damage to neurones was assessed with serum S-100 release, which correlated with the degree of memory impairment. In spite of all this, quality of life scores were improved. So, two philosophically similar studies produced conflicting results, although the individual tests and time points were different. As pointed out earlier, if the overwhelming factor in a patient's existence is angina or dyspnea, minor elements of post-operative cognitive dysfunction may be a reasonable trade.

More specifically relevant to general intensive care, Hopkins and colleagues [10] have conducted an extensive and rigorous study of 55 survivors of ARDS. At hospital discharge all patients exhibited affective and cognitive decline. At a year post discharge, 30 % of patients still exhibited generalized cognitive dysfunction, and overall 78 % of patients were impaired in one or all of: memory, attention, concentration and/or mental processing speed. SF-36 scores were still subnormal and overall many patients exhibited impaired health status, although HAD scale scores were back to normal. The investigators felt that the degree of cognitive decline reported would impair ability to take medication and follow post discharge instructions, as well as to function normally in a home, employment, and social sense. Indeed, 44 % of patients had not resumed normal activities or returned to work, although persisting physical disability was not recorded. Hopkins' group proposed a number of explanations for their findings including hypoxemia, but only initial PaO_2 correlated with outcome. Gas microemboli are possible, but so also are toxic and metabolic effects on the brain. An important limitation of the study, acknowledged by the authors, was the lack of a control group of similarly ill patients without ARDS. We still do not know the general effects of critical illness.

Rothenhäusler and colleagues [23] examined the relationship between cognitive dysfunction and quality of life in a series of 46 ARDS survivors studied a median of six years post recovery. The majority of patients did not demonstrate cognitive impairment, but quality of life, assessed with SF-36, was significantly impaired in the quarter that did. Two points are of particular interest: the degree of cognitive deficit was modest, and the SF-36 demonstrated reductions in 7 of 8 domains.

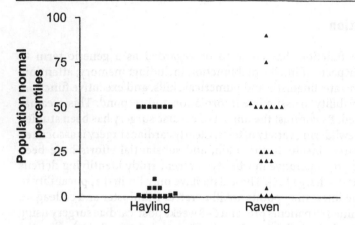

Fig. 3. Preliminary data from a study of neuropsychological consequences of critical illness. Patients studied at 3 months post ICU discharge. Very poor scores demonstrated in the Hayling assessment that examines so-called executive function. The data are not normally distributed and are skewed towards the lower performance end. Scores for Raven's progressive matrices, a test of general intelligence, are also generally poor. The poor scores are less dramatic; the results pass a normality test, although with low median (25) and mean (35) scores.

Furthermore there was a clear impact on the likelihood of returning to employment. Unfortunately, no independent assessment of affective state was made.

We are attempting to shed some further light on this area by using a battery of simple tests, including tests that examine executive function, in a study of general ICU survivors 3 and 9 months post ICU discharge. Preliminary results (Figure 3) at 3 months from this continuing study show poor scores on Raven's Progressive Matrices [24], a test of general intelligence, and extremely poor scores on the Hayling Sentence Completion Test [25–26], a specific test of executive function and mental agility. Limitations of these particular tests are that the results are presented as percentile performance of population derived normal data. We have to make the substantial assumption that the development data set does represent global population performance. The Hayling Test also only really works on people who are very fluent in English language and conversational idiom. Of interest, quality of life assessment, using SF-36 analysis (data not shown), shows decrements in most domains, although oddly not in Mental Health.

Why are there so few Data?

The issues outlined above are clearly extremely important for patient recovery, yet with a few notable exceptions there are very few published studies attempting to define and quantify the problem, let alone intervene. Why is this? The reasons are multi-factorial but include the following:

1. Few intensive care physicians see large numbers of their critical care patients for out of hospital follow-up, and these problems may not be obvious to

physicians undertaking such care. Physicians undertaking follow up are likely to be focused on physical aspects of health status. The concept of the intensive care clinic is still in its infancy in spite of isolated and committed centers of enthusiasm

2. The level of awareness of possible neuropsychological deficits post ICU discharge is generally low, and patterns of symptoms may not be recognized.
3. The deficits may be subtle and, although important, only identified with specialist testing.
4. The research is extremely difficult. Persuading large numbers of patients to return for testing is challenging. A bewildering variety of tests are available, and expert psychological help is required selecting and performing appropriate tests. A review of all the available tests is beyond the scope of this review but many are discussed in [27].
5. There seems to be an enthusiasm for developing new tests, which although doubtless of interest and amusement to psychologists, does leave the non-specialist struggling to compare the results of different studies.

Future Research Priorities

There appears to be a *prima facie* case that critical illness has neuropsychological consequences that stretch into and impair recovery. Additionally these consequences may have an independent effect on the ability of patients to return to work, and thus have a fiscal impact. This area has been inadequately explored and needs to be higher up the research priority list. A number of factors need to be considered:

1. Our understanding of, and ability to measure, the effect of critical illness on the brain needs to be improved. We need a better understanding of delirium, its causes and its natural history. This would include a study of sleep deprivation, and loss of diurnal rhythm.
2. A consensus is required on a group of neuropsychological tests to be used in assessing patients in the recovery phase. The lack of consistency of test selection, and constant development and validation of novel tests is somewhat confusing. The selection of a standard battery of tests will clearly require the advice of clinical psychologists experienced in the field, and sponsorship from the interested critical care parties.
3. Future studies need to be sufficiently large to allow meaningful interpretation of prospectively defined subgroup data, and the development of multiple regression models. The data sets will need to include clinical data from the critical illness phase, and will need to have some ethnic and cultural reference. Studies will have to continue for sufficient periods of time to allow repeat testing and elucidation of natural history.

All of the above factors need be addressed before serious intervention studies can start. For obvious reasons critical care has tended to concentrate on short-term goals, such as survival to 28 days or hospital discharge. Recently a paradigm shift has occurred and the results of large clinical trials are viewed with skepticism until long-term outcome data are published. Many of us have been ignorant of the fate of the patient post-ICU discharge, and the recent studies of post-discharge mortality on hospital ward areas have alerted us to this feature [28, 29]. Some excellent quality of life data have now been published. However, ICU follow-up clinics remain the exception rather than the rule; they can provide rather salutary lessons. The author was astounded after starting his own clinic to find that a significant number of patients, who had been discharged from ICU 'in good shape', were still in hospital 3 months post-discharge; furthermore, many of those at home were often in a very precarious and miserable state. Intensive care perhaps needs to be regarded as a phase in a health care process that also includes 'recovery'; currently we have no real idea of the resource implications, or indeed the size of the problem.

References

1. Kilminster S, Treasure T, McMillan T, Holt DW (1999) Neuropsychological change and S-100 protein release in 130 unselected patients undergoing cardiac surgery. Stroke 30:1869-1874
2. Trouillet JL, Scheimberg A, Vuagnat A, Fagon JY, Chastre J, Gibert C (1996) Long-term outcome and quality of life of patients requiring multidisciplinary intensive care unit admission after cardiac operations. J Thorac Cardiovasc Surg 112:926-934
3. Pearsall J (1999). Oxford Concise English Dictionary (10th Edition). Oxford University Press, Oxford
4. Papadopoulos MC, Davies DC, Moss RF, Tighe D, Bennett ED (2000) Pathophysiology of septic encephalopathy: a review. Crit Care Med 28:3019-3024
5. Ely EW, Margolin R, Francis J, et al (2001) Evaluation of delirium in critically ill patients: validation of the Confusion Assessment Method for the Intensive Care Unit (CAM-ICU). Crit Care Med 29:1370-1379
6. Hulsebos RG, Beltman FW, dos Reis Miranda D, Spangenberg JF (1991) Measuring quality of life with the sickness impact profile: a pilot study. Intensive Care Med 17:285-288
7. Ware JE (1993) SF-36 Health Survey Manuel and Interpretation Guide. The Medical Outcomes Trust, Boston
8. Chrispin PS, Scotton H, Rogers J, Lloyd D, Ridley SA (1997) Short Form 36 in the intensive care unit: assessment of acceptability, reliability and validity of the questionnaire. Anaesthesia 52:15-23
9. Ridley SA, Chrispin PS, Scotton H, Rogers J, Lloyd D (1997) Changes in quality of life after intensive care: comparison with normal data. Anaesthesia 52:195-202
10. Hopkins RO, Weaver LK, Pope D, Orme JF, Bigler ED, Larson-Lohr V (1999) Neuropsychological sequelae and impaired health status in survivors of severe acute respiratory distress syndrome. Am J Respir Crit Care Med 160:50-56
11. Bousquet J, Knani J, Dhivert H, et al (1994) Quality of life in asthma. I. Internal consistency and validity of the SF-36 questionnaire. Am J Respir Crit Care Med. 149:371-375
12. Davidson TA, Caldwell ES, Curtis JR, Hudson LD, Steinberg KP (1999) Reduced quality of life in survivors of acute respiratory distress syndrome compared with critically ill control patients. JAMA 281:354-360
13. Scragg P, Jones A, Fauvel N (2001) Psychological problems following ICU treatment. Anaesthesia 56:9-14
14. Ormel J, Kempen GI, Penninx BW, Brilman EI, Beekman AT, van Sonderen E. (1997) Chronic medical conditions and mental health in older people: disability and psychosocial resources mediate specific mental health effects. Psychol Med 27:1065-1077
15. Pochard F, Lanore JJ, Bellivier F, et al (1995) Subjective psychological status of severely ill patients discharged from mechanical ventilation. Clin Intensive Care 6:57-61

16. Roach MJ, Connors AF, Dawson NV, et al (1998) Depressed mood and survival in seriously ill hospitalized adults. The SUPPORT Investigators. Arch Intern Med 158:397–404
17. Schelling G, Stoll C, Haller M, et al (1998) Health-related quality of life and posttraumatic stress disorder in survivors of the acute respiratory distress syndrome. Crit Care Med 26:651–659
18. Briere J, Runtz M (1989) The trauma symptom checklist. Early data on a new scale (TSC-33). Journal of Interpersonal Violence 4:151–163
19. Briere J, Elliot DM (1998) Clinical utility of the Impact of Events Scale. Psychometrics in the general population. Assessment 5:171–180
20. Jones C, Griffiths RD, Humphris G, Skirrow PM (2001) Memory, delusions, and the development of acute posttraumatic stress disorder-related symptoms after intensive care. Crit Care Med 29:573–580
21. Stoll C, Kapfhammer HP, Rothenhausler HB, et al (1999) Sensitivity and specificity of a screening test to document traumatic experiences and to diagnose post-traumatic stress disorder in ARDS patients after intensive care treatment. Intensive Care Med. 25:697–704
22. Newman MF, Kirchner JL, Phillips-Bute B, et al (2001) Longitudinal assessment of neurocognitive function after coronary-artery bypass surgery. N Engl J Med 344:395–402
23. Rothenhausler HB, Ehrentraut S, Stoll C, Schelling G, Kapfhammer HP (2001) The relationship between cognitive performance and employment and health status in long-term survivors of the acute respiratory distress syndrome: results of an exploratory study. Gen Hosp Psychiatry 23:90–96
24. Raven J, Raven JC, Court JH (1998) Manuel for Raven's Progressive Matrices and Vocabulary Scales. Oxford Psychologists Press, Oxford
25. Burgess PW, Shallice T (1996) Response suppression, initiation and strategy use following frontal lobe lesions. Neuropsychologia 34:263–272
26. Burgess PW, Shallice T (1997) The Hayling Sentence Completion Test. The Thames Valley Test Company, Culford
27. Naugle RI, Cullum CM, Bigler ED (1998) Introduction to Clinical Neuropsychology: A Case Book. Pro-Ed, Austin
28. Goldhill DR, Sumner A (1998) Outcome of intensive care patients in a group of British intensive care units. Crit Care Med 26:1337–1345
29. Daly K, Beale R, Chang RW (2001) Reduction in mortality after inappropriate early discharge from intensive care unit: logistic regression triage model. Br Med J 322:1274–1276

The Burden of Caregiving on Families of ICU Survivors

M. M. Levy

Introduction

As a result of increasingly sophisticated therapies for critically ill patients, family members are caring for individuals with complex medical problems at home as the most financially feasible alternative to institutional care. These individuals include older adults with progressive dementia, children and adults who are technologically dependent, such as on home dialysis or respirators, individuals with stroke, survivors of traumatic brain injuries or spinal cord injuries, and individuals with chronic neurological disorders, such as multiple sclerosis. These patients may have survived life-threatening illnesses requiring ICU care, such as severe sepsis, septic shock, acute respiratory distress syndrome (ARDS), stroke, and multi-system organ failure. Patients who, even twenty years ago, most probably would have succumbed to a critical illness are now surviving in increasing numbers [14].

At the same time, third party payors and the current concepts in hospital remuneration are leading patients to be discharged from hospital more quickly than would have been true over the past twenty years. Earlier discharge and improved survival are two very important reasons why informal caregiving is becoming an ever more important aspect of, not only health care in general, but critical care in particular.

In a recent study [5] of seventy-five patients greater than seventy years old, with an ICU stay of longer than 30 days, 47 % were discharged alive from ICU and were found to have a median survival of 204 days. After ICU discharge, these patients were found to have a significant increase in dependence; this included disability in bathing (23 %), toileting (15 %), transfer (26 %), and continence (19 %). The study demonstrated 41 % one-year survival with good quality of life despite a moderate disability. Twenty-five of thirty survivors questioned felt they would want ICU care again. Also of note, the need for special equipment in activities of daily living was not felt to be an important disability by survivors, despite the fact that 16 to 23 % of patients needed some help in bathing. Of interest, in this study, there was no mention about family concerns or needs. The authors concluded that the acceptance of disability is better among elderly patients with good social conditions and with family or friends close to them.

This study points clearly to the importance of addressing the concerns and needs of families early in ICU stay, not just through discharge planning but seeing our curative attempts in the ICU in the true context of our patients lives. It is not enough for the patient alone to survive, the family must survive to health as well.

Many studies have documented the quality of life for ICU survivors [619]. Reports on the ability of ICU survivors to return to pre-hospitalization levels of function have varied widely in the literature, depending on the severity of illness. Several reports have found a low one-year level of functioning, even in patients less than fifty years old and without traumatic brain injury [10, 11, 16].

While improved survival from critical illness is certainly good news for our patients and demonstrates the ability to bring bench research to the bedside, leading to better care for patients, very little attention has been paid to the price paid for this improved survival – not solely in terms of financial costs, but also the global impact on families of ICU survivors. How do families cope with survivors of ICU care? What impact does critical illness have on the ongoing relationships for the families of these patients? Often the post-ICU and hospital recovery period is prolonged; although several studies document good quality of life after recovery from critical illness, the burden that families bear during this recovery period has long been overlooked. The demands of survival may be considerable, both physically and emotionally. Care for these survivors often falls to family members who then become informal caregivers with little training or preparation in caregiving skills. If our ultimate goal for ICU survivors is to return these patients to the best possible quality of life, the long-term impact on informal caregivers is important to understand. What are the effects of informal caregiving on caregivers, families, and patients? What are the determining factors that affect quality of life for all members of this informal team? Are there interventions that can brighten the long-term outlook of patients who survive critical illness?

For ICU survivors, there is limited available information to answer these important and difficult questions. Much of the available data is in survivors of traumatic brain injury and refers mostly to the parent/child relationship. The absence of good data in the literature on this topic speaks volumes to our lack of appreciation and understanding about the way in which survival from critical illness affects the everyday lives of our patients after they survive critical illness. In our excitement and rush to improve ICU care and survival for our patients, the problems which arise for the families left to care for their loved ones after ICU survival have been inadequately studied. Just as we have long ignored the problem of helping people *die* with dignity in the ICU, we have also ignored the problem of helping ICU survivors and their caregivers *live* with dignity after ICU care.

Although many questions are unanswered, it might be helpful to review some of the major areas identified in the literature, which may have a major impact on families who become caregivers to these survivors.

The Impact of Informal Caregiving

The high cost of long-term health care, combined with current trends to decrease healthcare costs, suggest that responsibility for the day-to-day care of ICU survivors will continue to fall on their families in the home setting. Families of survivors are expected to provide long-term continuous care, often without adequate resources. Families often lack nursing skills, coping skills, support systems, or knowledge of their own rights, available help or how to obtain help. Caregivers experience major psychological stress, including loneliness, social isolation and guilt. There are many reports in the literature that describe the impact of informal caregiving on families of patients who have sustained traumatic brain injury. As an example, in one such study, forty-two patients with traumatic brain injury and their caregivers were evaluated three months after discharge from a rehabilitation facility [20]. In this study, 50 % of the caregivers (most often women: mothers or wives) had quit their jobs to care for the person with traumatic brain injury; 42 % of caregivers reported a decrease in income; and 28.6 % reported that their loved ones required constant supervision. In the forty-two families surveyed, only two patients were able to live independently. The more physical and cognitive impairments the person with traumatic brain injury had, the greater the reported caregiver burden.

Caregiver Burden

The concept of family burden was first introduced by Grad and Sainsbury [21]. Burden was defined as any cost (negative consequences) to the family in which the patient is a member. Burden can be broadly viewed as a mediating force between the patient's impairment and the impact that caregiving has on the lives of the caregivers and their families. In order to understand the underpinnings of informal caregiving and the factors that may affect outcomes for caregivers, burden has been separated between events and activities that arise during caregiving, from emotions, feelings and attitudes associated with caregiving [22]. This means caregiving has been segregated into subjective and objective dimensions. Objective burden refers to the events and activities associated with negative caregiving experiences. Subjective burden refers to feelings aroused in caregivers as they fulfill their caregiving function.

Subjective burden [23-27] is defined as the caregiver's attitude towards or emotional reactions to the caregiving experience, or changes in various aspects of the caregiver's life and household. In this context, caregiver burden is not necessarily perceived as an unavoidable, negative consequence of providing care, but is defined by the subjective perceptions of caregivers related to the degree of problems experienced in relation to the patients specific impairments. This suggests that burden is processed through caregivers subjective perception.

Objective burden involves disruption to family life that is potentially verifiable and observable. More recently, instead of describing burden as a subjective/objective dichotomy, caregiver burden is viewed as multi-dimensional. This refers to the physical, psychological or emotional, social, and financial problems that can be experienced by family members caring for a chronically ill or impaired family member [28–31].

The Dimensions of Caregiver Burden

We must begin to quantify the factors that contribute to and describe informal caregiver burden so that appropriate outcome measures can be developed to assess the value of interventions with future initiatives and research. A recent conceptual model was introduced by Chou [32] and may provide a helpful context in which to look at the multiple factors that influence informal caregiver burden. This model of caregiver burden is based on delineation of:
1) critical attributes of burden
2) predisposing factors that influencing the occurrence of burden
3) mediating and or moderating factors and
4) consequences or outcomes.

Critical Attributes

The critical attributes of caregiver burden refer to the characteristics of the concept of burden. These factors could be considered the primary determinants of burden. In this model, the four primary attributes, or determinants of burden include: subjective perception, multidimensional phenomena, dynamic change and overload. Subjective perception has been described above. Many reports have described the process of burden as based on how the caregiver interprets the demands of the care-receiver. In this way, burden develops based on the caregivers subjective perception of the demands of caregiving.

Multidimensional phenomena: As already mentioned, the demand that arises out of caregiving is multi-faceted. Broadly speaking, the more objective aspects of caregiver burden appear to fall into four areas: physical, financial, psychological, and social [31].

Dynamic change: Most illness, whether chronic or acute, involves a dynamic process. Therefore, it follows that the burden arising for people caring for their loved ones at home will also be in flux. As the demands of care receivers change, whether because of intervening illness or due to deterioration in chronic disease, caregiver burden will also change. Clearly, burden will change as the demands and extent of caregiving involvement change. In fact, burden may change over time in both directions. Caregiver burden changes over time because of increasing disability of the impaired receiver, but it will also change as the caregiver adapts and discovers new coping mechanisms for new, and established, caregiving problems.

Overload: Another primary determinant of burden arises from the overload that may occur in the process of caregiving. This overload may lead to changes in the subjective perception of burden by the caregiver but is based on demands that may be easily recognized and that may provide opportunities for intervention to ease caregiver burden. These demands may come from the care receiver, work, family members, or society. It is really a matter of supply and demand. The caregiver will perceive burden to increase when demands are greater than available resources.

Predisposing Factors

For any illness, there are predisposing factors that may alter the course of disease. The same can be said for caregiver burden. In the same way that understanding the interaction between predisposing factors and the development of illness may inform the development of interventions that will alter the course of illness, identifying predisposing factors that affect the process of caregiver burden may allow for interventions that will attenuate burden. These factors increase the risk or vulnerability for perceiving burden, and are clearly primary determinants of burden. They include caregivers characteristics, demands of caregivers, and involvement in caregiving.

Caregivers characteristics: Pertinent characteristics of caregivers that are likely to affect the likelihood of burden include social situations, health status, and psychological factors.
1. *Social locations:* Social and economic class, race, ethnicity, gender have all been reported to affect the process of caregiver burden. Studies have demonstrated greater burden on female caregivers [29, 33–35]. Women often carry multiple roles including mother, wage earner, and household manager. The majority of reported caregivers are women (47–80 %), and several studies have reported that female caregivers perceived their burden to be greater than men [25, 26, 36–38].
2. *Economic resources* also play an important role in a family's perception of well-being. Income has been found to be the primary determinant of whether and how many services can be purchased to alleviate the burden of caregiving [21, 25, 35, 39]. Insufficient income reduces access to resources that might make caregiving more bearable. Financial expense of caregiving has been reported to correlate with burden.
3. *Race and culture* are important predisposing factors in the development of caregiver burden [36, 40]. Normal levels of intergenerational contact may affect perception of burden. Given the wide variation in this contact across cultures, cultural values [41] may also affect perceived burden.
4. *The health of a caregiver* will affect burden. For instance, two factors for human immunodeficiency virus (HIV) caregivers that may affect the context of caregiving and its outcomes is the caregiver's own HIV status and his or her perceptions of vulnerability to acquired immunodeficiency syndrome (AIDS) [42]. Caregiver health is a predisposing factor for burden and is also a dynamic factor, as burden itself may affect the health of caregivers [25, 29, 3335, 4345].
5. *Certain factors in the psychological makeup of the caregiver* will clearly impact the perception of burden. Some examples of these factors, as reported in the literature include: a sense of obligation and responsibility, affection and reciprocity in the caregiver/receiver relationship, and family history [25, 34, 38, 45–47]. In a study that evaluated the impact of caregiver-receiver relationship

on burden, Snyder [48] reported that the quality of the relationship between the caregiver and care-receiver, and the bonds established between caregiver and receiver, distinguished low burden and high satisfaction. Furthermore, this study found that the history of the parent/child relationship strongly impacts reciprocity in the aging parent/child relationship. In the burdened households, part of the frustration experienced by caregivers could be attributed to the absence of a reciprocal caregiver/receiver relationship and the lack of high quality interactions. These psychological factors may affect motivation for the caregiver as well as the level of burden experienced by the caregiver [33, 35, 43, 49, 50], and understanding these factors is essential to any process designed to moderate caregiver burden.

The demands of caregivers also provide important predisposing factors in the evolution of caregiver burden, and may be viewed as primary and secondary demands. Primary demands are determined by functional limitation and degree of disturbance behavior of care-receiver. The degree of functional limitation has been well documented in the literature to correlate with caregiver burden [40]. Other primary demands include the presence of disturbance behavior, which can lead to caregiver fatigue and anxiety [21, 22, 25, 26, 51, 52]. There are also secondary demands that may serve as predisposing factors for burden. These demands may come from family, work, or society. Demands such as the presence of other children in the house or single caregiver families have been reported to increase caregiver burden [20].

Involvement in caregiving: This is another predisposing factor and is defined as the number of caregiving tasks performed and the amount of time the caregiver spends performing them. The number of hours per day caregiving as well as the number of tasks involved has been positively correlated with burden [53]. A positive correlation between activities of care performed by the caregiver and caregiver burden has been reported, and includes both the provision of direct care such as bathing, transfer, continence-related measures, and indirect care such as running errands, preparing meals, helping with medicines and performing house-work [33].

Mediating and/or Moderating Factors

Having described the primary determinants, or attributes of burden and predisposing factors that may influence the development of burden, it is essential to incorporate the role of factors that may modify burden into any model of informal caregiving. These factors may alter the impact of the previously described factors significantly. This may account for contradictory reports on the impact of primary determinant caregiver burden. In some studies, some attributes are reported as major determinants of burden, while in others, the same element may be reported as playing a smaller role in the process of burden. For instance, the functioning level of the care-receiver, while viewed by many as a major determinant of caregiver burden, has been reported to have little impact on burden [20].

The burden experienced by a caregiver is in part determined by the caregiver's choice of coping strategies. Higher levels of interaction with family members, social and spiritual support seeking behaviors, and receiving help from family members have all been reported to decrease burden [28]. Other coping strategies, such as confidence in problem solving, reframing the problem, passivity, use of spiritual or social support, information seeking and extended families may lessen burden [28, 34, 52]. Turner and Catania [43] have reported that the association between objective demands and subjective burden is stronger among caregivers who receive little or no help than among caregivers who feel they have support. Receiving help with caregiving does appear to buffer the negative impact of high care giving demands on burden. Caregiver coping strategies are significantly related to caregiver burden, and may not always have a positive impact. Avoidance coping strategies, for example, have been shown to have a negative impact on burden [54].

Consequences/outcomes

Finally, any model of caregiver burden must also describe the consequences or outcomes of caregiver burden on the caregiver. Most studies are descriptive, so no precise predictions can be made about the impact of burden on various outcomes. However, impact can, and does, occur on the caregiver, care-receiver, family and health care system:

Caregiver: Deterioration in the health status of the informal caregiver has been extensively reported in the literature. These include somatic complaints such as chronic fatigue, sleeplessness, stomach problems, weight change, increase illness rate [33, 36]. Psychological symptoms are also well known in the caregiving population depression, anger, worry, discouragement, guilt, anxiety [23, 29, 51, 54]. A recent report [4] found depression much more common in stroke caregivers (3452 %) than in the normal matched population (1216 %). Using the Common-wealth Fund 1998 survey of womens health, a nationally representative sample of women and men, Donelan [36] reported that women caregivers are significantly more likely than other women to report having a serious health problem that requires medical care.

Obviously, restriction in the social activity of informal caregivers is another common outcome of caregiving, the role of which is often under-appreciated.

The care receiver may also suffer the consequences of caregiver burden. For children, personal distress in the caregiver has been correlated with an increase in withdrawn and apathetic behavior in the care-receiver child [55].

Family: In addition to the consequence of caregiving on the caregiver and receiver, families may also experience the negative outcomes of informal caregiving. Family/marital conflict is common when examining caregiver burden. It has been reported that 3056 % of caregivers experienced family or marital conflict as a result of burden. In families of patients with traumatic brain injury, problems with role functioning, marital relationships, drug or alcohol abuse and the physical health of individual family members become evident during the first few years after injury [23].

Healthcare system: Finally, no discussion of caregiver burden is complete without mentioning the enormous financial costs associated with informal caregiving. While healthcare systems may actually save considerable costs by moving care from institutions to families, these cost savings are not passed along to these families who suffer an enormous financial burden as a result.

Conclusion

Improved ICU survival and the transition to community-based care have increased awareness of the extent and importance of family caregiving. Many individuals are now cared for at home, who might otherwise have been institutionalized. This has placed increased attention on the need to address implications for family life and for the primary caregiver.

Further studies are needed to evaluate the long-term effects of ICU survival on the health and well being of relationships, and measurements of ICU outcomes must take much more than 28-day all cause mortality into consideration. While it is certainly good for ICU clinicians to feel good about the way in which survival is improving for critical illness, we must begin to look at a larger view of our patients' survival and ongoing health. As outcomes from critical illness continue to improve, it is inevitable that the number of informal caregivers will increase. As clinicians, it is important to recognize the impact of survival, not only on patients but on families as well. Given the enormous impact of caregiver burden on patients and their loved ones, evaluating and improving the burden placed on families of ICU survivors must be viewed as an essential aspect of the care we offer our patients who survive critical illness.

References

1. Bernard GR, Vincent JL, Laterre PF, et al (2001) for The Recombinant Human Activated Protein C Worldwide Evaluation in Severe Sepsis (PROWESS) Study Group. Efficacy and Safety of Recombinant Human Activated Protein C for Severe Sepsis. N Engl J Med 344:699–709
2. Rivers E, Nguyen B, Havstad S (2001) for the Early Goal-Directed Therapy Collaborative Group. Early goal-directed therapy in the treatment of severe sepsis and septic shock. N Engl J Med 345:1368–1377
3. Van den Berghe G, Wouters P, Weekers F, et al (2001) Intensive insulin therapy in critically ill patients. N Engl J Med 345:1359–1367
4. Han B, Haley WE (1999) Family caregiving for patients with stroke: Review and analysis. Stroke 30:1478–1485
5. Capuzzo M, Bianconi M, Contu P, Payoni V, Gritti G (1996). Survival and quality of life after intensive care. Intensive Care Med 22:947–953
6. Ridley SA, Wallace PGM (1990) Quality of life after intensive care. Anaesthesia 45:808–813
7. Wehler M, Martus P, Geise A, et al (2001) Changes in quality of life after medical intensive care. Intensive Care Med 27:154–159

8. Elliott D (1999) Measuring the health outcomes of general ICU patients: a systematic review of methods and findings. Aust Crit Care 12:132–140

9. Davidson TA, Rubenfeld GD, Caldwell ES, Hudson LD, Steinberg KP (1999) The effect of acute respiratory distress syndrome on long-term survival. Am J Respir Crit Care Med 160: 1838–1842

10. Davidson TA, Caldwell ES, Curtis JR, Hudson LD, Steinberg KP (1999) Reduced quality of life in survivors of acute respiratory distress syndrome compared with critically ill control patients. JAMA 28:354–360

11. Dragsted L, Qvist J (1989) Outcome from intensive care. I. A 5-year study of 1308 patients: methodology and patient population. Eur J Anaesthesiol 6:23–37

12. Brooks R, Kerridge R, Hillman K, Bauman A, Daffurn K (1997) Quality of life outcomes after intensive care. Intensive Care Med 23:581–586

13. Yinnon A, Zimran A, Hershko C (1989) Quality of life and survival following intensive medical care. Q J Med 71:347–357

14. Konopad E, Noseworthy T, Johnston R, Shustack A, Grace M (1995) Quality of life measures before and one year after admission to an intensive care unit. Crit Care Med 23:1653–1659

15. Parno JR, Teres D, Lemeshow S, Brown RB, Spitz Avrunin J (1984) Two-year outcome of adult intensive care patients. Med Care 22:167–176

16. Montuclard L, Garrouste-Orgeas M, Timsit JF, Misset B, De Jonghe B, Carlet J (2000) Outcome, functional autonomy, and quality of life of elderly patients with a long-term intensive care unit stay. Crit Care Med 28:3389–3395

17. Findlay JY, Plenderleith JL, Schroeder DR (2000) Influence of social deprivation on intensive care outcome. Intensive Care Med 26:929–933

18. Rivera-Fernández R, Sánchez-Cruz J, Abizanda-Campos R, Vázquez-Mata G (2001) Quality of life before intensive care unit admission and its influence on resource utilization and mortality rate. Crit Care Med 29:1701–1709

19. Capuzzo M, Grasselli C, Carrer S, Gritti G, Alvisi R (2000) Quality of life before intensive care admission: agreement between patient and relative assessment. Intensive Care Med 26:1288–1295

20. Smith AM, Schwirian PM (1998) The relationship between caregiver burden and TBI survivors cognition and functional ability after discharge. Rehabil Nurs 23:252–257

21. Grad J, Sainsbury P (1966) Problems of caring for the mentally ill at home. Proc R Soc Med 59:20–23

22. Kosberg JI, Caril R, Keller DM (1990) Components of burden: Interventive implications. Gerontologist 30:236–242

23. Schofield HL, Murphy B, Herrman HE, Block S, Singh B (1997) Family caregiving: measurement of emotional well-being and various aspects of the caregiving role. Psychol Med 27:647–657

24. Bull MJ (1990) Factors influencing family caregiver burden and health. West J Nurs Res 12:758–770

25. Carey PJ, Oberst MT, McCubbin MA, Hughes SH (1991) Appraisal and caregiving burden in family members caring for patients receiving chemotherapy. Oncol Nurs Forum 18:1341–1348

26. Chou KR, LaMontagne LL, Hepworth JT (1999) Burden experienced by caregivers of relatives with dementia in Taiwan. Nurs Res 48:206–214

27. Novak M, Guest C (1989) Application of a multidimensional caregiver burden inventory. Gerontologist 29:798–803

28. Kosciulek J (1999) A multidimensional longitudinal analysis of family coping with brain injury. Int J Rehabil Res 22:269–276

29. Kleinpell RM (1991) Needs of families of critically ill patients: a literature review. Crit Care Nurse 11:34, 38–40

30. McCubbin HI (1993) Culture, ethnicity, and the family: Critical factors in childhood chronic illness and disabilities. Pediatrics 116 (Suppl 5):1063–1070

31. Ostwald SK (1997) Caregiver exhaustion: Caring for the hidden patients. Adv Pract Nurs Q 3:29–35
32. Chou K-R (2000) Caregiver Burden: A Concept Analysis. J Pediatr Nurs 15:398–407
33. Faison K, Faria S, Frank D (1999) Caregivers of chronically ill elderly: Perceived burden. J Community Health Nurs 16:243–253
34. Kreutzer JS, Marwitz JH, Kepler K (1992) Traumatic brain injury: Family response and outcome. Arch Phys Med Rehabil 73:771–778
35. Braithwaite V (1992) Caregiving burden: Making the concept scientifically useful and policy relevant. Res Aging 14:327
36. Donelan K, Falik M, DesRoches C (2001) Caregiving: Challenges and Implications for Womens Health. Womens Health Issues 11:185–200
37. Fink SV (1995) The influence of family resources and family demands on the strains and well-being of caregiving families. Nurs Res 44:139–145
38. Coppel D, Burton C, Becker J, Fiore J (1985) Relationships of cognition associated with coping reactions to depression in spousal caregivers of Alzheimers disease patients. Cognitive Therapy and Research 9:253–266
39. Mastrian KG, Ritter RC, Deimling GT (1996) Predictors of caregiver health strain. Home Healthc Nurse 14:209–217
40. Lim PPJ, Sahadevan S, Choo GK, Anthony P (1999) Burden of Caregiving in Mild to Moderate Dementia: An Asian Experience. Int Psychogeriatr 11:411–420
41. Montgomery R, Stull D, Borgatta E (1985) Caregiving and experience of subjective and objective burden. Fam Relat 34:19–26
42. Turner H, Catania J (1997) Informal caregiving to persons with AIDS in the United States: Caregiver burden among central cities residents eighteen to forty-nine years old. Am J Community Psychol 25:35–59
43. Canam C, Acorn S (1999) Quality of life for family caregivers of people with chronic health problems. Rehab Nurs 24:292–300
44. Poulshock SW, Deimling GT (1984) Families caring for elders in residence: Issues in the measurement of burden. J Gerontol 39:230–239
45. Robinson K (1990) Relationship between social skills, social support, self-esteem and burden in adult caregivers. J Adv Nurs 5:788–795
46. Chakrabarti S, Kulhara P, Verma SK (1992) Extent and determinants of burden among families of patients with affective disorders. Acta Psychiatr Scand 86:247–252
47. Woods NF, Haberman MR, Packard NJ (1993) Demands of illness and individual, dyadic and family adaptations in chronic illness. West J Nurs Res 15:10–25
48. Snyder JR (2000) Impact of caregiver-receiver relationship quality on burden and satisfaction. J Women Aging 12:147–167
49. Elmstahl S, Malmberg B, Annerstedt L (1996) Caregivers burden of patients 3 years after stroke assessed by a novel caregiver burden scale. Arch Phys Med Rehabil 77:177–182
50. Dowler JM, Jordon-Simpson DA, Adams O (1992) Gender inequalities in caregiving in Canada. Health Rep 4:125–136
51. Wicks MN, Milstead EJ, Hathaway DK, Cetingok M (1998) Family caregivers burden, quality of life, and health following patients renal transplantation. J Transpl Coord 8:170–176
52. Davidhizar R (1994) Powerlessness of caregivers in home care. J Clin Nurs 3:155–158
53. Zarit SH, Reever KE, Bach-Peterson J (1980) Relatives of the impaired elderly: Correlates of feelings of burden. Gerontologist 20:649–655
54. Wade S, Borawski E, Taylor HG, Yeates K, Stancin T (2001) The relationship of caregiver coping to family outcomes during the initial year following pediatric traumatic injury. J Consult Clin Psychol 69:406–415
55. Sabbeth BF, Leventhal JB (1984) Marital adjustment to chronic illness: A critique of the literature. Pediatrics 73:762–768

Long-term Economic Consequences of Surviving Intensive Care

K. G. Kalassian and D. C. Angus

Introduction

Health care consumes an enormous amount of public spending. In the United States, the annual amount spent on health care reached $ 1.2 trillion in 1999 or 13.0 % of the gross domestic product (GDP) [1], of which $549 billion constituted public funds. This spending is expected to rise dramatically over the next decade with the projected national health expenditure increasing to $2.6 trillion or 15.9 % of GDP by the year 2010 [2]. The finite nature of societal resources available to meet this increased expenditure will mandate an evaluation of the cost effectiveness of all medical interventions. As one of the largest cost centers, intensive care will come under close scrutiny. Increasing costs of existing therapies, as well as new biopharmaceutical and other therapies for critical illness, will not only substantially raise the cost of acute medical care but will also produce ICU survivors who will have significant chronic health problems and associated long-term health care costs. In addition to direct medical expenditures, society will bear the burden of the indirect costs of the survivors, and of the caregivers of those survivors, such as reduced quality of life and lost productivity. We review the costs accrued after treatment in the intensive care unit (ICU) and propose a research agenda aimed at a better understanding of the economic consequences of surviving intensive care.

Data for Measuring the Costs of ICU Survival

The availability of data often determines the quality of research. Primary data collection for the investigation of a complex process such as the economic consequences of surviving intensive care would require extremely detailed measurement instruments, application of these instruments longitudinally over a prolonged period of time, and a large sample size. The logistical and cost considerations of such a study are usually prohibitive. Since primary data collection is rarely an option, public use survey data for general demography, health, and economics represent a more practical and affordable way of obtaining information [3]. Public use survey databases useful for investigation of the economic consequences of surviving intensive care are listed in Table 1. In addition, administrative databases such as the social security, federal and state workers compensation, and insurance industry databases may provide valuable information, particularly when linked to public use survey databases. The main obstacles to the utilization of these databases are:

1. Logistical concerns including rules of confidentiality, the dispersed locations of the data, and the proprietary nature of some of the information
2. Lack of an 'intensive care survivor' identifier among datasets
3. Comingling of cost data obscuring long-term cost differences between an intensive care survivor and hospital survivor, referred to as the attributable long-term cost
4. Case mix variation among datasets including age, diagnosis, and country of origin. Improved access and coordination of these data has become a priority in health services research and promises to facilitate investigation of the consequences of intensive care [4].

By convention, costs are classified as direct or indirect. Direct costs are defined as the value of all health care resources (e.g., medical facilities, personnel, tests, drugs) consumed in the provision of a medical intervention. Indirect costs are defined as non-medical costs (e.g., lost earnings, caregiver time, lost household productivity) associated with care of an individual suffering from illness. Indirect costs may be further subdivided into those arising from a disability directly affecting the ability to work (work-related disability), and those arising from a disability affecting non-work activities (work-unrelated disability). Assessment of these costs is de-

Table 1. Public Survey Databases. Modified from [3] with permission.

Survey	Description
Current Population Survey (CPS)	Monthly survey of 50,000 households includes questions regarding health of household members and effects of health on work.
Health and Retirement Study (HRS)	A nationally representative longitudinal survey focusing on retirement, aging, health insurance, and economic security
Medical Expenditure Panel Survey (MEPS)	A nationally representative probability survey of non-institutionalized US civilians on health care cost issues
National Health Interview Survey (NHIS)	A sample survey of 50,000 US civilians annually inquiring about the incidence and extent of illness and health services received.
National Longitudinal Survey of Youth	Longitudinal survey of youth ages 14–21 as of December 31, 1978. Inquires about health limitations to work.
National Health and Nutrition Evaluation Survey	A nationally representative probability survey of health care costs including information on nutrition and physical examinations

pendent on the purpose for which the costs are being obtained and the time frame of the cost analysis.

The perspective from which costs are determined and analyzed is of crucial importance because of its effect on what constitutes the appropriate components of a cost effectiveness analysis. As an example, health insurers may consider the economic impact of critical illness on family caregivers unimportant for their analysis of costs, whereas from the perspective of the patient and society, this impact may be profound. There has been general agreement within the discipline of healthcare economics that all stakeholders needed to be taken into account and that the concept of cost is therefore properly viewed from a societal perspective. From this viewpoint, healthcare expenditures are apportioned from available public capital in a way that maximizes the overall benefit to society [5].

Like perspective, the time frame of a cost analysis is a critical element in assessing healthcare costs. Critical illness, such as septic shock with multiorgan failure, may result in immediate post-ICU economic consequences. In contrast, certain manifestations of critical illness, for instance post-traumatic stress disorder after the acute respiratory distress syndrome (ARDS), may not become economically significant until a long period of time following the onset of the acute disease process.

Direct Medical Expenditures Following Intensive Care

Although significant effort has been directed at costing care provided within the ICI, a dearth of data exist on the cost of hospitalization after intensive care and the medical costs after hospitalization for intensive care survivors. The costs of medical care after discharge from intensive care and prior to hospital discharge can be estimated from hospital bills, which provide a registration of resource use for each patient at the patient level. Hospital charges do not reflect actual costs and, as a result, cost to charge ratios have been developed for all US hospitals. These cost to charge ratios are included in the Medicare Cost Report. The methods by which these ratios are formulated are subject to criticism. It is thus controversial as to whether true costs are being reflected [6]. Physician charges are not accounted for in hospital charges and actual costs of physician services are difficult to acquire. A standard multiplier technique has customarily been used to account for physician services as a percentage of total hospital costs [7]. Medical resource use at the patient level after hospital discharge is more difficult to calculate. Analyses of public use surveys that project annual medical expenditures as a function of age, are often used as a surrogate for costs at the patient level. Despite their limitations, these methods of cost estimation are now commonplace in formal cost analyses [8].

Formal cost analyses in fields such as cardiology, have been incorporated into large multinational randomized trials as well as many longitudinal cohort studies. In intensive care medicine, in contrast, investigations have been limited to studies utilizing such economic benchmarks as the cost of hospital readmissions and to studies informally examining the incremental cost of intensive care survivorship versus hospital survivorship to discharge [9–11]. These economic analyses however, in which the cost of one-year survivorship varied from approximately $60,000–$280,000, fall far short of a comprehensive cost accounting of the post-intensive care period. The need for such a comprehensive approach is underscored by studies suggesting that one third to one half of total hospital costs occur after discharge from the ICU [12, 13]. For example, diseases such as the acquired immune deficiency syndrome (AIDS) and organ failure requiring transplantation are much more likely to have on average higher non-hospital costs (e.g. large pharmacy expenditures) than hospital associated costs, hospitalization and intensive care notwithstanding.

Indirect Costs Following Intensive Care

Less apparent than direct medical expenditures are other costs to society such as, for example, death after surviving intensive care, decline in productivity of intensive care survivors and the economic impact upon their households. Although they may be less apparent and more difficult to quantify, indirect costs may be more important from an economic standpoint than direct medical expenditures. The indirect costs of care of the chronically debilitated, a population akin to many intensive care survivors, may make up as much 85 % of their total health care costs [14].

To consider these costs, we can adopt a taxonomy, such as that proposed by Weil for the cost analysis of traumatic injuries in the workplace (Fig. 1) [15]. In an adaptation of Weil')s model, critical illness results in a variety of discrete health states ranging from death to no lasting functional limitation. In between these limits are states of health defined in terms of work-related disability and work-unrelated disability. Each of these states produces economic consequences from a societal perspective.

The Cost of Fatal Illness

Not only does long-term intensive care survivorship entail a cost to society, but non-survivorship results in a tremendous cost to society as well. It is from the non-survivors that we can assign, while suspending ethical considerations, a monetary value to life. The economic cost to society of fatal illness may be conceptualized as the resources society is willing to expend to substantially reduce the risk of death. Three methods are commonly employed to estimate the cost of fatal illness to society: Foregone earnings, contingent valuation, and compensating wage differentials. The foregone earnings method uses an estimate of lost productivity based on prior ability, training, and experience discounted to the present value of lost future earnings. This method underestimates costs, however, in groups with low income or with limited time remaining in the workforce [16]. Contingent valuation utilizes surveys to assess how much an individual is willing to pay in exchange for a substantial reduction in mortality. The results of the surveys are used to arrive at a monetary estimate for the value of life. The survey instruments used in contingent valuation are, for a variety of reasons, plagued by inconsistency in their estimations [4, 17]. The compensating wage differentials method relies upon the distribution of wage premiums associated with increasing work-related risks of fatality to

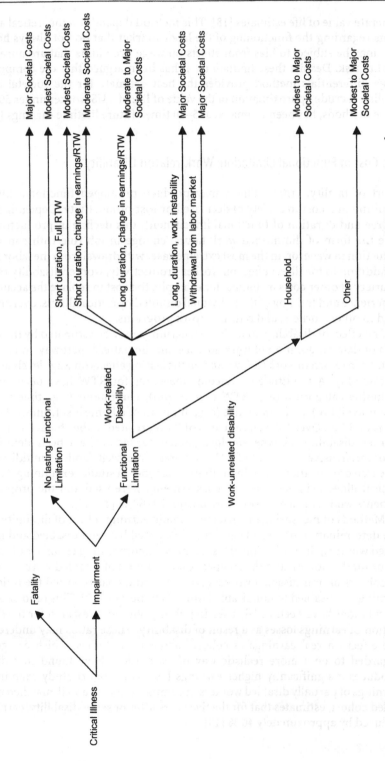

Fig. 1. Disability pathways from critical illness to economic outcomes. Adapted from [15] with permission. RTW: return to work

generate value of life estimates [18]. This method depends on theoretical assumptions regarding the functioning of the labor market that do not always hold true and may be subject to bias from effects on wage premiums that are unrelated to fatality risk. Despite these limitations, it has been argued that the compensating wage differentials method provides the best estimate for the societal costs of fatality. A crude approximation of the value of life of a US worker under 50, across these methods, has been estimated at 5–10 times future lifetime earnings [19].

The Cost of Functional Limitation: Work-related Disability

Short of fatality, critical illness may produce prolonged functional limitation resulting in a cost to society of decreased or lost productivity. Depending on the degree and duration of functional impairment, this decline in productivity may take the form of diminished work hours, change in job role with concomitant reduction in wage, or, in the most extreme case, withdrawal from the labor market. In addition to the direct effect on worker productivity, worker disability results in a variety of other costs including, for example, the cost to replace the accumulated experience and training of the individual disabled by critical illness, overtime costs paid to other workers, and return to work programs.

The effect of disability on individual earnings may be estimated by the integration of data on duration of work absence, on the pattern, pathway and economic result of a return to work (RTW), and on the lasting effects on wage levels as a result of disability. A multitude of outcome measures for RTW have been employed including categorical (e.g., RTW ever yes/no), continuous (e.g., time to first or sustained RTW), and cumulative (e.g., duration of all time lost from work) definitions of RTW. Over 100 determinants of RTW, related to the characteristics of the worker, disability, job type, employer, and other factors have been identified and a comprehensive treatment of RTW requires large, well-funded multidisciplinary research organizations [20]. In the limited number of studies examining RTW after critical illness, simple categorical assessments were used and the proportion of patients who returned to work varied from 20–80 % [21–24].

Methods of measuring the macroeconomic earnings effect of disability include the determination of a fixed earnings differential between disabled and non-disabled workers, the projection of lost earnings incorporating estimates of change in labor market forces, and the comparison of cohorts of disabled workers matched to cohorts of non-disabled workers [20]. One study has reported the ratio of real earnings of disabled to nondisabled workers to be 0.64 [25]. This ratio and similar calculations have been widely used in public policy and research for the determination of earnings losses as a result of disability. These ratios may underestimate the effect on real earnings as cohort comparison studies, which are generally regarded to be a more realistic way of estimation, have found that disability produces a significantly higher earnings loss. One cohort study examining the earnings of partially disabled workers in comparison with a well-matched non-disabled cohort, estimates that for the five years after onset of disability, earnings are reduced by approximately 40 % [15].

The Cost of Functional Limitation: Work-unrelated Disability

Work-unrelated disability greatly impacts upon the productivity and social functioning of those enlisted as caregivers. Work-unrelated disability is often left out of economic analyses because it is difficult to quantify and is often viewed as a free resource by policy makers. The costs resulting from work-unrelated disability have been examined in a variety of chronic illnesses [26–30].

A major problem in estimating the costs of work-unrelated disability is the accurate measurement of caregiver time. A number of validated disease-specific survey instruments have been developed, the majority of which ask caregivers to estimate the time spent on various activities on a typical day. These surveys are confounded by the inaccuracy of caregiver time estimates and by the intermingling of caregiver and non-caregiver, or what economists refer to as joint, activity. Detailed time and motion studies utilizing an observer to continuously record use of caregiver time, albeit complex and expensive, may be able to overcome such methodological problems [31].

Even if time allocation to caregiver activities is accurately assessed, the valuation of that time remains a challenge. The most common methods for valuing time include assessment of opportunity cost, frictional cost, replacement cost, and contingent valuation. In the opportunity cost method, caregivers are asked to identify the next-best use of their time and this foregone time is valued at their wage rate. The frictional cost method assumes that disability results in a temporary absence from the workplace, which entails a cost of a temporary absence from work and of worker replacement. The estimated cost of replacing an informal caregiver with professional allied health services is utilized in the replacement cost method. The contingent valuation method requires caregivers to estimate a cost they would be willing to pay for a substitute caregiver to assume their caregiver responsibilities. In one of the only studies examining the economic value of caregiver effort of patients who suffered a critical illness, the cost of caregiver time depended greatly on the choice of the method used for valuing that time [32].

Beyond caregiver time, there are numerous other direct and indirect costs to a household as a result of the disability of one member due to critical illness [33]. Costs of additional household expenses, for example heating, lighting, and other utilities, can be substantial. The impact on household non-work, social, and leisure activities is likewise significant. Methods examining overall effects on household income and household activity have been developed in order to more accurately capture the cost of these work-unrelated costs of disability [15].

Costs and Cost-Effectiveness Analysis

Cost-effectiveness analysis (CEA), the resource cost of a health intervention per unit measure of clinical outcome, has assumed greater importance as the demands on healthcare resources have increased. Examples of CEAs applied to intensive care are listed in Table 2. Few of these studies consider the long-term economic consequences of surviving intensive care. Furthermore, these studies vary widely in the manner in which costs were accounted for and in which CEA was performed, making them difficult to compare. National and international efforts have been mounted to standardize the methods of CEA to improve the quality and comparability of studies incorporating this technique, including satisfactory assessment of long-term economic consequences, so that it may effectively augment factors such as social equity and distributive justice when difficult decisions regarding resource allocation have to be made.

The ability of CEA to achieve this end is dependent upon accurate costing through comprehensive capture of all relevant costs. Ideally, this would occur through detailed 'micro-costing' approaches, but as described previously, this is rarely practical. General public use and administrative databases often allow for 'macro-costing' but may lack the detail for comprehensive capture of all costs relevant to assessing the long-term consequences of surviving intensive care.

Sensitivity analysis, in which a critical element (e.g., cost) of a CEA is varied from worst case to best case, can provide an indication of how sensitive a CEA might be to a substantial change in that element [34]. This method may aid in understanding uncertainty within a CEA but is not a substitute for detailed cost accounting. An activity-based costing method has been successfully implemented for tallying costs of patient care while in the ICU [35]. Activity-based costing relies on a limited number of labor-intensive primary data collection efforts to establish by micro-costing the cost of all the components (e.g., nursing, laboratory, consumables, etc.) of a particular patient care activity. This activity is then assigned a composite value that may obviate the need for repetitive, time-consuming cost accounting in subsequent CEAs. This proxy formation concept for critical care has yet to be applied outside of the ICU.

Future Directions

In recounting the difficulties in assessing the long-term economic consequences of intensive care, an agenda for further research may be generated:
- Management and linkage of databases to maximize the yield of high-quality data pertinent to cost assessment.
- Adoption of a structured approach to assessing post-ICU care to be included within increasingly standardized methods of cost-effectiveness analysis.
- Participation of intensivists in multidisciplinary research efforts to improve cost estimates of fatality as well as the factors affecting, and the cost of, work-related disability and work-unrelated disability.
- Increased emphasis on cost-effectiveness analysis, including long-term costs, as an integral part of clinical trials in intensive care.
- Large, detailed studies of the natural history of critical illness including micro-costing of long-term economic consequences of intensive care to allow the creation of valid cost proxies for use in further research.

Table 2. Examples of cost-effectiveness analyses in intensive care medicine. Adapted from [36] with permission.

1st Author	Study
Mascia	Pharmacoeconomic impact of rational use guidelines on the provision of analgesia, sedation, and neuromuscular blockade in critical care. Crit Care Med 28:2300–2306, 2000.
Lage	Association between abciximab and length of stay in intensive care for patients undergoing percutaneous coronary intervention. A 2-stage econometric model in a naturalistic setting. Pharmacoeconomics 18:581–589, 2000.
Dominguez	The impact of adverse patient occurrences on hospital costs in the pediatric intensive care unit. Crit Care Med 29:169–174, 2001.
Price	Financial impact of elimination of routine chest radiographs in a pediatric intensive care unit. Crit Care Med 27:1588–1593, 1999.
Thureen	Once versus twice-daily gentamycin dosing in neonates >34 weeks gestation: cost-effectiveness analyses. Pediatrics 103:594–98, 1999.
Shorr	Continuous subglottic suctioning for the prevention of ventilator-associated pneumonia: potential economic implications. Chest 119:228–235, 2001.
Veenstra	Cost-effectiveness of antiseptic impregnated central venous catheters for the prevention of catheter-related bloodstream infection. JAMA 282:554–560, 1999.
Saint	The clinical and economic consequences of nosocomial central venous catheter-related infection: are antimicrobial catheters useful? Infect Control Hosp Epidemiol 21:375–380, 2000.
Heikkinen	Percutaneous dilational tracheostomy or conventional surgical tracheostomy? Crit Care Med 28:1399–1402, 2000.
Angus	Epidemiology of severe sepsis in the united states: analysis of incidence, outcome, and associated costs of care. Crit Care Med, 29:1303–1309, 2001.
Heyland	Is it „worthwhile" to continue treating patients with a prolonged stay (>14 days) in the ICU?: an economic evaluation. Chest 114:192–198, 1998.
Sznajder	A cost-effectiveness analysis of stays in intensive care units. Intensive Care Med, 27:146–153, 2001
Roberts	Economic evaluation and randomized controlled trial of extracorporeal membrane oxygenation: UK collaborative trial. Br Med J 317:911–916, 1998.
Korkeila	Costs of care, long-term prognosis and quality of life in patients requiring renal replacement therapy during intensive care. Intensive Care Med 26:1824–1831, 2000.
Hamel	Outcomes and cost-effectiveness of ventilator support and aggressive care for patients with acute respiratory failure due to pneumonia or acute respiratory distress syndrome. Am J Med 109:614–620, 2000.

Conclusion

As the burden of healthcare costs to society grows, difficult choices will have to be made regarding the allocation of increasingly scarce public resources. Intensive care will be under increasing pressure to provide accurate estimates of costs, including both direct and indirect long-term costs, for standardized cost-effectiveness analysis. At present there are limited data regarding the cost of post-intensive care medical treatment and a paucity of information regarding the long-term economic consequences of intensive care. New methods to improve data management and to better describe this complex process are a priority within the field of health services research. To do our part, intensive care medicine should make it a priority to include formal cost analysis as an outcome in future clinical investigations so that the best decisions for our patients are made in the challenging economic environment ahead.

References

1. U. S. Department of Health and Human Services (2000) Health, United States, 2001. Centers for Disease Control and Prevention, National Center for Health Statistics, Hyattsville
2. National health expenditures projections: 2000–2010. (Last updated 2002) Available at: http://www.hcfa.gov/stats/nhe-proj/proj2000/default.htm.
3. Reville RT, Bhattacharya J, Sager WL (2001) New methods and data sources for measuring economic consequences of workplace injuries. Am J Ind Med 40:452–463
4. Boden LI, Biddle EA, Spieler EA (2001) Social and economic impacts of workplace illness and injury: current and future directions for research. Am J Ind Med 40:398–402
5. Russell LB, Gold MR, Siegel JE, Daniels N, Weinstein MC (1996) The role of cost-effectiveness analysis in health and medicine. Panel on Cost-Effectiveness in Health and Medicine. JAMA 276:1172–1177
6. Gyldmark M (1995) A review of cost studies of intensive care units: problems with the cost concept. Crit Care Med 23:964–972
7. Ellis SG, Miller DP, Brown KJ, et al (1995) In-hospital cost of percutaneous coronary revascularization. Critical determinants and implications. Circulation 92:741–747
8. Spillman BC, Lubitz J (2000) The effect of longevity on spending for acute and long-term care. N Engl J Med 342:1409–1415
9. Lipsett PA, Swoboda SM, Dickerson J, et al (2000) Survival and functional outcome after prolonged intensive care unit stay. Ann Surg 231:262–268
10. Heyland DK, Konopad E, Noseworthy TW, Johnston R, Gafni A (1998) Is it 'worthwhile' to continue treating patients with a prolonged stay (>14 days) in the ICU? An economic evaluation. Chest 114:192–198
11. Montuclard L, Garrouste-Orgeas M, Timsit JF, Misset B, De Jonghe B, Carlet J (2000) Outcome, functional autonomy, and quality of life of elderly patients with a long-term intensive care unit stay. Crit Care Med 28:3389–3395
12. Kanter RK (2000) Post-intensive care unit pediatric hospital stay and estimated costs. Crit Care Med 28:220–223
13. Bams JL, Miranda DR (1985) Outcome and costs of intensive care: a follow-up study on 238 ICU-patients. Intensive Care Med 11:234–241
14. McDaid D (2001) Estimating the costs of informal care for people with Alzheimer')s disease: methodological and practical challenges. Int J Geriatr Psychiatry 16:400–405
15. Weil D (2001) Valuing the economic consequences of work injury and illness: a comparison of methods and findings. Am J Ind Med 40:418–437

16. Leigh JP, Markowitz SB, Fahs M, Shin C, Landrigan PJ (1997) Occupational injury and illness in the United States. Estimates of costs, morbidity, and mortality. Arch Intern Med 157:1557–1568
17. Schumacher EJ, Whitehead JC (2000) The production of health and the valuation of medical inputs in wage-amenity models. Soc Sci Med 50:507–515
18. Viscusi WK (1978) Labor market valuations of life and limb: empirical evidence and policy implications. Public Policy 26:359–386
19. Keeler EB (2001) The value of remaining lifetime is close to estimated values of life. J Health Econ 20:141–143
20. Krause N, Frank JW, Dasinger LK, Sullivan TJ, Sinclair SJ (2001) Determinants of duration of disability and return-to-work after work-related injury and illness: challenges for future research. Am J Ind Med 40:464–484
21. Eddleston JM, White P, Guthrie E (2000) Survival, morbidity, and quality of life after discharge from intensive care. Crit Care Med 28:2293–2299
22. Grotz M, Hohensee A, Remmers D, Wagner TO, Regel G (1997) Rehabilitation results of patients with multiple injuries and multiple organ failure and long-term intensive care. J Trauma 42:919–926
23. Mundt DJ, Gage RW, Lemeshow S, Pastides H, Teres D, Avrunin JS (1989) Intensive care unit patient follow-up. Mortality, functional status, and return to work at six months. Arch Intern Med 149:68–72
24. Zaren B, Hedstrand U (1987) Quality of life among long-term survivors of intensive care. Crit Care Med 15:743–747
25. Haveman R, Wolfe B (1990) The economic well-being of the disabled, 1962–84. J Hum Resour 25:32–54
26. Birnbaum HG, Berger WE, Greenberg PE, et al (2002) Direct and indirect costs of asthma to an employer. J Allergy Clin Immunol 109:264–270
27. Fautrel B, Guillemin F (2002) Cost of illness studies in rheumatic diseases. Curr Opin Rheumatol 14:121–126
28. Brown ML, Lipscomb J, Snyder C (1902) The burden of illness of cancer: economic cost and quality of life. Annu Rev Public Health 22:91–113
29. Henriksson F, Fredrikson S, Masterman T, Jonsson B (2001) Costs, quality of life and disease severity in multiple sclerosis: a cross-sectional study in Sweden. Eur J Neurol 8:27–35
30. Katzelnick DJ, Kobak KA, DeLeire T, et al (2001) Impact of generalized social anxiety disorder in managed care. Am J Psychiatry 158:1999–2007
31. Finkler SA, Knickman JR, Hendrickson G, Lipkin MJ, Thompson WG (1993) A comparison of work-sampling and time-and-motion techniques for studies in health services research. Health Serv Res 28:577–597
32. Sevick MA, Bradham DD (1997) Economic value of caregiver effort in maintaining long-term ventilator-assisted individuals at home. Heart Lung 26:148–157
33. McKinlay JB, Crawford SL, Tennstedt SL (1995) The everyday impacts of providing informal care to dependent elders and their consequences for the care recipients. J Aging Health 7:497–528
34. Briggs A, Sculpher M (1995) Sensitivity analysis in economic evaluation: a review of published studies. Health Econ 4:355–371
35. Edbrooke DL, Stevens VG, Hibbert CL, Mann AJ, Wilson AJ (1997) A new method of accurately identifying costs of individual patients in intensive care: the initial results. Intensive Care Med 23:645–650
36. Chalfin DB (2001) Pharmacoeconomic investigations in intensive care. Curr Opin Crit Care 7:460–463

Understanding Outcomes of Critically Ill Older Patients

E. W. Ely

Introduction

As physicians in the 21st century, our approach to the care of intensive care unit (ICU) patients will be shaped dramatically by the most striking demographic population shift of modern time, termed the 'geriatric demographic imperative'. Many intensivists are already familiar with the 'graying of the ICU', which results from the fact that adults over 85 years old are the most rapidly growing segment of our population (Fig. 1). While the 'oldest old' (>85 years) are currently estimated at 4 million, this number is expected to double in the U.S. by the year 2030 (accounting for more than one-fifth of the entire population) [1], and by the year 2050 there will be an estimated 15.3 million persons in this age group [2]. More than half of all ICU days are incurred by those over 65 years old, and the number of days per year spent in the ICU (per 1000 person-years) is 7-fold higher above age 75 as compared to those less than 65 [3]. Among people older than 65, over 10 % have chronic lung disease [4] and these people are at particularly high risk for experiencing serious health complications [5]. The rate of hospitalization for pneumonia in the subgroup of elderly who have chronic lung disease, for example, is 2 to 7 times higher than for their counterparts without coexistent pulmonary disease [6].

Because of the increasing population of elderly patients in our society, issues pertinent to geriatrics are increasingly important to health care professionals who manage patients in the ICU. This chapter represents a sign of the priority that we as intensivists will need to place on these topics. Rather than cover the gamut of aspects of care that are unique to the elderly, this chapter will address the following especially challenging topics:
1. Sepsis in older patients
2. Respiratory failure in older patients and outcomes of mechanical ventilation
3. Cognitive outcomes following the ICU
4. Ethical decisions related to mechanical ventilation in older patients

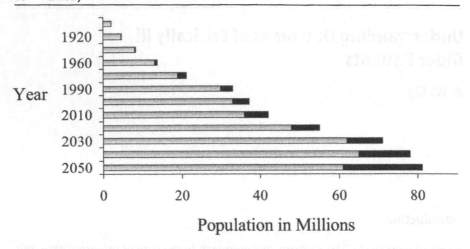

Fig. 1. Population 65 years and older: Historical data from US census bureau from year 1900 to year 2000 and then projected out to year 2050. Data for other continents, and especially from developed vs. developing countries were unavailable to the author at the time of this publication. Gray bars: 65–84 years old; black bars: over 85 years old

Severe Sepsis in Older Patients

Sepsis is an extremely important cause of morbidity and mortality in the older population, and its incidence has increased significantly in the last 10 years [7]. It is estimated that about 750,000 patients develop sepsis annually in the United States, 60 % of whom are over 65 years of age [8, 9]. Aging patients account for 40–50 % of all cases of bacteremia, and the overall case fatality rate for the older patient with bacteremia ranges from 40 to 60 % or more when due to Gram-negative organisms [10, 11].

The most recent observational cohort study conducted by Angus et al. [8] from seven state hospitals reported the incidence of severe sepsis according to the 1992 ACCP (American College of Chest Physicans) guidelines [12], i.e., sepsis associated with acute organ dysfunction. The estimated incidence of severe sepsis in this study was 3.0 cases per 1000 population. What is astounding is that the age-specific incidence of sepsis increased 100 fold with advanced age, to 26.2 cases per 1000 population in older patients. Mortality also steadily increased with comorbidity and advancing age, with a peak of 38.4 % in patients 85 years or older (Fig. 2) [8, 9].

In addition, sepsis consumes enormous healthcare resources, with an estimated annual cost of $16.7 billion in the United States in the year 2000 [8, 9]. With the advent of new and costly therapies for severe sepsis, such as drotrecogin alfa (activated) [11, 13], it will be important for the medical community to evaluate thoroughly the survival advantage and cost effectiveness of such interventions for older patients with severe sepsis. It is well documented that there is an age bias against aggressive care for older patients [14–16], and the appropriateness (or inappropriateness) of such a bias must be examined through future research. For

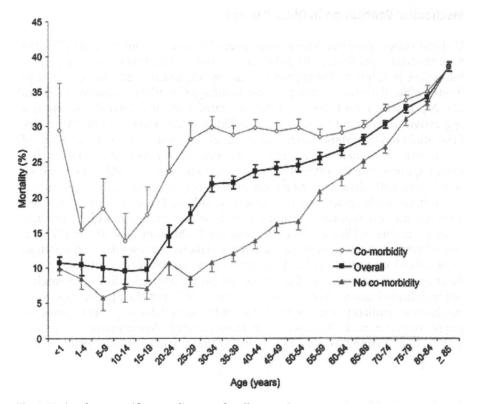

Fig. 2. National age-specific mortality rates for all cases of severe sepsis and for those with and without underlying comorbidity. Comorbidity is defined as a Charlson-Deyo score (23) >0. National estimates are generated from the seven-state cohort using state and national age- and gender-specific population estimates from the National Center for Health Statistics and the U.S. Census. Error bars represent 95 % confidence intervals. From [8] with permission

example, it is well known that the medical community exercised bias early on against the use of thrombolytics for acute myocardial infarction in older patients [17–19]. This may also occur with new sepsis treatments, though the available evidence does not support restricting use based on age alone. To use drotrecogin alfa (activated) as an example, PROWESS data demonstrated that the administration of recombinant activated protein C (rhAPC) was associated with a significant reduction in mortality (relative risk reduction =19.4 %; p=0.005) [11]. Mortality rates were 26 % and 49 % for placebo patients younger than 75 years and for those 75 years or older, respectively. The population of 386 patients 75 or older had a markedly high relative risk reduction of 31.7 %, and the number needed to treat to save a life in those 75 or older was six [20]. It was concluded from this analysis that the mortality benefit of drotrecogin alfa (activated) appears at least as high in older patients enrolled into PROWESS, with no increased risk of bleeding over the younger cohort.

Mechanical Ventilation in Older Patients

US health care expenditures for persons over 65 y/o are currently $1,740 billion (38 % of the total expenditure). By 2030, this amount is estimated to become $15,970 billion (74 % of total). One approach to decreasing health care costs might be to limit or ration the intensive care provided to the aged in order to conserve resources [21-24]. Indeed, recent data have demonstrated that the elderly do receive less aggressive management for some medical illnesses [25]. Data from the SUPPORT (The Study to Understand Prognoses and Preferences for Outcome and Risks of Treatments) investigators have shown that age (especially above 70 to 75 years) has great importance on the intensity of care given to patients [14-16] (Figs. 3 and 4). In addition, both physician and patient preferences for cardiopulmonary resuscitation influence hospital resource consumption [26]. There are surprisingly few 'expert consensus' reports regarding the decision to treat seniors with mechanical ventilation. One publication from the Office of Technology Assessment [27] discussed very reasonable perspectives, but few data were presented, and opinions were divided as to whether or not age should be a major determinant in the use of mechanical ventilation. One of the most limiting factors in this line of research is our inability to know with confidence the actual number of older patients in whom mechanical ventilation may be 'indicated' but bypassed due to patient, family, or physician preferences. Our inability to know the true 'denominator' should not stop us from learning what we can regarding the outcomes of older patients who

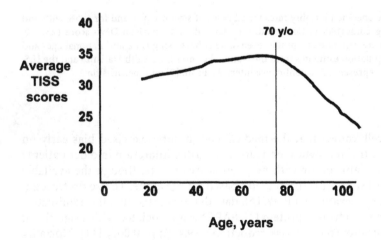

Fig. 3. The relationship between patient age and the intensity of care delivered to patients enrolled in the SUPPORT trial is depicted as patient age (x-axis) vs average Therapeutic Intervention Scoring System (TISS) on days 1 and 3 (y-axis). TISS is a valid and reliable method of measuring resource use in cohorts of patients. The solid line represents the TISS scores after adjustment for severity of illness and functional status, and shows that intensity of care was lower for older patients even after these adjustments. The reasons for this remain an important area for future research. Adapted from [14] with permission.

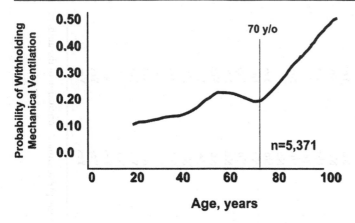

Fig. 4. The relationship between patient age and the adjusted probability of a decision to withhold mechanical ventilation by study day 30 in the SUPPORT investigation. At 70-79 years, relative risk 1.5 (1.2-1.9), and >80 relative risk 2.1 (1.6-2.7). Adapted from [14] with permission

succumb to respiratory failure, but must be acknowledged in academic discussions and also considered for future cohort investigations.

Age has been considered an important prognostic indicator of hospital outcome [23, 28], but many prior investigations of mechanical ventilation have been limited by their retrospective design and the absence of adjustment for confounding factors such as severity of illness [29–31]. Among 23 previously published reports (Table 1, [32, 33]), which included age-specific data on mechanically ventilated elderly patients, the authors' conclusions were divided regarding whether age influences outcome. Nineteen of these studies were restricted to mechanically ventilated patients, but only seven of them had prospective design. The diversity of the design and conclusions of these investigations has only served to fuel the controversy over the role of age on outcomes from mechanical ventilation.

Recent Cohorts of Older Patients Receiving Mechanical Ventilation

A recently published analysis of 902 patients from the National Heart, Lung and Blood Institute (NHLBI)-sponsored acute respiratory distress syndrome (ARDS) network's acute lung injury investigations in the US is the largest prospectively collected cohort to date. This investigation provided important insight into the outcomes of older patients with respiratory failure [32]. Patients 70 years and older had 28-day and 180-day mortality rates that were nearly twice those of patients less than 70, with steady reductions in survival by decile (Figs. 5 and 6). Even after adjusting for covariates, it was determined that age was a strong predictor of mortality. In fact, older persons had a hazard ratio of 2.5 for in-hospital mortality. Perhaps the most important findings of this report, with possible implications for patient management, were that surviving older persons achieved initial recovery landmarks at the same rate as their younger counterparts (i.e., they passed conven-

Table 1. Investigations describing outcomes after mechanical ventilation in older patients (references can be obtained from [32, 33])

Author/Year	Elderly (N) & Definition	Design of Study	Inclusion Criteria		Hospital Mortality (%)	Multivariate Analysis	Severity Adjustment	Age Influences Outcome**
Nunn, 1979	15 >75	Prospective	ICU	*	73	No	No	Yes
Campion, 1981	565 ≥75	Retrospective	ICU/CCU	16	No	No	No	
Fedullo, 1983	84 ≥70	Retrospective	MICU only	39	No	No	No	
Witek, 1985	51 >70	Prospective	ICU	*	51	No	No	Yes
McLean, 1985	49 ≥75	Prospective	ICU	*	43	No	No	No
Elpern, 1989	95 ≥60	Retrospective	ICU ≥ 3 days	*	66	No	No	Yes
Tran, 1990	92 >70	Retrospective	MICU only	46	No	No	Yes	
O'Donnell, 1991	17 >70	Retrospective	ICU	*	59	Yes	No	No
Pesau, 1992	99 ≥70	Retrospective	ICU	60	Yes	No	No	
Gracey, 1992	496 >65	Retrospective	ICU	*	46	No	No	Yes
Chelluri, 1992	34 ≥85	Retrospective	MICU only	*	38	No	No	No
Stauffer, 1993	118 >70	Retrospective	ICU	*	62	Yes	No	Yes
Swinburne, 1993	282 ≥80	Retrospective	ICU	*	69	No	No	No
Cohen, 1993	109 ≥80	Retrospective	ICU ≥ 3 days	*	62	No	No	Yes
Papadakis, 1993	138 ≥70	Retrospective	ICU	*	76	Yes	Yes	Yes
Dardaine, 1995	110 ≥70	Retrospective	ICU	*	38	No	No	No
Cohen, 1995	21,342 ≥70	Retrospective	ICU	*	59	No	No	Yes
Steiner, 1997	40 >65	Prospective	ICU/Stroke Pts	*	32 at 2 mo	Yes	No	Yes
Kurek, 1997	3,256 ≥70	Retrospective	Tracheostomy	*	64	No	No	Yes
Zilberberg, 1998	31 >65	Prospective	MICU	*	74	Yes	Yes	Yes
Kurek, 1998	4,101 ≥75	Retrospective	ICU	*	55	No	No	Yes
Ely, 1999	63 ≥75	Prospective	MICU/CCU	*	39	Yes	Yes	No
Ely, 2002	173 ≥70	Prospective	ARDS/ALI	*	50 at 28 days	Yes	Yes	Yes
Esteban, 2002	1038 ≥70	Prospective	ICU	*	52	Yes	Yes	Yes

MICU: medical intensive care unit; *Investigations including only mechanically ventilated patients; **Indicates the predominant conclusion of the authors as to whether or not age is independently important

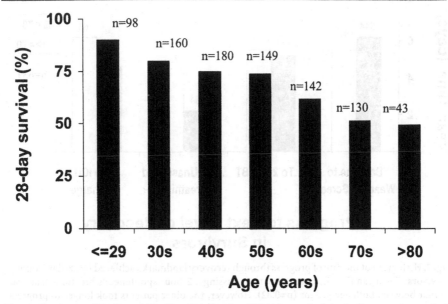

Fig. 5. Histogram of 28-day survival by decade of age: This figure depicts the decrease in survival seen in acute lung injury patients by decade of age (Spearman's rho=0.25, p<0.0001 across groups). The number of patients enrolled in each decade of age is listed above the bars, and the percentage of survivors at 28 days in each age group is plotted on the Y-axis. From [32] with permission.

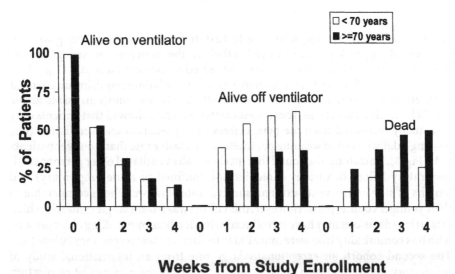

Fig. 6. Histogram of patient outcomes - time on ventilator and death: This plot shows the percentage of those <70 years old (white bars) vs. those 70 years and older (black bars) who were alive on the ventilator, alive off the ventilator, or dead at weekly intervals. At each time point, the percentages of younger and older patients alive and receiving mechanical ventilation (far left) were nearly identical (P=1.0), but the older patients were less often alive off the ventilator (center) and more often dead (far right). From [32] with permission.

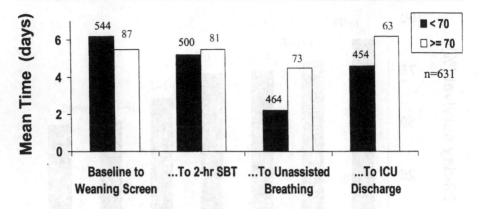

Progress to Next Level of Recovery in Survivors

Fig. 7. Histogram of the rate of progress through recovery landmarks achieved by 28-days among survivors: The mean time from enrollment to passing a 2-hour spontaneous breathing trial was similar between both age groups (p=0.82). However, the older patients took longer to progress from passing the 2-hour spontaneous breathing trial (SBT) to achieving 48 hours of unassisted breathing (p=0.002), as well as from this time point to being successfully discharged out of the ICU alive and off the ventilator (p=0.005). There were no differences seen in any of these time intervals among the nonsurvivors (data not shown, all p>0.2). From [32] with permission.

tional weaning criteria and were able to sustain spontaneous breathing without mechanical support), yet were delayed in their further progression through convalescence and much more likely to be reconnected to the ventilator [32] (Fig. 7).

Two additional cohorts of patients with respiratory failure requiring mechanical ventilation have particular relevance to the ARDS network cohort discussed above [33, 34]. The first report was from a medical ICU and also showed that patients over 75 actually recovered from the perspectives of oxygenation and ventilation (i.e., passing a daily screen of weaning parameters) at a faster rate than younger patients [33] (Fig. 8). This study also found that mechanically ventilated older persons (with respiratory failure of various etiologies not confined to acute lung injury) had lengths of stay on the ventilator and survival rates that were both comparable to their younger counterparts. However, this cohort was from a single center, in which local triage decisions may have introduced selection bias by enrolling older persons with less comorbidity who were more likely to survive their respiratory failure [33]. The second cohort, an exceptionally large one from an international study of respiratory failure that also enrolled patients with diverse causes of respiratory failure, showed that 1038 patients 75 years and older spent a similar amount of time on mechanical ventilation and in the hospital as compared to 4,118 patients less than 75 years old (both p>0.2) [34]. The older patients did have a higher ICU mortality than younger patients (38 vs. 30 %, p<0.001) and in-hospital mortality (52 vs. 37 %, p<0.001) [34].

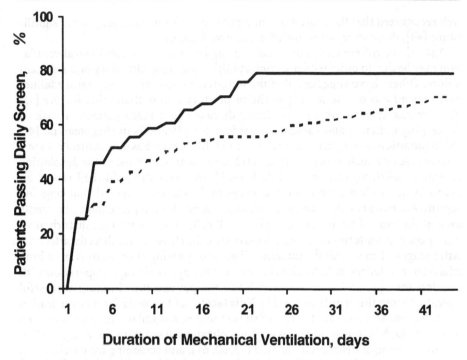

Fig. 8. Kaplan-Meier analysis of the days on mechanical ventilation versus the rate of recovery of respiratory failure (using the percent passing a daily screen of weaning parameters as a surrogate marker of 'recovery') after adjustment for sex, race, and severity of illness at baseline using a modified APACHE II score which excluded age. Using Cox proportional-hazards analysis to compare the proportions of patients who passed the daily screen in each group, elderly patients passed the daily screen earlier than younger patients [risk ratio 1.58 (95 % confidence interval, 1.13-2.22), p=0.03]. The solid line indicates patients >75 years old; dashed line indicates patients <75 years old. From [33] with permission.

Weaning in the Elderly

The duration of mechanical ventilation has been shown to be an independent predictor of mortality, even after adjusting for covariates such as severity of illness [35]. It is imperative that clinicians optimally time patients' liberation from the ventilator to reduce complications, pain and suffering, as well as expenses. The landmark most frequently used in ventilator weaning protocols to signify patients' readiness for extubation and independence from the ventilator has been the ability to breathe spontaneously [36–41]. In the ARDS network report [32], the most consistent message from the analyses was that older patients, regardless of their comparable rate of initial physiologic recovery, had a delay in successful liberation from the ventilator even after adjusting for survival status. Importantly, the reintubation rate for the older patients was more than twice that of the younger patients, which in itself has been found to increase independently the risk of adverse outcomes such as nosocomial pneumonia and mortality [39, 40, 42, 43]. While it is

well recognized that the cause and timing of reintubation have prognostic significance [44], these were not recorded in the investigation.

Age-related differences in outcomes during latter stages of mechanical ventilation may be due to older patients' comorbidities and nonpulmonary organ system
failure. Others have suggested that the long-term outcome of respiratory failure
may depend less on the severity of the respiratory failure than other factors [45,
46]. For example, occult cardiovascular disease could place patients at risk of
developing ischemia and subsequent cardiac complications during weaning [47,
48]. In addition, older patients are at great risk for having baseline central nervous
system diseases such as dementia or cerebrovascular accidents, or for developing
profound delirium while in the ICU [49–52]. In a recently published report on
delirium in mechanically ventilated patients, it was documented that ongoing
cognitive deficits and delirium were present in a substantial percentage of patients
even at the time of hospital discharge [53] (Fig. 9). Such neurologic disturbances
were poorly monitored in the ARDS network cohort, yet could directly affect the
latter stages of mechanical ventilation (i.e., after passing spontaneous breathing
trials) by interfering with the ability to protect the upper airway, cooperation with
physical therapy, and attempts to mobilize the patient, thus limiting successful
liberation from the ventilator [54–56]. This facet could prolong intubation, lead to
reintubation, and increase the risk of subsequent nosocomial pneumonia or even
death [39, 42, 57]. Recent advances in protocolization of sedation and analgesia [58,
59], monitoring of delirium in the ICU [53, 60, 61], and screening for baseline [62,
63] and long-term [64] cognitive impairment might enhance our ability to detect
and prevent such abnormalities and lead to improved quality of life [65] in older
survivors of acute lung injury.

The ACCP has recently published evidence-based guidelines for weaning [66]
including recommendations specific for the design and implementation of protocols driven by non-physician healthcare professionals [67]. It became evident
through the background research and writing of these guidelines, that specific

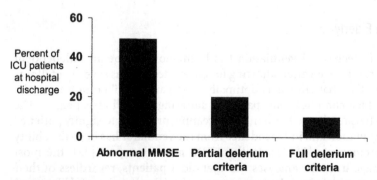

Fig. 9. Rate of ongoing cognitive deficits and delirium at hospital discharge following mechanical
ventilation. These data from survivors of ICU studied within 24 hours of leaving the hospital show
that 1 in 2 patients were significantly impaired by Folstein Mini-Mental State examination
(MMSE), 1 in 5 had partial delirium, and 1 in 10 met full delirium criteria at the time of hospital
discharge. From [53] with permission.

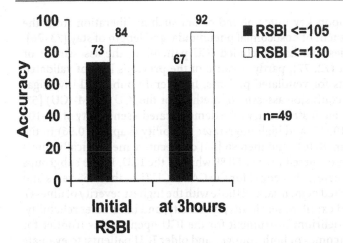

Fig. 10. The diagnostic accuracy of the rapid shallow breathing index (RSBI) in 49 patients over the age of 70 who were being weaned from mechanical ventilation. The highest accuracy of the RSBI in these patients was obtained by using a cutoff of 130 breaths/liter/minute at a delayed (3 hour) time point. Adapted from [69] with permission.

age-related decisions regarding the management of weaning from mechanical ventilation have been poorly studied. Gender, body habitus, and age are appropriate considerations, which may affect outcome from mechanical ventilation. Female gender, smaller endotracheal tube size (<7 mm), and age >70 have been associated with an elevated frequency/tidal volume (f/VT) ratio [68, 69], and it may be appropriate to adjust the 'passing' threshold for this measurement in these instances (Fig. 10). However, these age-related modifications of ventilator weaning parameters will require further prospective study prior to firm recommendations.

Cognitive Outcomes Following the ICU

Several other authors have contributed chapters directly related to this line of research. Therefore, this chapter will address the specific topic of delirium in the ICU and only briefly discuss neuropsychological deficits following ICU care.

The intensivist should think of delirium, or acute central nervous system dysfunction, as the brain's form of 'organ dysfunction' [60]. Delirium is extremely common in ICU patients due to factors such as age, critical illness, and medical management, and is associated with poor outcomes in hospitalized patients, including increased length of stay, the need for subsequent institutionalization, and higher mortality rates [51, 70]. While the frequency of delirium varies from 15 to 50 % among general medical or surgical patients [71], these rates apply to non-ICU patients, and few data exist concerning delirium in the ICU [60]. Mechanically ventilated ICU patients are at high risk for the development of delirium due to multi-system acute illnesses, comorbidities, medications, and numerous other risk factors [52, 60, 72]. In this population, 'cognitive impairment' has been reported to impact negatively upon key outcome indicators such as liberation from the ventilator, the development of nosocomial pneumonia, and length of stay [73–76].

There are few studies that have included ICU patients in the assessment or prevention of delirium [72, 77], partly because of the previous lack of validated assessment instruments for ventilated patients. In recently published investigations, we validated the confusion assessment method for the ICU (CAM-ICU) [53, 61], a 2-minute assessment instrument, which demonstrated a sensitivity of 93–100 %, a specificity of 98–100 %, and high inter-rater reliability (kappa = 0.96) in the detection of delirium. In 48 [61] and then 96 [53] consecutive mechanically ventilated patients, delirium occurred in over 80 % while in the ICU. In the subgroups expected to pose the greatest challenges for the CAM-ICU (i.e., those 65 years and older, those with suspected dementia, and those with the highest severity of illness), the instrument retained excellent sensitivity, specificity, and inter-rater reliability.

The validation of a delirium instrument for the ICU opens a new frontier for investigation of the outcomes of both younger and older ICU patients: to evaluate the impact of this important problem in the ICU. Important areas for future investigation include determination of risk factors for delirium in the ICU [72] and the impact of delirium in mechanically ventilated patients on clinical outcomes such as reintubation, nosocomial pneumonia, as well as broader outcomes such as quality of life [78–81]. While the use of psychoactive medications such as sedatives and analgesics in mechanically ventilated patients is intended to relieve anxiety and suffering, recent studies have suggested that these medications may be prescribed overzealously [58, 59, 82]. Interventional trials designed to reduce overuse of these medications and their attendant contributions to delirium and long-term cognitive deficits are greatly needed.

Cognitive impairment in the ICU may be independently related to prolonged neuropsychological deficits [64, 83–87], but studies specifically analyzing the interactions between delirium in the ICU and long-term neurocognitive function are lacking. A significant percentage of individuals developing delirium in the hospital continue to demonstrate symptoms of delirium after discharge [88]. Such patients demonstrate decreased cerebral activity and increased cognitive deterioration [89], and are more likely to develop dementia than patients without delirium [90]. Finally, patients who develop delirium have a greater rate of decline on cognitive tests than non-delirious patients [51, 91]. Importantly, future studies are needed to determine the prognostic significance of delirium in the ICU on long-term cognitive outcomes.

In conclusion regarding delirium, we have found that more than 8 of 10 mechanically ventilated adult medical ICU patients developed this complication. Indeed, ongoing delirium was present in 4 of 10 alert or easily arousable patients who are usually assumed to be 'cognitively intact' by ICU personnel. Unfortunately, delirium is often not recognized by clinicians [51, 91, 92]; and when noted in the ICU, it is often considered an 'expected' occurrence attributed to 'ICU psychosis' [94–96]. The most common type of delirium, hypoactive or 'quiet' delirium may be associated with a worse prognosis than hyperactive or 'agitated' delirium [70, 97–102]. It will be important for intensivists to be better versed in the distinguishing features of delirium as well as other common cognitive syndromes that are encountered in the ICU (Table 2).

Table 2. Definitions of cognitive syndromes

Confusion:
A characteristic occurring in delirium resulting in an altered state of consciousness, and characterized by deficits in attention, memory, visuconstructional ability, and executive functions.
Think: disturbed orientation with respect to person, place, and time.

Delirium:
A disturbance of consciousness characterized by an <u>acute</u> onset and fluctuating course of impaired cognitive functioning, so that a patient's ability to receive, process, store, and recall information is strikingly impaired. Delirium develops over a short period of time (hours to days), is usually reversible, and is a direct consequence of a medical condition, substance intoxication or withdrawal, use of a medication, toxin exposure, or a combination of these factors.
Think: rapid onset, clouded consciousness (bewildered/confused), often worse at night, fluctuating.

Dementia:
Development of a state of generalized cognitive deficits in which there is a deterioration of previously acquired intellectual abilities usually developing over weeks and months. The deficits include memory impairment and at least one of the following: aphasia, apraxia, agnosia, or a disturbance in executive functioning. The cognitive deficits must be sufficiently severe to cause impairment in occupational or social functioning, and they may be progressive, static, or reversible depending on the pathology and the availability of effective treatment.
Think: gradual onset, intellectual impairment, memory disturbance, personality/mood change, no clouding of consciousness.

Psychosis:
A major mental disorder characterized by hallucinations, delusions, or the inability to distinguish reality from fantasy, which lead to an inability to maintain interpersonal relations and to compromised daily functioning.
Think: hallucinations/delusions, impaired reality testing, inappropriate mood and impulse control.

According to the National Research Council, "For many people in good physical condition who succumb to an acute illness, cognitive decline is the main threat to their ability to recover and enjoy their favorite activities; for those whose physical activities were already limited, cognitive decline is a major additional threat to quality of life" [103]. We know that sepsis, ARDS, and other covariates result in profound neurologic injury during the course of a patient's illness [53, 56, 60, 104]. In fact, a prospective outcome study has demonstrated that cognitive abnormalities were present in all ARDS patients at hospital discharge, and in 80 % at one year [86]. Furthermore, in a general ICU population, it is remarkable that neuropsychological abnormalities were found to be present in over 50 % of survivors following mechanical ventilation at hospital discharge, and 1 in 3 have clinically relevant abnormalities in psychomotor speed, executive function and visuo-construction abilities, memory, and verbal fluency at 6 months [105]. It has recently been shown that neuropsychological sequelae of coronary artery bypass graft surgery have an important effect on outcomes up to 5 years later [87, 106], and in another cohort that up to 25 % of ICU survivors had deficits at 6 years following their ICU stay [64].

It is clear that both the lay public and health care professionals are becoming increasingly concerned not only with survival, but also with the quality of patients' lives, which is determined in large measure by their ability to return to baseline cognitive performance levels [107]. As the medical community strives to improve the outcomes of our older patients who succumb to critical illness and are cared for in the ICU, it is imperative that we better characterize the long-term cognitive function among survivors.

Ethical Decisions Related to Mechanical Ventilation in Older Patients

There is widespread belief that many patients do not want aggressive care at the end of life. Moreover, 78 % of healthcare professionals feel that the treatments they offer to patients are often overly burdensome [108]. In fact, more consistency in our attempts to obtain patients' preferences for do-not-resuscitate (DNR) orders might reduce the expense and burden of aggressive medical care in the elderly. While appropriate end-of-life care and patient preferences are being considered by some investigators [109, 110], relatively little is taught to most physicians in most medical schools or residency programs regarding this topic. Hamel et al. [16] recently reported data from the Support Study, which showed that physician error rates in approximating patients' preferences for mechanical ventilation increased from 36 % at age less than 50 to 79 % at age greater than 80. Furthermore, Support data also show that predicting death is very difficult for most illnesses [111]. At a time point of only seven days before death, experienced physicians prospectively estimated that 50 % of patients with congestive heart failure, chronic obstructive pulmonary disease (COPD), and cirrhosis would live for six months. For patients with acute respiratory failure and multiple organ dysfunction syndrome, the same physicians estimated that 20 % of the patients would live for six months, when in actuality they lived for only seven days [111].

Quality End-of-Life Care and Patients' Preferences

Considering the difficulty in estimating prognosis and the frequent misunderstanding and lack of communication between patients, families, and physicians, it is little wonder that we commonly err in establishing the appropriate end-of-life care plan for our critically ill patients [15, 16, 111–114]. In order to increase the quality of end-of-life care for our patients, it would be helpful to know what components of care patients consider most important, especially considering the huge economic burden placed onto society at the end of life in the ICU setting [115–117]. Singer et al. [118] recently sought to identify and describe elements of quality end-of-life care from patients' perspectives using in-depth, open-ended,

face-to-face interviews. This study showed that the following five domains of quality of end-of-life care were considered the most important by patients:
1. Receiving adequate pain and symptom management.
2. Avoiding inappropriate prolongation of death.
3. Achieving a sense of control.
4. Relieving burden.
5. Strengthening relationships with loved ones.

Regarding the first priority, it seems obvious that physicians ought to prioritize adequate pain and symptom management. In the SUPPORT project, four in ten family interviews reported serious pain (moderate to severe pain most or all of the time) during the last three days of life [119]. They did not report (nor were they asked) whether the pain was 'adequately relieved'. Physicians need to learn more and become appropriately aggressive in the use of sedatives and analgesics to relieve suffering in dying patients. The second priority, avoiding inappropriate prolongation of dying, has to do with patients' decisions to limit aggressive life support. Most patients say that they would prefer to forgo life-sustaining treatment if their quality of life after the treatment would be severely impaired [114, 120, 121]. Lo and Jonsen [122] discussed four reasons to limit treatment which included futility, patient refusal of therapy, excessive costs, and unacceptable quality of life. After careful consideration of these important concerns, clinical decisions to limit treatment will hopefully avoid unnecessary prolongation of death while providing compassionate terminal care. It is imperative that physicians and other health care professionals have discussions with patients and their families to determine their preferences for life-sustaining therapy and the options of ICU care vs. palliative care in the event of a life-threatening illness [115–117].

Many patients feel that DNR orders and advance directives help to achieve a sense of control over the possibility of dying in an unwanted environment such as the ICU [15, 113]. While patients prefer to participate actively in determining their 'code status', they often get confused by the precise treatment options [118]. In addition, once an acute illness occurs, the presence of associated delirium makes it very difficult to establish the patient's preferences with certainty if they are not already known. For these reasons, a surrogate decision maker for elderly persons should be established in advance.

The last two priorities listed by patients, relieving burden and strengthening relationships, seem to go hand in hand. Patients are often most worried about becoming a burden to their loved ones. This psychosocial burden includes the mental hardships, financial burdens, and time-intensive obligations placed on family members who care for their dying loved ones. Involving patients' loved ones in decisions about end-of-life care and treatment may lead to improved outcomes for everyone involved. In fact, the dying process frequently offers important opportunities for growth, intimacy, reconciliation, and closure of relationships [123].

Futility and Withdrawal of Care

In the course of caring for our critically ill patients it may become apparent to the patient, the family, or the healthcare professionals that further intervention would not be of benefit. While focus on the above outlined list of objectives is warranted, it is not always clear what constitutes a futile intervention. To aid in this complicated ethical dilemma we refer the reader to the recent report of the Council on Ethical and Judicial Affairs of the American Medical Association [124]. It is fair to say, however, that a strict definition of 'futility' is difficult due to the fact that each determination is dependent on people's values, which vary greatly. Therefore, the AMA recommends a standardized "fair process" rather than a strict definition of futility. As much as possible, physicians should base futility decisions on factors such as clinical efficacy of treatments, likelihood of mortality, and subsequent quality of life considerations rather than on chronological age alone [33, 122, 124].

In order to determine the frequency of withdrawal of life support in our country, a national survey of every American postgraduate training program with significant clinical exposure to critical care medicine was recently conducted [125]. Prendergast et al. [125] reviewed information on 6,303 ICU-related deaths which occurred under the following circumstances: 26 % (range 4 to 79 %) received full ICU care including failed cardiopulmonary resuscitation (CPR), 24 % (range 0 to 83 %) received full ICU care without CPR, 14 % (range 0 to 67 %) had life support withheld, and 36 % (the single largest group with a range across ICUs of 0 to 79 %) had life support actively withdrawn. While there was a wide variation in the practice pattern of the different ICUs, the authors concluded that limitation of life support prior to death is a common practice in our teaching ICUs across the country. The variable circumstances in the methods of withdrawal of life support in our ICUs does not seem to be explained by ICU, hospital type, mortality rates, or number of admissions per year [125–127]. While there is no recognized standard of practice in this important area of medicine, it is increasingly common for institutions to track their own end-of-life practices and even to rank the 'quality' of the dying experience [128, 129].

References

1. Hobbs F, Damon BL, Taeuber CM (1996) Sixty-Five Plus in the United States. Department of Commerce, Economics, and Statistics, Administration, Bureau of the Census, Washington
2. Randall T (1993) Demographers ponder the aging of the aged and await unprecendented looming elder boom. JAMA 269:2331–2332
3. Angus DC, Kelly MA, Schmitz RJ, White A, Popovich J, for the committee on manpower for pulmonary and critical care societies (COMPACCS) (2000) Current and projected workforce requirements for care of the critically ill and patients with pulmonary disease: Can we meet the requirements of an aging population? JAMA 284:2762–2770
4. Anonymous (1995) Assessing adult vaccination status at age 50 years. MMWR Morb Mortal Wkly Rep 44:561–563
5. Chan ED, Welsh CH (1998) Geriatric respiratory medicine. Chest 114:1704–1733
6. Ohmit SE, Monto AS (1995) Influenza vaccine effectiveness in preventing hospitalization among the elderly during influenza type A and type B seasons. Int J Epidemiol 24 :1240–1248

7. Martin GS, Mannino DM, Moss M (2002) Epidemiology shifts in sepsis in the United States. Am J Respir Crit Care Med (in press)
8. Angus DC, Linde-Zwirble WT, Clermonte G, Carcillo J, Pinsky MR (2001) Epidemiology of severe sepsis in the United States: Analysis of incidence, outcome, and associated costs of care. Crit Care Med 29:1303–1310
9. Angus D, Wax RS (2001) Epidemiology of sepsis: an update. Crit Care Med 29:109–116
10. Martin GS, Mannino DM, M Moss (2002) Sepsis, organ failure and mortality in the United States. Am J Respir Crit Care Med (in press)
11. Bernard G, Vincent JL, Laterre PF, et al for the recombinant human activated protein c worldwide evaluation in severe sepsis (PROWESS) Study Group (2001) Efficacy and safety of recombinant human activated protein C for severe sepsis. N Engl J Med 344:699–709
12. ACCP/SCCM consensus conference committee (1992) Definitions for sepsis and organ failure and guidelines for the use of innovative therapies in sepsis Chest 101:1644–1655
13. Bernard GR, Ely EW, Wright TJ, et al (2001) Safety and dose relationship of recombinant human activated protein C for coagulopathy in severe sepsis. Crit Care Med 29:2051–2059
14. Hamel MB, Philips RS, Teno JM, et al (1996) Seriously ill hospitalized adults: do we spend less on older patients? J Am Geriatr Soc 44:1043–1048
15. Hakim RB, Teno JM, Harrell FE, et al (1996) Factors associated with do-not-resuscitate orders: patients preferences, prognoses, and physicians judgments. SUPPORT Investigators. The Study to Understand Prognoses and Preferences for Outcome and Risks of Treatments. Ann Intern Med 125:284–293
16. Hamel MB, Teno JM, Goldman L,et al (1999) Patient age and decisions to withhold life-sustaining treatments from seriously ill, hospitalized adults. Ann Intern Med 130:116–125
17. Krumholz HM, Murillo JE, Chen J,et al (1997) Thrombolytic therapy for eligible elderly patients with acute myocardial infarction. JAMA 277:1683–1688
18. Thiemann DR, Coresh J, Schulman SP, Gerstenblith G, Oetgen WJ, Powe NR (2000) Lack of benefit for intravenous thrombolysis in patients with myocardial infarction who are older than 75 years. Circulation 101:2239–2246
19. Berger AK, Radford MJ, Krumholz H (2000) Factors associated with delay in reperfusion therapy in elderly patients with acute myocardial infarction: Analysis of the Cooperative Cardiovascular Project. Am Heart J 139:985–992
20. Ely EW, La Rosa SP, Helterbrand J, Bernard GR (2001) Effect of age on mortality reduction associated with recombinant human activated protein C in patients with severe sepsis. Am J Respir Crit Care Med 163:A459 (abst)
21. Shaw AB (1996) Age as a basis for healthcare rationing. Support for agist policies. Drugs Aging 9:403–405
22. Baltussen R, Leidl R, Ament A (1996) The impact of age on cost-effectiveness ratios and its control in decision making. Health Econ 5:227–239
23. Sage WM, Hurst CR, Silverman JF, Bortz WM (1987) Intensive care for the elderly: outcome of elective and nonelective admissions. J Am Geriatr Soc 35:312–318
24. Singer PA, Lowy FH (1992) Rationing, patient preferences, and cost of care at the end of life. Arch Intern Med 152:478–480
25. Giugliano RP, Camargo CA, Lloyd-Jones DM,et al (1998) Elderly patients receive less aggressive medical and invasive management of unstable angina. Arch Intern Med 158:1113–1120
26. Teno JM, Hakim RB, Knaus WA, et al (1995) Preferences for cardiopulmonary resuscitation: physician-patient agreement and hospital resource use. SUPPORT Investigators. J Gen Intern Med 10:179–186
27. Goldberg AI (1988) Life-sustaining technology and the elderly: prolonged mechanical ventilation factors influencing the treatment decision. Chest 94:1277–1282
28. Knaus WA, Draper EA, Wagner DP, Zimmerman JE (1986) An evaluation of outcome from intensive care in major medical centers. Ann Intern Med 104:410–418

29. Cohen IL, Lambrinos J (1995) Investigating the impact of age on outcome of mechanical ventilation using a population of 41,848 patients from a statewide database. Chest 107:1673–1680
30. Kurek CJ, Cohen IL, Lambrinos J, Minatoya K, Booth FV, Chalfin DB (1997) Clinical and economic outcome of patients undergoing tracheostomy for prolonged mechanical ventilation in New York state during 1993: analysis of 6,353 cases under diagnosis-related group 483. Crit Care Med 25:983–988
31. Kurek CJ, Dewar D, Lambrinos J, Booth FV, Cohen IL (1998) Clinical and economic outcome of mechanically ventilated patients in New York state during 1993. Chest 114:214–222
32. Ely EW, Wheeler A, Thompson T, Ancukiewicz M, Steinberg KP, Bernard G (2002) Recovery rate and prognosis in older persons who develop acute lung injury and the acute respiratory distress syndrome. Ann Intern Med 136:25–36
33. Ely EW, Evans GW, Haponik EF (1999) Mechanical ventilation in a cohort of elderly patients admitted to an intensive care unit. Ann Intern Med 131:96–104
34. Esteban A, Anzueto A, Alia I, et al for the International Mechanical Ventilation Study Group (2000) Indications for, complications from, and outcome of mechanical ventilation: effect of age. Am J Respir Crit Care Med 161:A385 (abst)
35. Ely EW, Baker AM, Evans GW, Haponik EF (1999) The prognostic significance of passing a daily screen of weaning parameters. Intensive Care Med. 25:581–587
36. Esteban A, Frutos F, Tobin MJ, et al (1995) A comparison of four methods of weaning patients from mechanical ventilation. N Engl J Med 332:345–350
37. Ely EW, Baker AM, Dunagan DP, et al (1996) Effect on the duration of mechanical ventilation of identifying patients capable of breathing spontaneously. N Engl J Med 335:1864–1869
38. Kollef MH, Shapiro SD, Silver P, et al (1997) A randomized, controlled trial of protocol-directed versus physician-directed weaning from mechanical ventilation. Crit Care Med 25:567–574
39. Esteban A, Alia I, Gordo F, et al and The Spanish Lung Failure Collaborative Group (1997) Extubation outcome after spontaneous breathing trials with T-tube or pressure support ventilation. Am J Respir Crit Care Med 156:459–465
40. Esteban A, Alia I, Tobin M, et al for the Spanish Lung Failure Collaborative Group (1999) Effect of spontaneous breathing trial duration on outcome of attempts to discontinue mechanical ventilation. Am J Respir Crit Care Med 159:512–518
41. Ely EW, Bennett PA, Bowton DL, Murphy SM, Haponik EF (1999) Large scale implementation of a respiratory therapist-driven protocol for ventilator weaning. Am J Respir Crit Care Med 159:439–446
42. Torres A, Gatell JM, Aznar E (1995) Re-intubation increases the risk of nosocomial pneumonia in patients needing mechanical ventilation. Am J Respir Crit Care Med 152:137–141
43. Epstein SK, Ciubotaru RL, Wong JB (1997) Effect of failed extubation on the outcome of mechanical ventilation. Chest 112:186–192
44. Epstein SK, Ciubotaru RL (1998) Independent effects of etiology of failure and time to reintubation on outcome for patients failing extubation. Am J Respir Crit Care Med 158:489–493
45. Gee MH, Gottleib JE, Albertine KH, Kubis JM, Peters SP, Fish JE (1990) Physiology of aging related to outcome in the adult respiratory distress syndrome. Am Physiol Soc 1:822–829
46. Luhr QR, Antonsen K, Karlsson M, et al (1999) Incidence and mortality after acute respiratory failure and acute respiratory distress syndrome in Sweden, Denmark, and Iceland. Am J Respir Crit Care Med 159:1849–1861
47. Chatila W, Ani S, Guaglianone D, Jacob B, Amoateng-Adjepong Y, Manthous CA (1996) Cardiac ischemia during weaning from mechanical ventilation. Chest 109:1577–1583
48. Srivastava S, Chatila W, Amoateng-Adjepong Y, et al (1999) Myocardial ischemia and weaning failure in patients with coronary artery disease: an update. Crit Care Med 27:2109–2112

49. Inouye SK, Viscoli C, Horwitz RI, Hurst LD, Tinetti ME (1993) A predictive model for delirium in hospitalized elderly medical patients based on admission characteristics. Ann Intern Med 474–481

50. Inouye SK, Charpentier PA (1996) Precipitating factors for delirium in hospitalized elderly persons: predictive model and interrelationship with baseline vulnerability. JAMA 275:852–857

51. Francis J, Martin D, Kapoor WN (1990) A prospective study of delirium in hospitalized elderly. JAMA 263:1097–1101

52. Marcantonio ER, Goldman L, Mangione CM,et al (1994) A clinical prediction rule for delirium after elective noncardiac surgery. JAMA 271:134–139

53. Ely EW, Inouye SK, Bernard GR, et al (2001) Delirium in mechanically ventilated patients: validity and reliability of the confusion assessment method for the intensive care unit (CAM-ICU). JAMA 286:2703–2710

54. Namen AM, Ely EW, Tatter S, et al (2001) Predictors of successful extubation in neurosurgical patients. Am J Respir Crit Care Med 163:658–664

55. Coplin WM, Pierson DJ, Cooley KD, Newell DW, Rubenfeld GD (2000) Implications of extubation delay in brain-injured. Patients meeting standard weaning criteria. Am J Respir Crit Care Med 161:1530–1536

56. Papadopoulos MC, Davies DC, Moss RF, Tighe D, Bennett ED (2000) Pathophysiology of septic encephalopathy: A review. Crit Care Med 28:3019–3024

57. OKeeffe S, Lavan J (1997) The prognostic significance of delirium in older hospital patients. J Am Geriatr Soc 45:174–178

58. Kress JP, Pohlman AS, OConnor MF, Hall JB (2000) Daily interruption of sedative infusions in critically ill patients undergoing mechanical ventilation. N Engl J Med 342:1471–1477

59. Brook AD, Ahrens TS, Schaiff R, et al (1999) Effect of a nursing implemented sedation protocol on the duration of mechanical ventilation. Crit Care Med 27:2609–2615

60. Ely EW, Siegel MD, Inouye S (2001) Delirium in the intensive care unit: An under-recognized syndrome of organ dysfunction. Semin Respir Crit Care Med 22:115–126

61. Ely EW, Margolin R, Francis J, et al (2001) Evaluation of delirium in critically ill patients: validation of the confusion assessment method for the intensive care unit (CAM-ICU). Crit Care Med 29:1370–1379

62. Jorm AF, Scott R, Cullen JS, MacKinnon AJ (1991) Performance of the Informant Questionnaire on Cognitive Decline in the Elderly (IQCODE) as a screening test for dementia. Psychol Med 21:785–790

63. Jorm AF (1994) A short form of the Informant Questionnaire on Cognitive Decline in the Elderly (IQCODE) development and cross validation. Psychol Med 24:145–153

64. Rothenhausler HB, Ehrentraut S, Stoll C, Schelling G, Kapfhammer HP (2001) The relationship between cognitive performance and employment and health status in long-term survivors of the acute respiratory distress syndrome: results of an exploratory study. Gen Hosp Psychiatry 23:90–96

65. Angus D, Musthafa AA, Clermonte G, et al (2001) Quality-adjusted survival in the first year after the acute respiratory distress syndrome. Am J Respir Crit Care Med 163:1389–1394

66. MacIntyre NR, Cook DJ, Ely EW, et al (2001) Evidence-based guidelines for weaning and discontinuing ventilatory support. Chest 120:375S–395S

67. Ely EW, OMeade M, Haponik E, et al (2001) Mechanical ventilator weaning protocols driven by non-physician health care professionals. Chest 120:454S–463S

68. Epstein SK, Ciubotaru RL (1997) Influence of gender and endotracheal tube size on preextubation breathing pattern. Am J Respir Crit Care Med 154:1647–1652

69. Krieger BP, Isber J, Breitenbucher A, Throop G, Ershowsky P (1997) Serial measurements of the rapid-shallow-breathing index as a predictor of weaning outcome in elderly medical patients. Chest 112:1029–1034

70. Inouye SK, Schlesinger MJ, Lyndon TJ (1999) Delirium: a symptom of how hospital care is failing older persons and a window to improve quality of hospital care. Am J Med 106:565–573

71. Inouye SK, Bogardus ST, Charpentier PA, et al (1999) A multicomponent intervention to prevent delirium in hospitalized older patients. N Engl J Med 340:669–676
72. Dubois MJ, Bergeron N, Dumont M, Dial S, Skrobik Y (2001) Delirium in an intensive care unit: A study of risk factors. Intensive Care Med 27:1297–1304
73. Vallverdu I, Calaf N, Subirana M, Net A, Benito S, Mancebo J (1999) Clinical characteristics, respiratory functional parameters, and outcome of a two-hour T-piece trial of patients weaning from mechanical ventilation. Am J Respir Crit Care Med 158:1855–1862
74. Cook DJ, Walter SD, Cook RJ, et al (1998) Incidence of and risk factors for ventilator-associated pneumonia in critically ill patients. Ann Intern Med 129:433–439
75. Ely EW, Margolin R, Francis J, et al (2000) Delirium in the ICU: measurement and outcomes. Am J Respir Crit Care Med 161:A506 (abst)
76. Ely EW, Gautam S, Margolin R, et al (2001) The impact of delirium in the intensive care unit on hospital length of stay. Intensive Care Med 27:1892–1900
77. Bergeron N, Dubois MJ, Dumont M, Dial S, Skrobik Y (2001) Intensive Care Delirium Screening Checklist: evaluation of a new screening tool. Intensive Care Med 27:859–864
78. Montuclard L, Garrouste-Orgeas M, Timsit JF, Misset B, Jonghe BD, Carlet J (2000) Outcome, functional autonomy, and quality of life of elderly patients with a long-term intensive care unit stay. Crit Care Med 28:3389–3395
79. Nelson BJ, Weinert CR, Bury CL, Marinelli WA, Gross CR (2000) Intensive care unit drug use and subsequent quality of life in acute lung injury patients. Crit Care Med 28:3626–3630
80. Orlando R III (2000) Quality of life in intensive care unit survivors: A place for outcomes research in critical care. Crit Care Med 28:3755–3756
81. Pronovost PJ, Miller MR, Dorman T, Berenholtz SM, Rubin H (2001) Developing and implementing measures of quality of care in the intensive care unit. Curr Opin Crit Care 7:297–303
82. Kollef MH, Levy NT, Ahrens T, Schaiff R, Prentice D, Sherman G (1999) The use of continuous IV sedation is associated with prolongation of mechanical ventilation. Chest 114:541–548
83. Moller J, Cluitmans P, Rasmussen L, et al (1998) Long-term postoperative cognitive dysfunction in the elderly:ISPOCD1 Study (International Study of Post-operative Cognitive Dysfunction investigators). Lancet 351:857–861
84. Williams-Russo P, Urquhart BL, Sharrock NE, Charlson ME (1992) Post-operative delirium: predictors and prognosis in elderly orthopedic patients. J Am Geriatr Soc 40:759–767
85. Brandl KM, Langley KA, Riker R, Dork LA, Qualls CR, Levy H (2001) Confirming the reliability of the sedation-agitation scale administered by ICU nurses without experience in its use. Pharmacotherapy 21:431–436
86. Hopkins RO, Weaver LK, Pope D, Orme JF, Bigler ED, Larson-Lohr V (1999) Neuropsychological sequelae and impaired health status in survivors of severe acute respiratory distress syndrome. Am J Respir Crit Care Med 160:50–56
87. Newman MF, Kirchner JL, Phillips-Bute B, et al (2001) Longitudinal assessment of neurocognitive function after coronary-artery bypass surgery. N Engl J Med 344:395–402
88. Levkoff SE, Evans DA, Liptzin B, et al (1992). Delirium: The occurrence and persistence of symptoms among elderly hospitalized patients. Arch Intern Med 152:334–340
89. Katz IR, Curyto KJ, TenHave T, Mossey J, Sands L, Kallan MJ (2001) Validating the diagnosis of delirium and evaluating its association with deterioration over a one-year period. Am J Geriatr Psychiatry 9:148–159
90. Rockwood K, Cosway S, Carver D (2001) The risk of dementia and death after delirium. Age and Ageing 28:551–556
91. Francis J, Kapoor WN (1992) Prognosis after hospital discharge of older medical patients with delirium. J Am Geriatr Soc 40:601–606
92. Inouye SK (1994) The dilemma of delirium: clinical and research controversies regarding diagnosis and evaluation of delirium in hospitalized elderly medical patients. Am J Med 97:278–288
93. Armstrong SC, Cozza KL, Watanabe KS (1997) The misdiagnosis of delirium. Psychosomatics 38:433–439

94. Geary SM (1994) Intensive care unit psychosis revisited: understanding and managing delirium in the critical care setting. Crit Care Nurse 17:51–63
95. Justic M (2000) Does "ICU psychosis" really exist? Crit Care Nurse 20:28–37
96. Nuttall GA, Kumar M, Murray MJ (1998) No difference exists in the alteration of circadian rhythm between patients with and without intensive care unit psychosis. Crit Care Med 26:1351–1355
97. Lipowski ZJ (1983) Transient cognitive disorders (delirium, acute confusional states) in the elderly. Am J Psychiatry 140:1426–1436
98. Lipowski ZJ (1989) Delirium in the elderly patient. N Engl J Med 320:578–582
99. Lipowski ZJ (1987) Delirium (acute confusional states). JAMA 258:1789–1792
100. Meagher DJ, Hanlon DO, Mahony EO, Casey PR, Trzepacz PT (2000) Relationship between symptoms and motoric subtype of delirium. J Neuropsychiatry Clin Neurosci 12:51–56
101. Francis J (1992) Delirium in older patients. J Am Geriatr Soc829–838
102. Francis J, Kapoor WN (1990) Delirium in hospitalized elderly. J Gen Intern Med 65–79
103. Stern PC, Carstensen LL 1ˢᵗ (2000) National Research Council. The Aging Mind: Opportunities in Cognitive Research. National Academy of Press, Washington
104. Eidelman LA, Putterman D, Putterman C, Sprung CL (1996) The spectrum of septic encephalopathy: definitions, etiologies, and mortalities. JAMA 275:470–473
105. Ely EW, Jackson J, Gordon S, et al (2002) Long-term neuropsychological deficits following delirium in mechanically ventilated ICU patients. Am J Respir Crit Care Med (abst, in press)
106. Newman MF, Grocott HP, Mathew JP, et al (2001) Report of the substudy assessing the impact of neurocognitive function on quality of life 5 years after cardiac surgery. Stroke 32:2874–2881
107. Scragg P, Jones A, Fauvel N (2001) Psychological problems following ICU treatment. Anaesthesia 56:9–14
108. Solomon MZ, ODonnell L, Jennings B, et al (1993) Decisions near the end of life: professional views on life-sustaining treatments. Am J Public Health 83:14–23
109. Council on Ethical and Judicial Affairs, AMA (1992) Decisions near the end of life. JAMA 268:1859–1860
110. Hofmann JC, Wenger NS, Davis RB, et al (1997) Patient preferences for communication with physicians about end-of-life decisions. Ann Intern Med 127:1–12
111. Lynn J, Harrell FE, Cohn F, Wagner D, Connors AF (1997) Prognoses of seriously ill hospitalized patients on the days before death: implications for patient care and public policy. New Horiz 5:56–61
112. Seckler AB, Meier DE, Mulvihill M, Cammer-Paris BE (1997) Substituted judgement: how accurate are proxy predictions? Ann Intern Med 115:92–28
113. Teno JM, Lynn J (1996) Putting advanced-care planning into action. J Clin Ethics 7:205–213
114. Lynn J, Ely EW, Zhong Z, et al (2000) Living and dying with chronic obstructive pulmonary disease. J Am Geriatr Soc 48:S91–S100
115. Provonost P, Angus D (2001) Economics of end-of-life care in the intensive care unit. Crit Care Med 29 (suppl 2):N46–N51
116. Truog RD, Cist AFM, Brackett ES, et al (2001) Recommendations for end-of-life care in the intensive care unit: the ethics committee of the society of critical care medicine. Crit Care Med 29:2332–2348
117. Hall RI, Rocker GM (2000) End-of-life care in the ICU: treatments provided when life support was or was not withdrawn. Chest 118:1424–1430
118. Singer PA, Martin DK, Merrijoy K (1999) Quality end-of-life-care: patients perspectives. JAMA 281:163–168
119. Lynn J, Teno JM, Phillips RS, et al (1997) Perceptions by family members of the dying experience of older and seriously ill patients. Ann Intern Med 126:97–106
120. Murphy DJ, Burrows D, Santilli S, et al (1994) The influence of the probability of survival on patients preferences regarding cardiopulmonary resuscitation. N Engl J Med 330:545–549

121. Gerety MB, Chiodo LK, Kanten DB, Tuley MR, Cornell JE (1993) Medical treatment preferences of nursing home residents: relationship to function and concordance with surrogate decision-makers. J Am Geriatr Soc 41:953–960
122. Lo B, Jonsen AR (1980) Clinical decisions to limit treatment. Ann Intern Med 93:764–768
123. Byock I (1997) Dying Well: Peace and Possibilities at the End of Life. Riverhead Books, New York
124. Council on Ethical and Judicial Affairs, American Medical Association (1999) Medical futility in end-of-life care: report of the council on ethical and judicial affairs. JAMA 281: 937–941
125. Prendergast TJ, Luce JM (1998) A national survey of end-of-life care for critically ill patients. Am J Respir Crit Care Med 158:1163–1167
126. Campbell ML, Bizek KS, Thill M (1999) Patient responses during rapid terminal weaning from mechanical ventilation: a prospective study. Crit Care Med 27:73–77
127. Faber-Langendoen K (1994) The clinical management of dying patients receiving mechanical ventilation. Chest 106:880–888
128. Loss CR, Ely EW, Bowman C, et al (2001) Quality of death in the ICU: comparing the perceptions of family with multiple professional care providers. Am J Respir Crit Care Med 163:A896 (abst)
129. Curtis JR, Rubenfeld GD (2001) Managing death in the intensive care unit: the transition from care to comfort. Oxford University Press, New York

Measuring the Health Status of Pediatric Intensive Care Unit Survivors

A.G. Randolph and R. Graham

Introduction

Pediatric intensive care is designed to serve the needs of neonates, infants, children and adolescents. In relative years, the age range is rather narrow. With respect to the developmental spectrum, the patient population varies dramatically. The majority of patients in most pediatric intensive care units (ICUs) are less than five years old, thus the impact of disease and medical intervention occurs during crucial periods of socialization and neurological development. Normal adults are independent in major functional areas and the resumption of that independence during recovery is a reasonable goal. In young children, measurement of health status is more challenging because independence is gradually achieved through normal development. This development is dynamic and nonlinear with broad individual variation.

Complete independence in activities of daily living, ability to be productive at work or regular school, and evaluation of cognitive skills using written materials are not relevant until after children are well into their school-age years. In addition, motor and cognitive skills develop quite rapidly in the first years of life. This complicates the association between pre-ICU status and follow-up at six months or beyond. A patient admitted at two months of age would be expected to do many more things at eight months of age. Therefore, the impact of the ICU stay on functional status must be dissected out from the normal variability in achieving developmental milestones.

Despite these challenges, measurement of the extent and nature of pediatric neurodevelopmental deficits and impairments and their associated functional limitations is being increasingly promoted. The reason for this growth in support is partially due to dramatic declines in the mortality rates for infants born prematurely and for high-risk procedures, such as open-heart surgery [1]. Overall pediatric intensive care mortality rates are relatively low at 5–6 % [2]. Evidence of brain injury during surgical correction of heart defects [1] and in the survivors of neonatal intensive care [3] has led to emphasis on assessment of neurological impairment. However, identification of impairment, defined as an anatomic, biochemical or physiologic abnormality, is not equivalent to evaluation of functional status [3] because all abnormalities do not impact a child's ability to function. Given that most pediatric ICU survivors have long life expectancies, it is important to measure morbidity, functional health status, and the impact on the family over time.

Figure 1 shows the relationship among measures of patient outcome in a health-related quality of life conceptual model. As shown in the Figure, impairment (biological or physical variables) leads to symptoms that can limit the patient's ability to function. Functional status influences the patient's general health perceptions and overall quality of life. Characteristics of the individual and of the environment influence many of these patient outcome measures. In addition, these outcome measures are multidimensional (e.g., functional status includes self-care, mobility, play, communication, social function and others). In children, measurement of functional status can be challenging because functional capacity may exceed performance in the evaluation environment. Because of this, many measurement instruments rely on parental report of the child's abilities and baseline status.

In this chapter, we will review multiple health status measurement instruments that have been or could be used in pediatric ICU survivors. These include instruments that were developed specifically for the pediatric ICU population, scoring systems to evaluate severity of illness and resource use, instruments that can be used to evaluate impairment and functional status during infancy, instruments developed for use in young children, and health-related quality-of-life scales. We will highlight only those health status instruments that have been previously used in the pediatric ICU and other relevant populations. This is not a comprehensive review and does not include any disease specific measures. Finally, we will report how some of these tools have been used as an outcome measure in clinical trials evaluating interventions in critically ill children.

Outcome Measurement Instruments Developed for Pediatric ICU Patients

The only instruments developed specifically to measure the health status of pediatric ICU survivors are the Pediatric Cerebral Performance Category Scale (PCPC) and the Pediatric Overall Performance Category Scale (POPC), both developed by Fiser [4]. These scales were based on the Glasgow Outcomes Scale [5] with childhood based operational definitions. The PCPC scoring from 1 to 6 is as follows: 1 = Normal (at age appropriate level; school age child attending regular school); 2 = Mild disability (conscious, alert, and able to interact at age appropriate level; school age child attending regular school classroom but grade perhaps not appropriate for age; possibility of mild neurological deficit); 3 = Moderate disability (conscious; sufficient cerebral function for age-appropriate activities of daily life; school-age child attending special education classroom and/or learning deficit present; 4 = Severe disability (conscious; dependent on others for daily support because of impaired brain function); 5 = Coma or Vegetative State; 6 = Brain death. The POPC Scale also ranges from 1-6 and is very similar to the PCPC but focuses on physical function. Due to their focus on school performance, the PCPC and the POPC are not as useful in very young children. Because they do not comprehensively assess

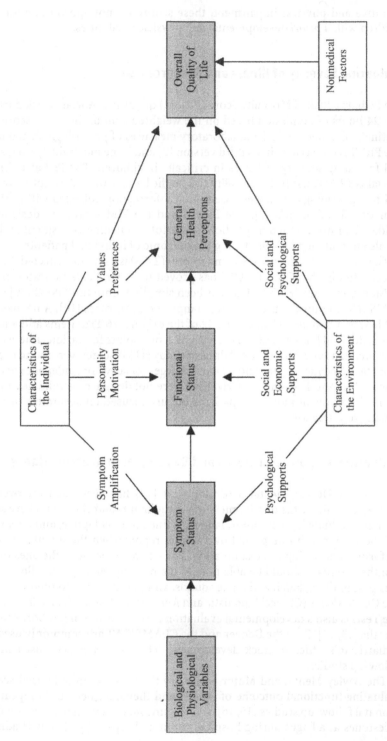

Fig. 1. Relationships among measures of patient outcome in a health-related quality of life conceptual model. From [44] with permission

cognitive and physical impairment, these scores are not appropriate for use in children with *a priori* developmental and physical disabilities.

Evaluating Severity of Illness and Resource Use

The Pediatric Risk of Mortality Score (PRISM) quantifies mortality risk during the first 24 hours of admission based on the weighted sum of the worst score for 14 routinely obtained clinical and laboratory measures of physiologic instability [6]. The PRISM score is now in its third version [2] and is the most widely used scoring tool for rating severity of illness in critically ill children. The Pediatric Index of Mortality (PIM) quantifies mortality risk on the basis of three descriptive variables and five physiologic variables based upon information collected within the first hour of ICU admission [7]. The PRISM and the PIM scores are designed and validated for use as outcome predictors and not as outcome assessment tools; they are also not intended for predicting the outcome of individual patients.

The Therapeutic Intensity Scoring System (TISS) is a set of 76 selected therapeutic activities in the ICU. The TISS has proved to be a reliable indicator of use of nursing manpower [8]. The TISS has been simplified into the TISS-28 [9] and the NEMS (Nine Equivalents of nursing Manpower Use) scores [10]. A neonatal TISS (NTISS) was developed by deleting 42 of the original 76 TISS items and adding 28 new factors [11]. Like TISS, NTISS assigns score points for various intensive care therapies that range from 1 to 4. Admission-day NTISS scores were found to predict neonatal ICU length of stay and hospital charges for survivors independent of birth weight [11]. The TISS and its derivatives were not designed or validated to assess the health status of individual patients but are focused on accurately measuring nursing resource use.

Evaluating Neurological Status and Development in Early Infancy

The Denver Developmental Screening Test [12] has been used for over three decades to evaluate the development of young infants and children. There are four domains evaluated: gross motor, language, fine motor-adaptive, and personal-social. Some items can be passed by parental report when the infant is unable to perform them during the examination. For example, between the ages of 2 to 4 months, an infant should be able to hold the head up 90 degrees, follow with the eyes past midline, laugh and make sounds, and pay attention to their own hands. The CLAMS/CAT (Clinical Linguistic and Auditory Milestone Scale/Clinical Adaptive Test) is also a developmental evaluation system for use in newborns to age 36 months [13, 14]. Both the Denver and the CLAMS/CAT are commonly used in the pediatrician's office to track development. They have not been used in infant follow-up studies.

The Bayley Mental and Motor Scales are the most commonly used scales for evaluating functional outcome of infants and they have been used repeatedly in neonatal follow-up studies [15, 16]. It is not unusual to see regression or halting of milestones at all ages during hospitalization and especially after ICU admission (e.g., loss of normal bowel and bladder continence). The Bayley Scales can be used to track return to baseline and development over time.

Evaluating Functional Status in Older Infants and Young Children

The Wee-Functional Independence Measure (Wee-FIM) [17] is a generic instrument to measure disability that is used mainly in rehabilitation settings. It was derived from the adult FIM [18] for use in children aged 6 months to 8 years. Like the adult tool, the Wee-FIM assesses burden-of-care across multiple domains, including self-care, sphincter control, mobility, locomotion, communication, and social cognition. The Wee-FIM can be administered through either trained observation or interview. The National Pediatric Trauma Registry included Wee-FIM scores as part of their follow-up assessment [19].

The Vineland Adaptive Behavioral Scales (VABS) [20] can be used in all pediatric patients from birth to 19 years. It focuses on multiple performance domains, including communication, activities of daily living, socialization, and motor skills. Implementation options include a survey form, an expanded version, and a classroom edition. Unfortunately, the emphasis on performance detracts from the sensitivity of the VABS when assessing infants or toddlers. It is best used for older school-aged children and adolescents. While not an ICU based study, Limperopoulos and colleagues utilized both the VABS and Wee-FIM to evaluate children with congenital heart disease following open heart surgery [1]

The Wee-FIM and VABS are generic and can be used across population case-mixes. Both scores are useful mainly for long term follow-up. Immediate measurement after ICU discharge may not be feasible and there will not be a baseline measurement for comparison when illness is acute. The farther out from ICU discharge, the more environmental and personal adaptive factors may influence performance and perception scores.

Measuring Health-Related Quality-of-Life (HRQL) in Children

HRQL incorporates functional status, an individual's perceptions of well-being, and satisfaction with life. HRQL measures support the World Health Organization's definition of health as "a state of complete physical, mental and social well-being" [21]. The Health Utilities Index (HUI) was developed to measure health status and HRQL. Three versions of the HUI have been developed called Mark I, II, and III. The MARK I is a four attribute system initially used to evaluate survivors of neonatal intensive care [22]. The MARK I has been used in pediatric intensive care to evaluate the outcome of children after severe head injury in a clinical trial of decompressive craniectomy [23]. The Mark II is a seven attribute system (sensation, mobility, emotion, cognition, self-care, pain, and fertility) with three or more levels of each attribute, that was initially devised to measure health status in survivors of childhood cancer [24]. The Mark II has been used also to evaluate the outcome of pediatric intensive care [25]. The Mark III was developed to be applicable across a broader age range and encompasses eight attributes (vision, hearing, speech, ambulation, dexterity, emotion, cognition and pain) [26]. The Mark II and III complement each other and can be used together. All three versions of the HUI have been used as part of the Canadian National Population Health Survey, providing a potential comparison group for ICU outcome studies in those regions (http://www-fhs.mcmaster.ca/hug/).

The Child Health Questionnaires (CHQ) developed by Landgraf and colleagues examines the child's health, functioning and behavior and its impact on the parent and family activities and has been validated for use across many cultures [27]. Two questionnaires are available: One is for parents (CHQPF50) and the other is for their children 5 to 15 years old (CHQ87). The parents answer questions about the child's global health including growth and development, temperament, moods, general health perceptions, and mental health.

Measurement of HRQL in infants and young children is dependent on parental report. Waters and colleagues found that maternal report is influenced by the parent's own health status [28]. Other HRQL measures have been used in teenagers with the teen as the respondent. The Short-Form 36 (SF-36) used widely in adult patients, has been used to evaluate HRQL in pediatric patients who survived massive burns [29]. Interestingly, the HRQL of these patients was similar to the normal population. The Adolescent Child Health Illness Profile is a self-administered questionnaire for teenagers and includes six domains (activity, comfort, satisfaction, disorder, achievement and resilience) that are rated on a Likert Scale [30]. This profile has been used to evaluate the outcome of neonates born at very low birth weight (< 750 grams) when they reach adolescence [3].

Outcomes Evaluated in Clinical Trials in Critically Ill Children

Neurologic function has been evaluated in clinical trials comparing different cardiac bypass strategies. All of these patients were critically ill and admitted to the pediatric ICU pre and post-operatively. Assessment was made both during the acute and convalescent phase. The increased seizure activity found in the acute phase when one bypass strategy was compared to another [31, 32] did not necessarily lead to differences in neurological development at long-term follow-up [33, 34]. Intelligence tests such as the Wechsler IQ test have been used to evaluate one aspect of neurological function in children after major heart surgery [34, 35] and the VABS has also been used [35]

Long-term follow-up of survivors who had undergone extracorporeal membrane oxygenation (ECMO) support during the neonatal period has included neurological evaluation. Neurological evaluation is extremely important for veno-arterial ECMO where one carotid artery must be used for cannulation and then at decannulation it is ligated permanently or repaired. Neurological evaluation in the one large randomized trial of ECMO in neonates included evaluation of hearing, vision, developmental level and functional ability [36, 37].

As mentioned previously, HRQL using the HUI Mark I has been used as an outcome measure in one clinical trial of surgical decompression after closed head injury in children [23]. The POPC has been used in one trial evaluating a drug called recombinant bactericidal/permeability increasing protein (BPI) for treatment of meningococcemia [38]. These authors found no significant differences in mortality. However, in the treatment group, the POPC measured at day 60 was more similar to the pre-illness POPC showing less deterioration in functional status in patients receiving the drug.

All of the measurement instruments described above are useful after hospital discharge but not during the ICU stay. Short-term morbidity as evidenced by multiple organ dysfunction syndrome (MODS) has been advocated for use as a surrogate outcome for death in critically ill adults and three scores have been developed and validated for use in adult patients [39-41]. The incidence of MODS in critically ill children (approximately 18 %) is at least three times more frequent than death [42]. A pediatric MODS score has been created (the Pediatric Logistic Organ Dysfunction or PELOD score) [43] and is being used in a multicenter trial evaluating transfusion for high versus low hematocrit goals in critically ill children (personal communication, J Lacroix, Montreal, Canada).

Conclusion

Due to developmental changes and limitations, pediatric patients require specialized instruments to measure health status. Many reliable, valid instruments are available to evaluate the various dimensions of health status in children. However, even tools with a developmental framework may not be responsive enough to measure change after ICU stay in children who have baseline developmental disabilities. This is important because a recent randomized clinical trial in pediatric ICU patients showed that almost half of the children eligible for a study evaluating methods of weaning from mechanical ventilator support had one or more chronic disabling health problems (unpublished data, AG Randolph). Enabling and disabling social and environmental factors must be considered when evaluating health status, especially as the duration from discharge to outcome assessment increases. No measurement instrument exists that will evaluate multiple dimensions of health status during the acute and recovery phases of illness. Use of multiple tools may be time-consuming but is required for comprehensive assessment. Measurement of neurological, developmental and functional status is becoming increasingly important for evaluating the quality of pediatric ICU care and the efficacy of therapies in critically ill infants and children.

References

1. Limperopoulos C, Majnemer A, Shevell MI et al. (2001) Functional limitations in young children with congenital heart defects after cardiac surgery. Pediatrics 108:1325–1331
2. Pollack MM, Patel KM, Ruttimann UE (1996) PRISM III: an updated Pediatric Risk of Mortality score. Crit Care Med 24:743–752
3. Hack M (1999) Consideration of the use of health status, functional outcome, and quality-of-life to monitor neonatal intensive care practice. Pediatrics 103:319–328
4. Fiser DH (1992) Assessing the outcome of pediatric intensive care. J Pediatr 121:68–74
5. Jennett B, Bond M (1975) Assessment of outcome after severe brain damage. Lancet 1:480–484

6. Pollack MM, Ruttimann UE, Getson PR (1988) Pediatric risk of mortality (PRISM) score. Crit Care Med 16:1110–1116
7. Shann F, Pearson G, Slater A, Wilkinson K (1997) Paediatric index of mortality (PIM): a mortality prediction model for children in intensive care. Intensive Care Med 23:201–207
8. Cullen DJ, Civetta JM, Briggs BA, Ferrara LC (1974) Therapeutic intervention scoring system: a method for quantitative comparison of patient care. Crit Care Med 2:57–60
9. Miranda DR, de Rijk A, Schaufeli W (1996) Simplified Therapeutic Intervention Scoring System: the TISS-28 items – results from a multicenter study. Crit Care Med 24:64–73
10. Miranda DR, Moreno R, Iapichino G (1997) Nine equivalent of nursing manpower use score (NEMS). Intensive Care Med. 23:760–5
11. Gray JE, Richardson DK, McCormick MC, Workman-Daniels K, Goldmann DA (1992) Neonatal therapeutic intervention scoring system: a therapy-based severity-of-illness index. Pediatrics 90:561–567
12. Frankenburg WK, Dodds JB (1967) The Denver developmental screening test. J Pediatr 71:181–191
13. Capute AJ, Accardo PJ (1996) The infant neurodevelopmental assessment: a clinical interpretive manual for CAT-CLAMS in the first two years of life, Part 2. Curr Probl Pediatr 26:279–306
14. Capute AJ, Accardo PJ (1996) The infant neurodevelopmental assessment: a clinical interpretive manual for CAT-CLAMS in the first two years of life, part 1. Curr Probl Pediatr 26:238–257
15. Hack M, Wilson-Costello D, Friedman H, Taylor GH, Schluchter M, Fanaroff AA (2000) Neurodevelopment and predictors of outcomes of children with birth weights of less than 1000 g: 1992–1995. Arch Pediatr Adolesc Med 154:725–731
16. Harris SR, Langkamp DL (1994) Predictive value of the Bayley mental scale in the early detection of cognitive delays in high-risk infants. J Perinatol 14:275–279
17. Msall ME, DiGaudio K, Rogers BT, et al (1994) The Functional Independence Measure for Children (WeeFIM). Conceptual basis and pilot use in children with developmental disabilities. Clin Pediatr (Phila) 33:421–430
18. Keith RA, Granger CV, Hamilton BB, Sherwin FS (1987) The functional independence measure: a new tool for rehabilitation. Adv Clin Rehabil 1:6–18
19. Sanchez JI, Paidas CN (1999) Childhood trauma. Now and in the new millennium. Surg Clin North Am 79:1503–1535
20. Sparrow S, Balla DA, Cichetti DV (1984) Vineland Adaptive Behavior Scales. Interview Edition, Survey Form Manual. A revision of the Vineland Social Maturity Scale by E. A. Doll. American Guidance Service, Circle Pines
21. World Health Organization (1958) Constitution of the World Health Organization. In: The first ten years of the World Health Organization. World Health Organization, Geneva
22. Torrance GW, Boyle MH, Horwood SP (1982) Application of multi-attribute utility theory to measure social preferences for health states. Oper Res 30:1043–1069
23. Taylor A, Butt W, Rosenfeld J, et al (2001) A randomized trial of very early decompressive craniectomy in children with traumatic brain injury and sustained intracranial hypertension. Childs Nerv Syst 17:154–162
24. Feeny D, Furlong W, Barr RD, Torrance GW, Rosenbaum P, Weitzman S (1992) A comprehensive multiattribute system for classifying the health status of survivors of childhood cancer. J Clin Oncol 10:923–928
25. Gemke RJ, Bonsel GJ (1996) Reliability and validity of a comprehensive health status measure in a heterogeneous population of children admitted to intensive care. J Clin Epidemiol 49:327–333
26. Feeny D, Furlong W, Boyle M, Torrance GW (1995) Multi-attribute health status classification systems. Health Utilities Index. Pharmacoeconomics. 7:490–502
27. Landgraf JM, Maunsell E, Speechley KN, et al (1998) Canadian-French, German and UK versions of the Child Health Questionnaire: methodology and preliminary item scaling results. Qual Life Res 7:433–445

28. Waters E, Doyle J, Wolfe R, Wright M, Wake M, Salmon L (2000) Influence of parental gender and self-reported health and illness on parent-reported child health. Pediatrics 106:1422–1428
29. Sheridan RL, Hinson MI, Liang MH, et al. (2000) Long-term outcome of children surviving massive burns. JAMA 283:69–73
30. Starfield B, Riley AW, Green BF, et al (1995) The adolescent child health and illness profile. A population-based measure of health. Med Care 33:553–566
31. du Plessis AJ, Jonas RA, Wypij D, et al (1997) Perioperative effects of alpha-stat versus pH-stat strategies for deep hypothermic cardiopulmonary bypass in infants. J Thorac Cardiovasc Surg 114:991–1000
32. Newburger JW, Jonas RA, Wernovsky G, et al (1993) A comparison of the perioperative neurologic effects of hypothermic circulatory arrest versus low-flow cardiopulmonary bypass in infant heart surgery. N Engl J Med 329:1057–1064
33. Bellinger DC, Wypij D, du Plessis AJ, et al (2001) Developmental and neurologic effects of alpha-stat versus pH-stat strategies for deep hypothermic cardiopulmonary bypass in infants. J Thorac Cardiovasc Surg 121:374–383
34. Bellinger DC, Wypij D, Kuban KC, et al (1999) Developmental and neurological status of children at 4 years of age after heart surgery with hypothermic circulatory arrest or low-flow cardiopulmonary bypass. Circulation 100:526–532
35. Goldberg CS, Schwartz EM, Brunberg JA, et al (2000) Neurodevelopmental outcome of patients after the fontan operation: A comparison between children with hypoplastic left heart syndrome and other functional single ventricle lesions. J Pediatr 137:646–652
36. UK Collaborative ECMO Group (1998) The collaborative UK ECMO (Extracorporeal Membrane Oxygenation) trial: follow-up to 1 year of age. Pediatrics 101:E1
37. Neonatal Inhaled Nitric Oxide Study Group (2000) Inhaled nitric oxide in term and near-term infants: neurodevelopmental follow-up of the neonatal inhaled nitric oxide study group (NINOS). J Pediatr 136:611–617
38. Levin M, Quint PA, Goldstein B, et al (2000) Recombinant bactericidal/permeability-increasing protein (rBPI21) as adjunctive treatment for children with severe meningococcal sepsis: a randomised trial. Lancet 356:961–967
39. Le Gall JR, Klar J, Lemeshow S, et al (1996) The Logistic Organ Dysfunction system. A new way to assess organ dysfunction in the intensive care unit. ICU Scoring Group. JAMA 276: 802–810
40. Marshall JC, Cook DJ, Christou NV, Bernard GR, Sprung CL, Sibbald WJ (1995) Multiple organ dysfunction score: a reliable descriptor of a complex clinical outcome. Crit Care Med. 23:1638–1652
41. Vincent JL, Moreno R, Takala J, et al (1996) The SOFA (Sepsis-related Organ Failure Assessment) score to describe organ dysfunction/failure. Intensive Care Med 22:707710
42. Proulx F, Fayon M, Farrell CA, Lacroix J, Gauthier M (1996) Epidemiology of sepsis and multiple organ dysfunction syndrome in children. Chest 109:1033–1037
43. Leteurtre S, Martinot A, Duhamel A, et al (1999) Development of a pediatric multiple organ dysfunction score: use of two strategies. Med Decis Making 19:399–410
44. Wilson IB, Cleary PD (1995) Linking clinical variables with health-related quality of life: a conceptual model of patient outcomes. JAMA 273:59–65

Predictors and Modifiers of Long-term Outcomes

Pre-ICU Factors

R. Moreno, R. Matos, and P.G.H. Metnitz

Introduction

In the modern hospital, the intensive care unit (ICU) plays a small but very important part in the continuum of care. Although the majority of patients do not need ICU admission, a small but significant percentage (about 5 % in most series) will be admitted to the ICU as part of their overall care. Time spent in the ICU represents the investment of a significant portion of community resources in hospital care [1].

This situation is likely to change in the next few years. Already, there is a clear trend to move most of the provision of health care out of the hospital and to reserve hospital admission for severely ill patients and those requiring invasive procedures. As a result of these changes, the percentage of hospitalized patients with severe and/or complicated diseases will increase, with a corresponding increase in the need for intensive care.

Improved strategies for identifying those patients who will need intensive care as part of their hospital stay will allow communities to make better use of the available resources and to reduce the morbidity and mortality of acute disease.

Effect of Preexisting Conditions and Diseases

Genetic Susceptibility to Critical Illness

The significance of genetic susceptibility to critical illness has been studied extensively in recent years. An association between some genetic markers, e.g., tumor necrosis factor (TNF) polymorphism associations, and the outcome from severe community-acquired pneumonia has been reported [2], as well as genetic influences on the level of acquired immunity to endotoxin [3] and the inflammatory versus anti-inflammatory response to severe injury [4]. Unfortunately, no genetic marker has yet proved to be of use in the prospective evaluation of severity of illness or as an aid in making ICU triage decisions.

The study of genetic markers is clearly a field that we will hear more about in the coming years. It is probable that practical methods of genetic profiling will soon appear, helping those involved in the complex process of clinical decision making about ICU admission to choose the appropriate therapy.

The Effect of Age, Chronic Disease, and Previous Quality of Life

Survival from critical illness is strongly linked to age. In the EURICUS-I study, age showed a significant relationship with ICU and hospital mortality: hospital mortality rates varied from 6.2 % in patients 18 to 24 years of age to 33.0 % in patients 85 years of age (Fig. 1) [5]. This effect can be partially explained by severity of illness [6] but remained significant even after correction for the severity of illness with the new Simplified Acute Physiology Score (SAPS II) [7] or by the Mortality Probability Models (MPM II) [8].

For this reason, chronological age is a major component in all general outcome prediction models. For example, in the SAPS II, age > 80 years has a greater effect on prognosis than does the presence of acquired immunodeficiency syndrome (AIDS) (18 versus 17 points) and is surpassed only by a low (< 6) Glasgow Coma Score (GCS). However, no existing model is able to assess or quantify biological age.

The presence and type of chronic disease at hospital admission have an effect on survival from acute illness. The importance of chronic disease was recognized and incorporated in the process of clinical decision making in the 1970s with the development of the physical status score by the American Society of Anesthesiologists [9]. This factor was subsequently incorporated in most general severity scores.

Recently, the effect of co-morbidities before hospital admission was demon-

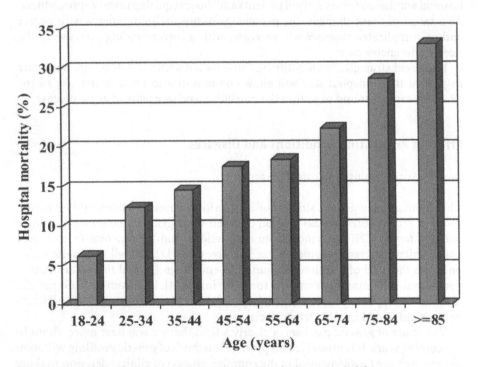

Fig. 1. Relationship of age to hospital mortality in the EURICUS-I study [5].

strated by the European Sepsis Group. In patients with a length of stay in the ICU longer than 24 hours, patients with no co-morbidities had a total admission infection rate of 26.8 %, compared with 36.9 % in patients with at least one co-morbidity. In some situations, such as immuno-compromised state, this value increased up to 55.1 % [10].

Quality of life before ICU admission has been shown to be related to ICU mortality but to have little influence on ICU resource utilization, as measured by length of stay in the ICU or extent of therapeutic interventions [11].

These preexisting factors – age, chronic disease, and quality of life – are related to two types of conditions: those that are linked to immunodeficiency (e.g., poor nutritional status, AIDS, metastatic neoplasia, chemotherapy) and those that are linked to poor cardiovascular status (e.g., a history of cardiac insufficiency).

Surgical Morbidity and Mortality

A high proportion of patients are admitted to the ICU after scheduled surgery. These patients, who usually have a lower mortality rate than non-operative patients or unscheduled surgery patients (Figure 2) [5], nonetheless have significant mortality in the ICU and in the hospital (7.4 %); this population is therefore a clear target for strategies aimed at reducing preventable mortality. Some studies have shown that patients who die after surgery tend to be older, have more preexist-

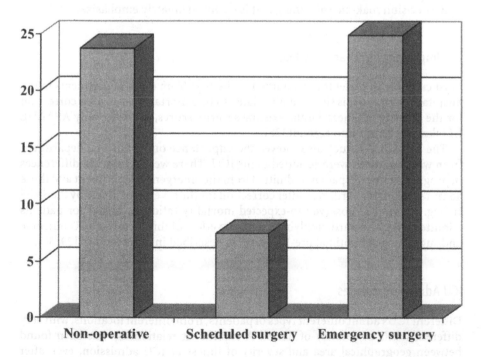

Fig. 2. Relationship of type of patient to hospital mortality in the EURICUS-I study [5].

ing medical disorders, and undergo abdominal, colorectal, or orthopedic surgery [12].

Several efforts have been made to identify patients at risk for complications and/or mortality after surgery. Overall, it seems that postoperative complications and mortality occur mainly in patients who are unable to mount a normal physiological response, particularly those unable to increase cardiac output [13] and those with a low anaerobic threshold [14]. Other factors, such as the expertise of the surgeon, the reduction of perioperative cardiac ischemia, and the preoperative optimization of physiological variables, are probably also important [15, 16].

Identifying Patients at Risk for Critical Illness

Given the importance of pre-ICU factors on ICU mortality, many efforts have been made toward the early identification of patients at high risk for developing complications and needing ICU care. Several scores and methods have been described [17–24], but they are usually directed at surgical patients. These efforts should be supplemented by better prediction and decision rules for hospital and ICU admission [25], since a significant number of patients can be identified in advance [26].

Of the existing general outcome models, only the $MPMII_0$ [8] was designed to be applied at ICU admission. However, this model was developed and calibrated on the assumption that the patient would subsequently be treated in the ICU. This fact, together with its probabilistic nature, makes the MPM unsuitable for ICU triage decision making, something that is rarely adequately emphasized [27].

The Importance of Lead-time Bias

Most critically ill patients are admitted to the ICU from other departments in the hospital, a factor that is significantly related to ICU mortality, even after correction for the severity of illness. Of the existing severity scores, however, only APACHE III takes this factor into account [28].

The EURICUS-I study also showed the importance of the hospital department from which patients were admitted to the ICU. There were significant differences in prognosis between patients admitted from the emergency department and those admitted from the ward, even after correction for the severity of illness by the SAPS II (Fig. 3) [6]. The observed-to-expected mortality ratio was higher for patients admitted from the ward, implying a negative effect of this factor on ICU outcome and suggesting suboptimal pre-ICU care, as described in other studies [29, 30].

ICU Admission Policies

Different ICUs admit different types of patients, from different locations, with very different levels of severity of illness. A significant relationship has been found between geographical area and severity of illness at ICU admission, even after correction for the severity of illness [31]. This is probably related to the availability

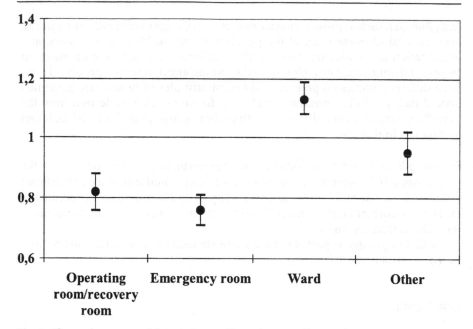

Fig. 3. Observed-to-expected hospital mortality ratios according to the SAPS II model in the EURICUS-I study [5]. Patients were classified by the hospital department from which they were admitted to the ICU.

of ICU beds. Other factors, such as length of stay in the ICU, type of admission, and institutional characteristics also vary between different countries and even within the same country [32].

The decision to refuse a patient admission to the ICU can have significant consequences [33]. Patients who are first refused ICU admission and later admitted to the ICU have a higher mortality, a fact that stresses the need for clear and objective rules for ICU triage decision making [34].

Alternative explanations for differences between geographical areas should also be considered. These differences can be grouped according to individual characteristics, collective characteristics, and sampling bias [31].

Individual characteristics: One of the possible explanations for geographical differences in outcomes is that geographical region is a surrogate marker for differences among patients, revealing, for example, differences in nutritional status, use of tobacco, alcohol consumption, and prevalence of chronic diseases. In other words, geographical area acts as an effect modifier, changing the relation between severity of illness and mortality. It has yet to be shown, however, that there are great differences between populations in neighboring countries.

Collective characteristics: The second possible explanation is that geographical area is a surrogate marker for collective characteristics in a given country or area (e.g., Europe), such as gross national product, percentage of expenditure on health care, cultural characteristics of the population and health care personnel, and organization of health care. Some of these differences could have an effect on clinical and nonclinical variables, since they would affect the entire process of care, from different admission policies to different attitudes of health care personnel toward their work. The positive correlations found for all data derived from the same European area should affect (positively or negatively) all the individuals and institutions in that area.

Sampling bias: In almost all outcome studies performed in Europe to date, the participating ICUs were not randomly chosen. This could introduce a significant sampling bias. The problem has not been adequately addressed, mostly because of the lack of information about the ICUs in each country, such as the number of units, their characteristics, and so on.

All three hypotheses probably have some elements of truth and must be subjected to further research.

Conclusion

A revolution is needed in the organization of the delivery of care to critically ill patients independently of their in-hospital location. The delivery of pre-ICU care should be coordinated with the choice of the appropriate hospital environment for the provision of care. Developments such as the patient-at-risk team [21] and outreach care are gigantic steps toward the delivery of better care to hospitalized patients, because they permit the early identification of patients with impending or established critical illness and encourage the education of ward staff and the sharing of critical care skills [35]. Multidisciplinary educational programs intended for non-intensivists who may be faced with unstable patients should also be mentioned here, since they too permit better identification and better initial treatment of the patient at risk who is not in the ICU. Examples of such ongoing programs are the Fundamentals of Critical Care Support (FCCS) course and the Patient-Centered Acute Care Training (PACT) package.

These measures will ensure that:

- patients who do not require intensive care will remain in the ward, reducing the use of scarce ICU resources [36], and
- patients who need intensive care will be treated in the appropriate environment – the ICU – thus reducing morbidity and mortality as well as costs [37].

These changes will also encourage intensivists to abandon a reactive posture in favor of a proactive posture [38]. This change will in turn provide better coordination of efforts and improvement in the outcomes of patients with a lower level of resource use.

References

1. Reis Miranda D, Gyldmark M (1996) Evaluating and understanding of costs in the intensive care unit. In: Ryan DW (ed) Current Practice in Critical Illness. Chapman & Hall, London, pp 129–149
2. Waterer GW, Quasney MW, Cantor RM, Wunderink RG (2001) Septic shock and respiratory failure in community-acquired pneumonia have different TNF polymorphism associations. Am J Respir Crit Care Med 163:1599–604
3. Riddington DW, Venkatesh B, Boivin C, et al (1996) Intestinal permeability, gastric intramucosal pH and systemic endotoxaemia in patients undergoing cardiopulmonary bypass. JAMA 275:1007–1012.
4. Westendorp RGJ, Langermans JAM, Huizinga TWJ, et al (1997) Genetic influence on cytokine production and fatal meningococcal disease. Lancet 349:170–173
5. Moreno R, Reis Miranda D, Fidler V, Van Schilfgaarde R (1998) Evaluation of two outcome prediction models on an independent database. Crit Care Med 26:50–61
6. Moreno R, Apolone G, Reis Miranda D (1998) Evaluation of the uniformity of fit of general outcome prediction models. Intensive Care Med 24:40–47
7. Le Gall JR, Lemeshow S, Saulnier F (1993) A new simplified acute physiology score (SAPS II) based on a European / North American multicenter study. JAMA 270:2957–2963
8. Lemeshow S, Teres D, Klar J, Avrunin JS, Gehlbach SH, Rapoport J (1993) Mortality Probability Models (MPM II) based on an international cohort of intensive care unit patients. JAMA 270:2478–2486
9. Vacanti CJ, VanHouten RJ, Hill RC (1970) A statistical analysis of the relationship of physical status to postoperative mortality in 68,388 cases. Anesth Analg 49:564–566
10. Alberti C, Brun-Buisson C, Burchardi H, et al (2002) Epidemiology of sepsis and infection in ICU patients from an international multicentre cohort study. Intensive Care Med 28:525–526
11. Rivera-Fernandez R, Sánchez-Cruz J, Abizanda-Campos R, Vazquez-Mata G (2001) Quality of life before intensive care unit admission and its influence on resource utilization and mortality rate. Crit Care Med 29:1701–1709
12. Sherry KM (2000) Demographics: National Confidential Enquiry in Perioperative Deaths (NCEPOD). Clin Intensive Care 11:2–3
13. Grounds RM, Rhodes A, Bennett ED (2001) Reducing surgical mortality and complications. In: Vincent J-L (ed) 2001 Yearbook of Intensive Care and Emergency Medicine. Springer, Heidelberg, pp 57–67
14. Older P, Smith R, Courtney P, Hone R (1993) Preoperative evaluation of cardiac reserve and ischemia in elderly patients by cardiopulmonary exercise. Chest 104:701–704
15. Shoemaker WC, Appel PL, Kram HB, Waxmann K, Lee TS (1988) Prospective trial of supranormal values of survivors as therapeutic goals in high risk surgical patients. Chest 94:1176–1186
16. Boyd O, Grounds RM, Bennet ED (1993) A randomized clinical trial of the effect of deliberate perioperative increase of oxygen delivery on mortality in high risk surgical patients. JAMA 270:2699–2707
17. Bone RC, McElwee NE, Eubanks DH, Gluck EH (1993) Analysis of indications for early discharge from the intensive care unit. Clinical efficacy assessment project: American College of Physicians. Chest 104:1812–1817
18. Hourihan F, Bishop GF, Hillman KM, Daffurn K, Lee AJ (1995) The medical emergency team: a new strategy to identify and intervene in high-risk patients. Clin Intensive Care 6:269–272
19. Morgan RJ, Williams F, Wright MM (1997) An early warning scoring system for detecting developing critical illness. Clin Intensive Care 8:100 (abst)
20. Hickey C, Allen MJ (1998) A critical care liaison service. Br J Anaesth 81:650P (abst)
21. Goldhill DR, Worthington L, Mulcahy A, et al. (1999) The patient-at-risk team: identifying and managing seriously ill ward patients. Anaesthesia 54:854–860

22. Stenhouse CW, Coates S, Tivey M, Allsop P, Parker T (2000) Prospective evaluation of a modified early warning score to aid earlier detection of patients developing critical illness on a surgical ward. Br J Anaesth 84:663P (abst)
23. Cioffi J (2000) Recognition of patients who require emergency assistance: a descriptive study. Heart Lung 29:262–268
24. Hillman KM, Flabouris A, Parr M (2001) A hospital-wide system for managing the seriously ill: a model of applied health systems research. In: Sibbald WJ, Bion JF (eds) Evaluating Critical Care. Using Health Services Research to Improve Quality. Springer, Heidelberg, pp 140–154
25. Fine MJ, Albe TE, Yealy DM, et al (1997) A prediction rule to identify low-risk patients with community-acquired pneumonia. N Engl J Med 336:243–250
26. Goldhill DR, White SA, Sumner A (1999) Physiological values and procedures in the 24 h before ICU admission from the ward. Anaesthesia 54:529–534
27. Lemeshow S, Klar J, Teres D (1995) Outcome prediction for individual intensive care patients: useful, misused, or abused ? Intensive Care Med 21:770–776
28. Knaus WA, Wagner DP, Draper EA, et al (1991) The APACHE III prognostic system. Risk prediction of hospital mortality for critically ill hospitalized adults. Chest 100:1619–1636
29. McQuillan P, Pilkington SN, Allan A, et al (1998) Confidential inquiry into quality of care before admission to intensive care. Br Med J 316:1853–1858
30. Goldhill DR, Sumner A (1998) Outcome of intensive care patients in a group of British intensive care units. Crit Care Med 26:1337–1345
31. Reis Miranda D, Ryan DW, Schaufeli WB, Fidler V (1997) Organization and Management of Intensive Care: a Prospective Study in 12 European Countries. Springer-Verlag, Berlin.
32. Thijs LG (2001). Geographical differences in outcomes. In: Sibbald WJ, Bion JF (eds) Evaluating Critical Care. Using Health Services Research to Improve Quality. Springer, Heidelberg, pp 292–308
33. Metcalfe MA, Sloggett A, McPherson K (1997) Mortality among appropriately referred patients refused admission to intensive-care units. Lancet 350:7–11
34. Sprung CL, Geber D, Eidelman LA, et al (1999) Evaluation of triage decisions for intensive care admission. Crit Care Med 27:1073–1079
35. Stenhouse CW, Bion JF (2001) Outreach: a hospital-wide approach to critical illness. In: Vincent J-L (ed) 2001 Yearbook of Intensive Care and Emergency Medicine. Springer, Heidelberg, pp 661–675
36. Zimmerman JE, Wagner DP, Knaus WA, Williams JF, Kolakowski D, Draper EA (1995) The use of risk predictors to identify candidates for intermediate care units. Implications for intensive care unit utilization. Chest 108:490–499
37. Lundberg JS, Perl TM, Wiblin T, et al (1998) Septic shock: an analysis of outcomes for patients with onset on hospital wards versus intensive care units. Crit Care Med 26:1020–1024
38. Bion JF (2000) Susceptibility to critical illness: reserve, response and therapy. Intensive Care Med 26:S57–S63

Intra-ICU patient factors

J.-L. Vincent

Introduction

Relatively little information is available regarding the intra-intensive care unit (ICU) patient factors that can determine long-term outcome of the ICU patient. Indeed, ICU physicians are usually happy to see their patient leaving the ICU alive, but there are few data on long-term survival and outcome. Few ICU physicians systematically follow their patients after ICU discharge; although this would be interesting, time constraints mean that once discharged from the ICU, the patient's course generally progresses unknown to the intensivist except by a chance meeting with the physician-in-charge in the elevator or cafeteria, or perhaps a note of thanks (or complaint) from the patient.

There are perhaps two key factors why data on the long-term effects of intra-ICU factors are scarce: The first is the difficulty in determining how an event occurring during the ICU stay can impact on survival or outcome some 6 or more months later; the second is which definition is used for 'long-term outcome'. Taking this second factor first, mortality has long been regarded the 'standard of reference' in terms of outcome; indeed the two terms mortality and outcome are often used interchangeably. However, survival is not the only outcome of interest; some knowledge of the quality of life of patients treated in an ICU is central to judging the benefits, medical and human, of that treatment [1]. While mortality data are clear and easily interpreted, they do not provide a full picture of the benefits of intensive care; a previously healthy and independent patient who is discharged with no, or poor, functional capacity can hardly be called an ICU 'success'.

This chapter will summarize the results from the few available studies and suggest areas of research for the future.

Specific Disease States

There are some studies reporting on the long-term outcome of patients with specifically defined acute disease states that required ICU admission and treatment including renal failure, acute respiratory distress syndrome (ARDS), pancreatitis, trauma, or post cardiac surgery [2–8]. Most of these studies have focused on outcome in terms of mortality, but some have included attempts to assess outcome in terms of quality of life. Angus et al. [4] reported that in 200 patients treated for

ARDS, who had had high functional status and minimal comorbid illness prior to their admission, quality-adjusted survival was poor with a quality-adjusted survival of 36 quality-adjusted life years (QALYs) per 100 patients. In 1048 trauma patients admitted to the ICU with normal pre-injury quality of well-being (QWB) scores, high levels of functional limitation were reported at 12 and 18-month follow-up; at the 18-month follow-up 80 % of patients had QWB scores below the healthy norm [7]. Such studies thus suggest that long-term outcomes after intensive care are often poor for a variety of disease processes.

Severity of Disease Factors

It has been shown that long-term outcome is related more to the prognosis of underlying disease processes than to the severity of the acute episode necessitating the ICU admission [9]. As the prognosis of chronic diseases, such as acute respiratory failure and acquired immune deficiency syndrome (AIDS), has improved with time, with advances in diagnosis and therapeutics, the survival of patients with one of these diseases will therefore be inherently better than a few years ago, regardless of the severity of their acute admitting illness. Nevertheless, disease severity can impact on long-term outcomes; the difficulty lies in how best to assess severity and how to relate it to outcome data.

Organ Dysfunction Scores

The traditional severity of disease scores, such as APACHE II and SAPS, were developed to be used once on admission; as such, they give no information regarding the pattern of disease during the ICU stay and do not allow for intra-ICU events that may influence outcome. During the ICU stay, the degree of severity is best assessed by repeated measures of the degree of organ dysfunction/failure. Several scores have been developed to monitor organ function, including the multiple organ dysfunction score (MODS) [10], the Brussels score [11], and the sequential organ failure assessment score (SOFA) [12]. The idea behind all these scores is that organ dysfunction is not an all-or-none phenomenon, rather a range of severity can occur from very mild to full blown organ failure, and importantly this severity can alter, in both directions, with time. The scores all employ the same six organ systems (cardiovascular, respiratory, renal, hepatic, neurological, hematological) but vary slightly in the components used to assess each of the systems. The key difference between the three scores is in the evaluation of the cardiovascular system. The MODS score uses a calculated measure, the pressure adjusted heart rate (heart rate multiplied by right atrial pressure divided by the mean arterial pressure). This parameter makes the score more difficult to calculate, and, being independent of therapy, can give acceptable values in patients whose cardiovascular status is only apparently good because of the large amounts of vasopressor support they are receiving. The Brussels score bases its evaluation of cardiovascular function on hypotension and acidemia, but acidemia can be caused by many conditions other than circulatory failure. The SOFA score uses a treatment-related variable for the cardiovascular system, and while this is perhaps not ideal, it must be accepted that therapeutic interventions influence markers of severity, as seen with the MODS score. However, the development of a new vasopressor, not allowed for in the SOFA score, could cause erroneously low cardiovascular scores, giving the impression that the patient's cardiovascular function was improving, whereas in fact it was just that the doses of the conventional agents were being replaced by the new agent. Thus, all these systems have their own quirks and drawbacks. Nevertheless, the MODS and the SOFA have been widely validated in large populations of critically ill patients and provide valuable information on the ongoing disease status of patients during their ICU stay [10, 13–17].

ICU Discharge Score?

We thus have scores to describe patient prognosis at ICU admission and scores to characterize patient morbidity and prognosis during the ICU stay, but as yet there is no good means of evaluating the patient at the time of ICU discharge. Such an evaluation would need to take into account not only the patient's organ failure status, but also many other aspects of pre- and co-morbid disease, as well as mental state and perhaps other quality-of-life factors. A prognostic ICU discharge score could be very important for several reasons. First, being able to evaluate likely outcome at ICU discharge may assist in determining the optimum time for a patient to be discharged, thus reducing the risk of re-admission. Second, such a system would facilitate in establishing the need for - or need to transfer to - an intermediate care unit.

We are currently working on a score that could be calculated at the time of ICU discharge (Table 1). A high score would indicate a high risk of death, prolonged hospital stay, and re-admission to the ICU. The proposed score is relatively long and complex, but could be computerized. Nevertheless, it will remain quite a gross evaluation. Ideally, we should evaluate the degree of impairment at the time of ICU discharge in view of the condition at the time of ICU admission. As an example, two patients may be discharged with chronic renal failure requiring hemodialysis; but one was admitted with this diagnosis, while the other developed the condition during their ICU stay - in essence the same discharge data, but, in fact, two very different outcomes. The patient with new renal failure will have a considerably worse functional status than when admitted; while for the other patient nothing much will have changed (at least in terms of renal status). Similarly for two patients discharged with a hemiparesis due to a stroke; one had the stroke prior to admission, while for the other patient the stroke occurred during their ICU stay. This latter patient will have reduced functional outcome as a direct result of their ICU stay. Pre-morbid factors thus need to be considered in the development of any system evaluating long-term outcomes.

Importantly, for all the scoring systems used, a model developed in one hospital or country may not be reliable in another hospital or area. The models used, therefore, need to be calibrated for any given environment, and in particular for different countries where populations and policies may differ.

Table 1. Prototype for ICU discharge score

	0	1 = mild	2 = moderate	3 = severe
Respiratory	Normal RR, no support	Oxygen therapy	Oxygen therapy + regular medication	Major lung disease. Continuous mechanical ventilation.
Cardiovascular	Normal, no medication	NYHA I	NYHA II	NYHA III
Renal/metabolic	Normal	Mild renal failure	Severe renal failure	Extracorporeal renal epuration
Liver/pancreas	Normal	Moderately abnormal liver function tests	Major alteration in liver function	Severe hyperbilirubinemia Liver or pancreatic cancer Established cirrhosis
Gastrointestinal/ nutrition	Normal, oral diet	Peptic ulcer disease Nausea, diarrhea, vomiting	Enteral nutrition Malabsorption syndrome	Parenteral nutrition Gastro-jejunostomy
Endocrine	Normal	Mild, diet-controlled diabetes Osteoporosis	Diabetes requiring regular sc insulin Morbid obesity Anti-thyroid medication	Severe complicated diabetes
Neurological	Normal	Depression Medication for anxiety or epilepsy	Altered mental status/confusion Severe depression Severe epilepsy	Coma Dementia Cerebral cancer
Locomotor/ psychiatric	Normal	Paresis Sedation	Plegia Polytrauma High dependency	Tetraplegia Severe polytrauma Polyneuropathy Bone metastases
Hematological/ immunological	Normal	Increased white blood cell count Moderate anemia Low platelet count	Anemia requiring transfusion Anticoagulation Systemic disease	Hematologic cancer AIDS Immunotherapy/chemotherapy
Infectious status	No infection	Oral antibiotics Fever	IV antibiotics	Invasive fungal or opportunistic infection

Time Factors

Another aspect of intra-ICU disease that may influence long-term outcomes is the time at which disease occurs. While this has not been studied over the long-term, the timing of certain conditions has been shown to affect short-term outcomes, principally survival. Knaus et al. [18] reported that mortality was increased in patients with a longer lead-time, i.e., a longer hospital or ICU stay before developing sepsis. Indeed, patients who develop septic shock early during the course of their stay may have improved outcome despite higher severity scores (Roman-Marchant et al., unpublished data). In patients with renal failure, those diagnosed within two days of admission had a hospital mortality rate of 66 % compared to 81 % in those developing renal failure after day 7 [19]. Respiratory failure may also show the same pattern with late onset being associated with a greater mortality rate than early onset respiratory failure. Whether these effects translate into differences in long-term outcomes remains to be determined.

Conclusion

Various intra-ICU factors, including disease severity and time of onset of disease, may impact on long-term outcomes. However, determining the effects of these factors on outcome is difficult and there are few data available. Evaluation of the process of disease and of ICU care is very important, yet few studies have been done in this field, and there are few tools available to assist. While organ dysfunction scores provide valuable information, they confront just one aspect of this complex area and more work needs to be done before we can really determine those intra-ICU patient factors that affect patient mortality and quality of life.

References

1. Konopad E, Noseworthy TW, Johnston R, Shustack A, Grace M (1995) Quality of life measures before and one year after admission to an intensive care unit. Crit Care Med 23: 1653–1659
2. Korkeila M, Ruokonen E, Takala J (2000) Costs of care, long-term prognosis and quality of life in patients requiring renal replacement therapy during intensive care. Intensive Care Med 26: 1824–1831
3. Hamel MB, Phillips RS, Davis RB, et al (2000) Outcomes and cost-effectiveness of ventilator support and aggressive care for patients with acute respiratory failure due to pneumonia or acute respiratory distress syndrome. Am J Med 109: 614–620
4. Angus DC, Musthafa AA, Clermont G, et al (2001) Quality-adjusted survival in the first year after the acute respiratory distress syndrome. Am J Respir Crit Care Med 163: 1389–1394
5. Bashour CA, Yared JP, Ryan TA, et al (2000) Long-term survival and functional capacity in cardiac surgery patients after prolonged intensive care. Crit Care Med 28: 3847–3853
6. Soran A, Chelluri L, Lee KK, Tisherman SA (2000) Outcome and quality of life of patients with acute pancreatitis requiring intensive care. J Surg Res 91: 89–94
7. Holbrook TL, Anderson JP, Sieber WJ, Browner D, Hoyt DB (1999) Outcome after major trauma: 12-month and 18-month follow-up results from the Trauma Recovery Project. J Trauma 46: 765–771

8. Gopal I, Bhonagiri S, Ronco C, Bellomo R (1997) Out of hospital outcome and quality of life in survivors of combined acute multiple organ and renal failure treated with continuous venovenous hemofiltration/hemodiafiltration. Intensive Care Med 23: 766–772
9. Short TG, Buckley TA, Rowbottom MY, Wong E, Oh TE (1999) Long-term outcome and functional health status following intensive care in Hong Kong. Crit Care Med 27: 51–57
10. Marshall JC, Cook DJ, Christou NV, Bernard GR, Sprung CL, Sibbald WJ (1995) Multiple organ dysfunction score: A reliable descriptor of a complex clinical outcome. Crit Care Med 23: 1638–1652
11. Bernard GR, Doig BG, Hudson G, et al (1995) Quantification of organ failure for clinical trials and clinical practice. Am J Respir Crit Care Med 151:A323 (abst)
12. Vincent JL, Moreno R, Takala J, et al (1996) The SOFA (Sepsis-related Organ Failure Assessment) score to describe organ dysfunction/failure. Intensive Care Med 22: 707–710
13. Jacobs S, Zuleika M, Mphansa T (1999) The multiple organ dysfunction score as a descriptor of patient outcome in septic shock compared with two other scoring systems. Crit Care Med 27: 741–744
14. Barie PS, Hydo LJ, Fischer E (1996) Utility of illness severity scoring for prediction of prolonged surgical critical care. J Trauma 40: 513–518
15. Vincent JL, de Mendonça A, Cantraine F, et al (1998) Use of the SOFA score to assess the incidence of organ dysfunction/failure in intensive care units: Results of a multicenter, prospective study. Crit Care Med 26: 1793–1800
16. Janssens U, Graf C, Graf J, et al (2000) Evaluation of the SOFA score: A single centre experience of a medical intensive care unit in 303 consecutive patients with predom inantly cardiovascular disorders. Intensive Care Med 26: 1037–1045
17. Antonelli M, Moreno R, Vincent JL, et al (1999) Application of SOFA score to trauma patients. Sequential Organ Failure Assessment. Intensive Care Med 25: 389–394
18. Knaus WA, Harrell FE, Fisher CJ, et al (1993) The clinical evaluation of new drugs for sepsis: A prospective study design based on survival analysis. JAMA 270: 1233–1241
19. Guerin C, Girard R, Selli JM, Perdrix JP, Ayzac L (2000) Initial versus delayed acute renal failure in the intensive care unit. A multicenter prospective epidemiological study. Rhone-Alpes Area Study Group on Acute Renal Failure. Am J Respir Crit Care Med 161: 872–879

ICU Environmental Factors and Quality of Sleep in Critically Ill Patients

S. Grasso, L. Mascia, and V. M. Ranieri

Introduction

The intensive care unit (ICU) represents a hostile environment for the patient, the family and all personnel. Pain, forced positioning, physical constraints, nursing and medical procedures, noise, light pollution and sleep deprivation are the most common sources of patient discomfort [1], representing a major source of physical and psychological stress that heightens the depersonalizing effects of the ICU environment and potentially leads to anxiety and depression [2].

Quantitative and qualitative sleep disruption is commonly seen in ICU patients [3]. Sleep disruption is however a multi-factorial phenomenon and underlying disease, pain, anxiety, and medications, together with environmental factors, are all potentially able to contribute to sleep disruption. Under these circumstances, it is not clear whether sleep deprivation and altered circadian rhythm causes emotional/physical distress or is caused by emotional/physical distress [3, 4]. If the patient is mechanically ventilated, asynchronous patient-ventilator interaction may be a further potentially important source of patient stress and sleep disruption.

Sleep abnormality could have an influence on morbidity and mortality in ICU patients through various mechanisms including disorientation psychological disturbances and fatigue, increase in oxygen consumption and carbon dioxide production both potentially leading to delayed weaning from mechanical ventilation and reduced immune response to endogenous and exogenous pathogens [3–5]. In the present chapter we will review available clinical data, discuss the potential mechanisms involved, and evaluate the potential clinical implications of sleep disruption in the critically ill.

Sleep Pattern in the Critically Ill

Normal sleep architecture consists of two kinds of sleep: non rapid eye movement (NREM) sleep and rapid eye movement (REM) sleep. NREM sleep is characterized by synchronized electroencephalograph (EEG) pattern and loss of skeletal muscle tone, and can be arbitrarily divided into four stages of increasing deepness. REM sleep is characterized by rapid bilaterally synchronous eye movements, desynchronized EEG pattern and loss of skeletal muscle tone [6]. Sleep onset occurs with a transient stage 1 that quickly progresses to stage 2, which consists of small amplitude brain waves together with sleep spindles and K complexes. Stage 2 can either progress to stages 3 and 4 (that are also known as 'deep sleep' or slow-wave sleep [SWS] stages due to their EEG characteristics of synchronized very slow brain waves) or into a REM phase. SWS stages (15-20 % of the total sleep time) and REM sleep (20-25 % of total sleep time) are both considered the phases of most restful sleep (although during REM phases the brain is much more active than during slow wave sleep stages).

Polisomnography (PSG) is the gold standard to assess sleep architecture [7]. Briefly, it consists of the simultaneous recording of four or more channels of EEG, including two central channels (C4/A1, C3/A2) and one occipital (O1/A2 or O2/A1), right and left electro-oculograms [EOG], sub mental and anterior limb elec-tromyography [EMG], pulse oximetry and electrocardiograph (EKG) signals. The analysis of PSG data is an important topic especially for studies involving critically ill patients, as several confounding factors such as movements, electrical noises from other equipment connected to the patient, nurse interventions are typical of the ICU environment [8].

Both quantitative sleep deprivation ('wakefulness') and qualitative sleep disrup-tion ('architectural') were already recognized as peculiar characteristics of ICU patients 30 years ago [9,10]. In clinical practice, however, the importance of sleep deprivation has been largely underestimated probably because nurses and medical staff overestimate sleep as compared to PSG recordings [11]. A recent study clearly defined the typical pattern of sleep alteration in ICU patients [8]. Sleep was studied for a 24 h period in 26 mechanically ventilated patients. None of the patients included in the study showed a 'normal' sleep pattern. Based on the PSG findings, the patients were classified as having a "disrupted" or an "atypical" sleep. Patients with "disrupted" sleep had all the stages of normal NREM and REM sleep, but their temporal distribution was clearly abnormal. In all patients, stage 1 sleep was predominant while stage 2, SWS and REM sleep were severely reduced as compared with age-matched control subjects. This pattern of sleep disruption was similar during day and night periods. Daytime sleep was 54±14.2 % of total sleep time indicating loss of the circadian rhythm of sleep. A very high frequency of arousals and awakenings was recorded during day and night periods. Patients with "atypi-cal" sleep had virtually absent stage 2 and REM sleep; a unique feature of these patients was the finding of pathological wakefulness, i.e., the recording of behav-ioral correlates of wakefulness together with an EEG pattern indicating a deep SWS sleep. Dosages of sedative drugs, uremia, and APACHE II score were higher in the "atypical" than in the "disrupted" sleep patients [8].

The pattern of "atypical" sleep seems to be typical in ICU patients [11-16]. In a postoperative non cardiac ICU, the total sleep time during the first postoperative night was greatly reduced in all patients when compared with normal controls (83 min vs 402 min) and, in the limited amount of residual sleep, stages 3 and 4 [SWS] and REM sleep were severely or even completely suppressed [11]. Rosemberg et al. showed suppression of REM and SWS sleep in the early postoperative period (the first two nights after the operation), with a subsequent 'rebound effect' in the late postoperative period in a group of 10 postoperative patient [13]. In a recent 24 hour PSG study on 17 mechanically ventilated medical ICU patients Freedman and coworkers found that although the total mean sleep time was within the normal

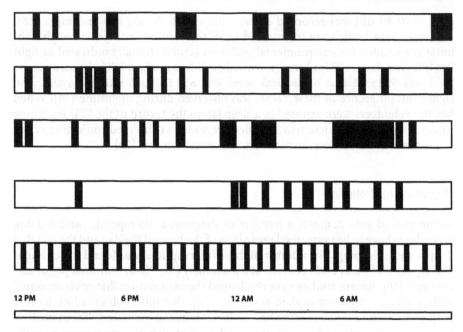

Fig. 1. Representation of sleep distribution in 10 critically ill patients during a 24 hr. period of observation. From [14] with permission

range (8 hours) the standard deviation among patients was very high with large individual variations in total sleep time from 1.7 to 19.4 hours [14] (Fig. 1). Again, the architecture of sleep was strongly disrupted with a predominance of stage 1 sleep, decreased or absent stages 2, 3, 4, and virtually absent REM sleep [14]. Therefore, the quality of sleep was poor, showing a clear pattern of frequent, short and non-consolidated sleep periods abnormally distributed over the 24 hours in all patients; the mean number of sleep periods per 24 h study period was 41±28, with the mean length of each sleep bout being 15±9 min.

Etiologies of Sleep Disruption in Critically Ill Patients

Noise and Light Pollution

The most obvious cause of sleep disruption is sound and light pollution, a peculiar feature of the ICU environment [14–20]. Mejer and coworkers [16] recorded light and sound levels for a minimum of 7 days in different hospital locations: three-bed medical ICU, three-bed respiratory care unit room (BRCU), single bed respiratory care unit room (RCU) and a private room on a general medical floor (PR). The overall average sound peak levels were very high in all settings, well above the American Environmental Protection Agency recommendations for the hospital setting (of 45 dB in the day and 35 dB at night). Heavy noise pollution (a sound peak > 70–80 dB) was recorded several times both during day and night [16]. Circadian light levels were maintained in all the studied settings, although light burst responsible for environmental pollution (conventionally indicated as light levels higher than 1000 lux) were recorded [16]. In a medical ICU, the mean noise level was 59.1±6.1 and mean peak level was 85.1±5.1 dB during daytime; no significant difference in these values was observed during nighttime [14]. When healthy volunteers were exposed in a sleep lab to the record of the ICU nighttime sound, a significant reduction in REM sleep periods was observed, indicating a clear influence of noise on sleep architecture in normal subjects [20].

Interventional Pollution

In the critical care context, a number of diagnostic, therapeutic, and nursing procedures have to be performed regardless of the hour of the day and the fact that the patient is sleeping. The number of these interruptions was found to be similar during day and night and occurred at least hourly (the "interventional pollution" concept) [16]. Recent studies have challenged the assumption that environmental pollution can completely explain *per se* the sleep disruption observed in the ICU [14]. Indeed, simultaneous recording of environmental noise and PSG in medical mechanically ventilated ICU patients has allowed an objective measurement of the effects of noise on sleep; environmental noise was found to be responsible for only 11.5 % of arousals and 17 % of awakening from sleep [14]. In addition, sleep was found to be severely disrupted in a postoperative ICU despite a specific effort of medical and nursing staff directed toward almost complete reduction of sound and light noise and reduction of disturbing interventions on patients [11]. Indeed, from a subjective point of view, patients do not perceive ICU noise as the most disruptive environmental stimulus [21]; recent data show that human interventions and diagnostic tests are perceived to be as sleep disturbing as environmental noise [21, 22].

Patient-ventilator Asynchrony

Asynchrony between patient and ventilator is a potentially important source of sleep disruption in mechanically ventilated patients [23, 24]. During NREM sleep the control of breathing is dominated by chemical feedback; experiments on normal volunteers showed that when mechanical ventilation reduces PCO_2 by a few mmHg below the eupneic threshold, apnea develops [23]. Under these circumstances, mechanical ventilation may compromise a patient's control on CO_2 levels and central apnea is likely to occur. This may, therefore, destabilize breathing patterns and lead to arousal, hypoxia, and sleep fragmentation [25].

The concept of 'patient ventilator interactions' (PVI) describes the matching of the triggering, flow delivering, and inspiratory-to-expiratory cycling functions of the ventilator with the patient's ventilatory drive, spontaneous inspiratory flow demand, and spontaneous 'neural' inspiratory time, respectively [25]. Only preliminary investigations on the influences of patient ventilator interactions and sleep are available [26–30]. In a recent study, Meza and coworkers showed that normal sleeping subjects systematically develop periodic breathing when ventilated with pressure support ventilation (PSV); these normal subjects appeared to be quite resistant to developing periodic breathing when ventilated with proportional assist ventilation (PAV) [24].

Underlying Disease

A patient's acute and/or chronic illness may directly or indirectly affect sleep quality. A recent study showed that 50 % of patients with heart failure suffer from sleep-related disorders; these patients are characterized by a high prevalence of atrial fibrillation and ventricular arrhythmias [31]. In addition, sleep disorders are ubiquitous in patients with chronic obstructive pulmonary disease (COPD) [32].

The role of the central nervous system (CNS) in the host response to infection and inflammation and modulation of these responses by the hypothalamic-pituitary-adrenal (HPA) system are well established [5, 33]. Activation of host defense mechanisms increases NREM sleep, which is thought to support host defense [33]. In humans, administration of endotoxin before nocturnal sleep onset increased plasma levels of tumor necrosis factor (TNF)-alpha, soluble TNF receptors, interleukin (IL)-1 receptor antagonist (IL-1ra), IL-6, and cortisol in a dose dependent fashion. At low doses, endotoxin increased circulating levels of cytokines and soluble cytokine receptors, but it did not affect cortisol levels; this subtle host defense activation increased NREM sleep. Conversely, sleep disruption was observed when the highest dose of endotoxin increased cytokines and cortisol plasma levels [34].

Medication

Studies on ambulatory patients have shown that opiates decrease REM sleep, and benzodiapines can reduce SWS [35, 36]. It is, however, difficult to directly extrapolate these findings to ICU patients since pharmacodynamics and pharmacokinetics in critically ill patients are different from normal and difficult to predict. Anesthesia can also result in severe sleep disruption [37, 38]. A list of common drugs that can be associated with sleep disruption is shown in Table 1 [2].

Clinical Consequences of Sleep Disruption in the Critically Ill

Can the consequences of sleep disruption have an impact on morbidity and mortality in critically ill patients? It has been suggested that sleep fragmentation can alter the process of weaning from mechanical ventilation [16]. Sleep abnormalities in healthy subjects are associated with attenuated ventilatory responses to hypoxia and hypercapnia [39], increases in oxygen consumption and carbon dioxide production [40], abnormalities of cognitive functions, such as significant reduction in attention, short-term memory, verbal recall and problem solving

Table 1. Common drugs associated with sleep disruption.

Anesthetics	Propofol
	Clonazepam
	Pentobarbital
Local anesthetics	Lidocaine
	Bupivacaine
Analgesic	Fentanyl
Antibiotics	Penicillins
	Cephalosporins
	Quinolones (ciprofloxacin)
	Aminoglycosides
	Carbapenems (imipemen)
Anticholinergics	Atropine
Antihypertensives	Enalapri
	Diltiazem
	Verapamil
Antiarrhythmics	Mexiletine
Anticonvulsants	Carbamazepine
	Phenytoin
H₁ and H₂ antagonists	Ranitidine
	Cimetidine

Modified from [2] with permission

activity ('ICU psychosis') [41,42]. It follows that sleep disorders may potentially influence long-term outcomes in the critically ill.

Sleep and the Immune System

A strong trend in the literature indicates that sleep is essential for optimal functioning of the immune system [5]. Through comparative research, specific physical effects and underlying mechanisms altered by sleep deprivation are being elucidated [43]. Rats that are chronically sleep deprived show various physiological derangements including negative energy balance, weight loss and finally death; a fatal bloodstream infection without an infectious focus was demonstrated in such model [44–46]. Recently, Everson and coworkers investigated the conditions antecedent to advanced morbidity in sleep-deprived rats by determining the time course and distribution of live microorganisms in body tissues that are normally sterile; they found early infection of the mesenteric lymph nodes by bacteria and transient infection of extra-intestinal sites. Bacterial translocation and pathogenic sequelae may, therefore, represent the underlying mechanisms by which sleep deprivation appears to adversely affect health [47]. Indeed, the brain and the host defense system seem capable of bi-directional communication: neurons and glial cells have specific receptors for regulatory substances produced by the host defense system, whereas the immune system has a direct innervation and host defense cells have specific surface receptors for neurotransmitters [45–47]. It follows that sleep loss could impact on host defense indirectly, through an impairment of CNS regulatory effects on immune response [48]. These data may therefore support the hypothesis that sleep disruption in the ICU context can contribute to overall ICU morbidity and mortality through a reduced immune response to endogenous and exogenous pathogens and further research on this topic is required.

Sleep and Metabolism

Bonnet and coworkers showed that brief and extended arousals are accompanied by increased oxygen consumption and carbon dioxide production that are both related to the length of arousal [40]. Sleep disturbances may adversely affect glucose tolerance since glucose and insulin secretion rate during sleep deprivation remained essentially stable during the first part of the night and then decreased significantly, despite bed rest and a constant glucose infusion [49]. Everson and Wehr showed that sleep deprivation causes malnutrition due to increased energy expenditure. Levels of plasma cholesterol, triglycerides or glucose were normal when animals were fed with a hyper caloric, high fat diet, thus indicating accelerated turnover of nutrients [50].

Scule and coworkers evaluated the consequences of sleep deprivation on the HPA axis activity using the dexamethasone-suppression/corticotropin-releasing hormone-stimulation, and the dexamethasone suppression (DST) tests. They found that partial sleep deprivation was associated with a negative feedback of the HPA system as reflected by the DST status [51].

The extra cellular matrix is of central importance to the structure and function of several tissues including the lung, the gut, and the brain [52]. The composition of the extra cellular matrix is in a dynamic flux that represents a balance between synthesis and degradation both regulated by matrix metalloproteinase-9 (MMP-9). Taishi and coworkers recently showed that sleep loss down regulates MMP-9mRNA expression [52].

Sleep and Cardiovascular Function

Normal spontaneous arousals from sleep are associated with transient increases in blood pressure, heart rate, and ventilation caused by large transient changes in autonomic output [53]. These autonomic changes are out of proportion to obvious physiological need and are in excess of those observed in later periods of quiet wakefulness. Based on this observation, sleep disruption was hypothesized to be accompanied by a specific hemodynamic response similar to the cardiovascular defense reaction. Iliac vaso-dilation associated with renal vasoconstriction, tachycardia, and minimal changes in mean arterial blood pressure were the most common pattern of arousal response [54]. Measurements of regional blood flow show that an impaired central nervous regulation underlies the disruption of peripheral circulation patterns observed during sleep disruption [55]. The lack of adaptive vasomotor adjustments, which has little consequence in normal conditions, may become relevant in cardiovascular pathophysiology when blood flow redistribution becomes a major compensating mechanism.

Sleep and Muscle Function

Chen and Tang [56] found that respiratory muscle endurance decreases after 30 hours of sleep deprivation, and Leiter et al. [57] observed a blunted EMG response to CO_2. Others have reported decreased ventilatory responsiveness to hypercapnia following sleep deprivation [58].

Sleep and "ICU Psychosis"

Delirium is a disturbance of consciousness characterized by an acute onset and fluctuating course of impaired cognitive functioning so that a patient's ability to receive, process, store, and recall information is strikingly impaired [59]. Agitation and/or hallucinations are characteristic of hyperactive delirium and are features not required for the diagnosis since recent data show that hyperactive delirium contributes to only 5 % of observed episodes of delirium [60]. Table 2 summarizes perceptions of 76 patients during their ICU stay [1]. Sleep deprivation may certainly contribute to delirium although it is not conclusive that the lack of sleep precedes and causes delirium rather than being a consequence of delirium [2].

Conclusion

Sleep deprivation and sleep disruption are major problems in the ICU context. It is important for the ICU caregiver to become aware of the potentially devastating

Table 2. Perception of ICU stay in 76 patients.

Analgesic request not giving the expected pain relief	94 %
Sleep deprivation	63 %
Anxiety	62 %
Isolation	46 %
Pain	43 %
Lack of information	33 %

Modified from [1] with permission

effect of ICU sleep abnormalities. Sleep disruption is linked to ICU environmental pollution but other factors are important too, and more studies are needed to completely assess its etiology, particularly in mechanically ventilated patients. Similarly, a better knowledge of the impact of sleep deprivation on the immune system function is required to evaluate the effect of sleep deprivation on outcome in ICU patients.

References

1. Simini B (1999) Patients' perceptions of intensive care. Lancet 354:571–572
2. McGuire BE, Basten CJ, Ryan CJ, Gallagher J (2000) Intensive care unit syndrome: a dangerous misnomer. Arch Intern Med 160:906–909
3. Treggiari-Venzi M, Borgeat A, Fuchs-Buder T, Gachoud J-P, Suter PM (1996) Overnight sedation with midazolam or propofol in the ICU: effects on sleep quality, anxiety and depression. Intensive Care Med 22:1186–1190
4. Weber RJ, Oszko MA, Bolender BJ (1985) The ICU syndrome: causes, treatment and prevention. Drug Intelligence Clin Pharm 19:13–20
5. Benca RM, Quintans J (1997) Sleep and host defenses: a review. Sleep 20:1027–1037
6. Association ASD (1992) EEG arousals: scoring rules and examples. Sleep 15:173–184
7. Carkskadon M, Dement W (1994) Normal human sleep, an overview. In: Kryger MH, Roth T, Dement WC (eds) Principles and Practice of Sleep Medicine. WB Saunders Company, Philadelphia, pp 16–25
8. Cooper AB, Thornley KS, Young GB, Slutsky AS, Stewart TE, Hanly PJ (2000) Sleep in critically ill patients requiring mechanical ventilation. Chest 117:809–819
9. Dlin BM, Rosen H, Dickstein K, Lyons JW, Fischer HK (1971) The problem of sleep and rest in the intensive care unit. Psychosomatics 12:241–249
10. Broughton R, Baron R (1978) Sleep pattern in the intensive care unit and on the ward after acute myocardial infarction. Electroencephalogr Clin Neurophysiol 45:348–360
11. Aurell T, Elmquist D (1985) Sleep in the surgical intensive care unit: continuous polygraphic recording of sleep in nine patients receiving postoperative care. Br Med J 290:1029–1032
12. Young GB, McLachlan RS, Kreeft JH, Demelo JD (1997) An electroencelographic classification for coma. Can J Neurol Sci 24:320–325
13. Rosemberg J, Wildschodtz M, Pedersen MH, Von Jessen F, Kelhet H (1994) Late postoperative nocturnal episodic hypoxemia and associated sleep pattern. Br J Anaesth 72:145–150
14. Freedman NS, Gazednam J, Levan L, Pack A, Schwab RJ (2001) Abnormal sleep-wake cycles and the effects of environmental noise on sleep disruption in the intensive care unit. Am J Respir Crit Care Med 163:451–457
15. Schwab RJ (1994) Disturbances of sleep in the intensive care unit. Crit Care Clin 10:681–694
16. Mejer TJ, Eveloff SE, Bauer MS, Schwartz WA, Hill NS, Millman RP (1994) Adverse environmental conditions in the respiratory and medical ICU settings. Chest 105:1211–1216
17. Balogh D, Kittinger E, Benzer A, Hackl JM. (1993) Noise in the ICU. Intensive Care Med 19:343–346
18. Topf M, Bookman M, Arand D (1996) Effects of critical care unit noise on the subjective quality of sleep. J Adv Nurs 24: 545–551
19. Topf M, Davis JE (1993) Critical care unit noise and rapid eye movement (REM) sleep. Heart Lung 22: 252–258
20. Walder B, Francioli D, Meyer JJ, Lancon M, Romand JA (2000) Effects of guidelines implementation in a surgical intensive care unit to control nighttime light and noise level. Crit Care Med 28:2242–2247
21. Freedman NS, Kotzer N, Schwab RJ (1999) Patient perception of sleep quality and etiology of sleep disruption in the intensive care unit. Am J Respir Crit Care Med 159:1155–1162

22. Wooten V (1995) Sleep disorders in psychiatric illness. In: Chokroverty S (ed) Sleep Disorders Medicine: Basic Science, Technical Considerations and Clinical Aspects. Butterworth-Heineman, Boston, pp 337–347

23. Meza S, Giannouli E, Younes M (1998) Control of breathing during sleep assessed by proportional assist ventilation. J Appl Physiol 84: 3–12

24. Meza S, Mendez M, Ostrowski M, Younes M (1998) Susceptibility to periodic breathing with assisted ventilation during sleep in normal subjects. J Appl Physiol 85: 1929–1940

25. Mcintyre NR (1996) New modes of mechanical ventilation. Clin Chest Med 17: 411–421

26. Grasso S, Ancona G, Ranieri VM (1998) New modes of mechanical ventilation. Curr Opin Crit Care 4:1–5

27. Ranieri VM (1997) Optimization of patient-ventilator interactions: closed-loop technology to turn the century. Intensive Care Med 23:936–939

28. Cooper AB, Stewart TE, Thornley K (1998) Sleep patterns in critically ill, mechanically ventilated patients. Am J Respir Crit Care Med 157:A108 (abst)

29. Parthasarathy S, Malik I, Jubran A, Tobin MJ (2001) Does ventilator mode influence sleep quality in critically ill patients? Am J Respir Crit Care Med 163:A180 (Abst)

30. Parthasarathy S, Jubran A, Tobin MJ (2001) Does addition of dead space alter sleep quality during pressure support ventilation. Am J Respir Crit Care Med 163:A483 (abst)

31. Parker JS, Liming JD, Corbett WS, Nishiyama H, Wexler L, Roselle GA (1999) Sleep apnea in 81 ambulatory male patients with stable heart failure. Types and their prevalence, consequences, and presentations. Circulation 99: 2711–2712

32. Brown LK (1988) Sleep-related disorders and chronic obstructive pulmonary disease. Respir Care Clin N Am 3:493–512

33. Uthgenannt D, Schoolmann D, Pietrowsky R, Fehm HL, Born (1955) Effects of sleep on the production of cytokines in humans. J.Psychosom Med 57: 97–104

34. Mullington J, Korth C, Hermann DM, et al (2000) Dose-dependent effects of endotoxin on human sleep. Am J Physiol 278:R947–R955

35. Bradley CM, Nicholson AN, Viveash JP (1991) Opioids and non-opioids. In: Klepper ID, Saunders LD, Rosen M (eds) Ambulatory Anaesthesia and Sedation. Blackwell Science, Oxford, pp 218–34

36. Gallard JM, Blois R (1983) Effect of benzodiazepine antagonist R:15–1788 on flunitazepam-induced sleep changes. Br J Clin Pharmacol 15: 529–536

37. Moote CA, Knill RL (1988) Isoflurane anesthesia causes a transient alteration in nocturnal sleep. Anesthesiology 69: 327–331

38. Knill RL, Moote CA, Skinner MI, Rose EA (1990) Anesthesia and abdominal surgery leads to intense REM sleep during the first postoperative week. Anesthesiology 73:52–61

39. White DP, Douglas NJ, Pickett CK, et al (1983) Sleep deprivation and the control of ventilation. Am Rev Respir Dis 128: 984–986

40. Bonnet MH, Berry RB, Arand DL (1991) Metabolism during normal, fragmented and recovery sleep. J Appl Physiol 71:1112–1118

41. Bonnet LH (1989) Infrequent periodic sleep disruption: effects on sleep, performance and mood. Physiol Behav 45:1049–1055

42. Helton MC, Gordon SH, Nunnery SL (1980) The correlation between sleep deprivation and the intensive care unit syndrome. Heart Lung 9:464–468

43. Rechtschaffen A, Bergmann BM (1995) Sleep deprivation in the rat with the disk-over-water method. Behav Brain Res 69:55–63

44. Brown R, PangG, Husband AJ, King MG (1989) Suppression of immunity to influenza virus in the respiratory tract following sleep disturbance. Reg Immunol 2:321–325

45. Brown R, Price RJ, King MG, Husband AJ (1989) Interleukin 1 and muramil peptide can prevent decreased antibody response associated with sleep deprivation. Brain Behav Immun 3:320–330

46. Madden KS, Felten DL (1995) Experimental basis for neural-immune interactions. Physiol Rev 75:77–106

47. Everson CA, Toth LA (2000) Systemic bacterial invasion induced by sleep deprivation. Am J Physiol 278: R905–R916
48. Dinges DF, Douglas SD, Zaugg L, et al (1994) Leukocytosis and natural killer cells functions parallel neurobehavioural fatigue induced by 64 hours of sleep deprivation. J Clin Invest 93:1930–1939
49. Scheen AJ, Byrne MM, Plat L, Leproult R, Van Cauter E (1996) Relationships between sleep quality and glucose regulation in normal humans. Am J Physiol 271: E261–E270
50. Everson CA, Wehr TA (1993) Nutritional and metabolic adaptations to prolonged sleep deprivation in the rat. Am J Physiol 264: R376–E387
51. Schule C, Baghai T, Zwanzger P, Minov C, Padberg F, Rupprecht R (2001) Sleep deprivation and hypothalamic-pituitary-adrenal (HPA) axis activity in depressed patients. J Psychiatr Res 35: 239–47
52. Taishi P, Sanchez C, Wang Y, Fang J, Harding JW, Krueger JM (2001) Conditions that affect sleep alter the expression of molecules associated with synaptic plasticity. Am J Physiol 281: R839–R845
53. Horner RL (1996) Autonomic consequences of arousal from sleep: mechanisms and implications. Sleep 19: S193–S195
54. Launois SH, Abraham JH, Weiss JW, Kirby DA (1998) Patterned cardiovascular responses to sleep and non-respiratory arousals in a porcine model. J Appl Physiol 85: 1285–1291
55. Cianci T, Zoccoli G, Lenzi P, Franzini C (1991) Loss of integrative control of peripheral circulation during desynchronized sleep. Am J Physiol 261:R373–R377
56. Chen H, Tang Y (1989) Sleep loss impairs inspiratory muscle endurance. Am Rev Respir Dis 140:907–909
57. Leiter JC, Knuth SL, Bartlett D (1985) The effect of sleep deprivation on the activity of the genioglossus muscle. Am Rev Respir Dis 132:1242–1245
58. White DP, Douglas NJ, Pickett CK, Zwillich CW, Weil JV (1983) Sleep deprivation and the control of ventilation. Am Rev Respir Dis 128:984–986
59. Ely EW, Inouye SK, Bernard GR, et al (2001) Delirium in mechanically ventilated patients. Validity and reliability of the confusion assessment method for the intensive care unit (CAM-ICU). JAMA 286:2703–2710
60. Ely EW, Gautam S, Margolin R, et al (2001) The impact of delirium in the intensive care unit on hospital length of stay. Intensive Care Med 27:1892–1900

The Impact of Routine ICU Supportive Care on Long-term Outcomes of Critical Illness

J. B. Hall and J. Kress

Introduction

As critical care medicine has matured as a discipline, clinical investigation and scholarship in this area has expanded beyond its initial focus on the pathophysiology of specific disorders and the utility of specific diagnostics and treatments to include long-term consequences of critical illness and its treatment. This expanded vision is of extraordinary importance since it can yield information essential in helping us most prudently weigh risk-benefit, in assessing more completely the consequences of current therapeutics, in counseling patients and families about the wisdom of limiting or withdrawing therapy, in determining the usefulness of critical care interventions vis-à-vis other healthcare interventions and allocating resources appropriately, and in providing more comprehensive assessment of new therapies in the future. These studies of long-term outcome have gone well beyond information concerning survival alone and now attempt to characterize quality of life, functional status, requirement for additional health care interventions beyond the critical care unit, and psychiatric and social consequences of critical illness on patients, families, and society.

Many examples of this type of research are beginning to appear in the literature, and include emphasis on special groups such as the elderly [1, 2]; specific disorders such as post-cardiac arrest [3], sepsis [4] or acute respiratory distress syndrome (ARDS) [5]; or specific interventions such as renal replacement therapy [6]. Other studies have described long-term outcome in heterogeneous patient groups admitted to medical or surgical intensive care units (ICUs) [7]. Others have described fairly specific long-term endpoints, such as memories, delusions, and posttraumatic stress symptoms following ICU discharge [8–11].

Regardless of the focus of these studies, study of long-term outcomes of critical illness tends to be confounded by a number of factors that include but are not limited to:

1) that in many care environments, patients are referred considerable distances or across health care systems for critical care, and if data collection systems do not span these various systems, extensive data collection after ICU and hospital discharge can be difficult if not impossible;

2) that many tools developed to assess quality of life, functional status, or psychiatric condition have not been well validated in this patient population;

3) that the sudden nature and unpredictability of critical illness make it nearly impossible to have baseline evaluations of patients and thus it is difficult to assess changes that may occur longitudinally over time;

4) that critical care is not highly standardized, and determining which aspect or aspects of care may be operative when differences in long-term outcome are measured can be difficult;

5) that the patient populations admitted to critical care units likely do not reflect the general population or even a subset of the population with a specific disorder, and hence referencing outcome differences to populations not sustaining critical illness is inherently flawed.

Given these substantial impediments to study of long-term outcomes of critical illness, clinical investigators have sought a number of approaches to expand knowledge in this area. We offer one approach in this brief monograph – the extension of data collection from a randomized control trial of sedative strategy in the ICU to describe long-term psychiatric consequences of these strategies.

Long-term Outcomes from Critical Illness: The Example of Sedation

Critically ill patients who are mechanically ventilated often require sedative drugs to assure their comfort while in the ICU. When these drugs are used by continuous infusion or are given frequently by bolus the possibility of drug accumulation is large, and the result can be a protracted drug-induced delirium [12]. This in turn could delay the time to the performance of a spontaneous breathing trial for mechanically ventilated patients which would in turn likely protract the duration of mechanical ventilation [13].

In an earlier study [14], we sought to determine if the simple strategy of discontinuing sedation infusions on a daily basis and allowing patients to awaken and interact with an examiner would impact ICU outcome as compared to routine sedation administration. In this study, 150 patients admitted to a University medical ICU and undergoing mechanical ventilation were randomized to a daily 'Stop' of sedatives or routine care. In the 'Stop' group, sedative and opiate infusions were discontinued in all patients each day, until the patient was alert and following simple commands, or became agitated. At that point, opiate and sedative infusions were restarted at one-half of the dose at the 'Stop' point and titrated as required by the bedside nurse. Demographics and outcome data concerning the ICU and hospital stay were collected for both groups.

The results of this simple approach to sedation were striking. As shown in Table 1, the duration of mechanical ventilation and duration of ICU stay were decreased by more than two and three days respectively.

In addition to these effects on duration of ICU care, patients undergoing a daily interruption of sedatives underwent less diagnostic testing for neurological dysfunction and when that testing was performed, it had a higher likelihood of yielding a meaningful result. The percentage of days during which patients were awake (defined as able to perform three or more simple commands) while receiving a

Table 1. Results of study [14] assessing effects of discontinuing (Stop) sedation

	Stop	Control	p value
Duration of mechanical ventilation (days)	4.9 (2.5–8.6)	7.3 (3.4–16.1)	.004
ICU length of stay (days)	6.4 (3.9–12.0)	9.9 (4.7–17.9)	.02

sedative infusion was greater in the intervention group than in the control group (85.5 vs 9.0 %, p<.001). There were no differences in complications such as unintentional extubation between the groups. Finally, there was a strong trend toward a greater percentage of patients in the stop group being discharged to home (rather than dying or being transferred to a chronic care facility) than in the control group.

While these appeared to be uniformly salutary effects upon the index hospitalization, we and others [15] were concerned that the abrupt cessation of sedation could have adverse neuropsychiatric effects that would become apparent after patients had made a more complete recovery from respiratory failure. Previous studies have reported pain and anxiety as common experiences for patients during their ICU stay, especially after invasive procedures such as arterial puncture and endotracheal suctioning [16, 17]. Some patients who recover from critical illness suffer from long term psychological disturbances such as depression, anxiety and other chronic stress syndromes [18, 19]. Post traumatic stress disorder has been described in patients who have recovered from critical illness [11], but it is not clear if 'awakening' in the ICU or amnesia secondary to sedatives would be a greater risk factor for its development [8]. It seemed important to follow-up patients enrolled in this initial study for a number of reasons: 1) since the intervention we described had an effect to reduce duration of mechanical ventilation and ICU stay, pressures were large to implement this approach; 2) further randomization of patients to follow long-term endpoints was not favored by many clinicians, given the short-term benefits; and 3) if long-term adverse neuropsychiatric consequences resulted, it would be necessary to utilize metrics not initally anticipated in the original study and to perform follow-up well after the resolution of critical illness when patients had recovered to a point that such phenomena could be detected and their impact assessed.

Thus, we proceeded to study patients enrolled in our earlier study; to date, these data have been published only in abstract form [20].

Methods

We interviewed patients previously admitted to our medical ICU who were mechanically ventilated and enrolled and randomized to either a daily discontinuation of sedatives or not. Long term psychological functioning of this cohort was assessed a minimum of six months after hospital discharge. Patients were initially contacted by mail, followed by a phone call inviting them to participate in the study. Those who agreed to participate were interviewed by clinical psychologists experienced in assessing psychological adjustment of patients hospitalized for acute medical illnesses.

The original database was expanded with additional information including occupation, marital status, number of medications prescribed, and number of new medical conditions since hospital discharge. All patients were queried about previous psychiatric illnesses and psychiatric treatments since hospital discharge. All patients were initially asked if they recalled being in the ICU. Those with ICU recall were subsequently questioned for spontaneous recall ("What exactly do you recall?") as well as cued recall (multiple choice questions). Patients were asked whether they remembered being awakened in the ICU. Those who recalled being awakened in the ICU were asked if they were instructed to do anything when being awakened.

All patients underwent a detailed psychological evaluation by a clinical psychologist who was blinded to patient randomization (stop vs. control). The psychological evaluation included an assessment of overall perceived health and psychological well-being as measured by the Medical Outcomes Study 36 item short-form health survey (SF-36) [21], the Psychosocial Adjustment to Illness (PAIS) Score [22], the revised Impact Of Event Scale [23], and a State-Trait Anxiety Inventory [24–27].

Results

A total of 74 patients from the original study survived to hospital discharge. From this group, 18 (8 control, 10 intervention) had died since hospital discharge and 21 (13 control, 8 intervention) could not be reached. Three patients declined the invitation to be interviewed (1 control, 2 intervention). A total of 32 patients agreed to participate in the interview, and the evaluation of these patients is ongoing.

The majority of patients in both groups recalled being present in the ICU during their hospital stay (65 % control vs. 69 % intervention; p = 1.0). In spite of this, very few patients in either group actually recalled the experience of awakening in the ICU at the time of this follow up interview (26 % control vs. 0 % intervention; p = 0.06). Interestingly, fewer patients in the intervention group recalled awakening in the ICU, despite daily attempts to awaken them. Indeed, no patient in the intervention group recalled this routine awakening.

As assessed by SF-36 evaluation, overall perceived health and psychological well-being was lower in both groups in all categories when compared to normative values from the United States population. These results are graphically depicted in Figure 1. Nevertheless, patients in the intervention group fared substantially better than control patients with regard to their general health assessment (mean transformed SF-36 score 28.4 vs. 9.0; p = 0.02). There was also a trend toward better physical role functioning (i.e., physical functioning with regard to work or other daily activities) in the intervention group (median transformed SF-36 score 50 vs.

0; p = 0.3), as well as a trend toward better mental health in the intervention group (mean transformed SF-36 score 66.8 vs. 59.3; p = 0.29).

Four of the first 12 patients interviewed had intrusive thoughts as a result of their ICU stay but were equally distributed between the two study groups and no patient had sought psychiatric help after hospital discharge. No patient had post-traumatic stress disorder diagnosed by the impact of event scale and no differences between the groups were noted. Anxiety was high and mild depression common across both patient groups but not different between the groups. At this point of interim analysis, the data support the following conclusions: 1) patients subjected to daily discontinuation of sedatives during mechanical ventilation rarely recall this experience; 2) these patients have acceptable psychological health; 3) they do not suffer from post-traumatic stress disorder; and 4) they suffer anxiety and depression at rates similar to patients undergoing mechanical ventilatory support but not subjected to daily discontinuation of sedation.

Comment

The data presented are at an interim analysis and are offered not for firm conclusions to be drawn but for points to be made about studying long-term outcomes from critical illness.

Many of the impediments to study of long-term outcomes are represented. Our hospital is a typical tertiary care University facility. Accordingly, many patients are referred from other hospitals and physicians and return to care elsewhere following discharge from our site. Thus, this follow-up study required extensive telephone and mail contact of patients and study subjects had to be willing to return to our site for interviews. This of course creates a potential selection bias in the study population, and acting jointly with the mortality and morbidity of critical illness, can result in even large populations of patients entering an ICU-based study dwindling to the point that the power to detect various differences is limited.

The tools we selected to characterize neuropsychiatric and functional status in our patients are well standardized in general but admittedly their use in our patient population is somewhat limited, at least based upon current publications. While it is not reasonable to expect every parameter to be re-validated in slightly modified clinical settings, it is at a minimum advisable that further study of these tools in critically ill patients be performed. It will also be necessary for clinical investigators of long-term outcomes of critical illness to master these metrics and to forge collaborative relationships with those using them routinely to assure the highest level of clinical science.

Another set of problems relate to the fact that the central data collected here – interview-based assessments of function at one point in time after an episode of critical illness – can be compared across the two groups of interest but are otherwise difficult to understand in relationship to other patient populations or the general population. We have offered a comparison of the SF-36 data to US population norms (Fig. 1), but are unable to speak to the baseline function of our patients, prior to the onset of their critical illness. This of course makes it difficult to determine if

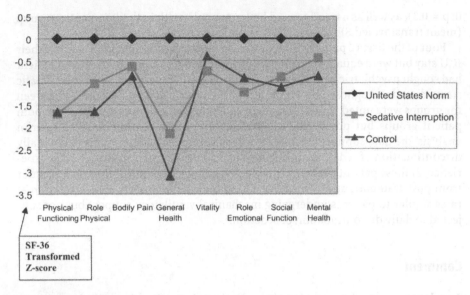

Fig. 1. Differences in SF-36 scores of control patients and those in the sedative interruption group, compared to normative values.

the patient groups were comparable at baseline, a general tenet of data analysis in prospective randomized trials.

Finally, these data, at least upon preliminary analysis, do not point to glaring differences in neuropsychiatric outcome when daily discontinuation of sedative use is employed as a strategy to reduce the duration of mechanical ventilation. If these early trends are supported by further data collection and analysis, we would be reasonably confident that this is true when this strategy is used in our hands. However, since so many elements of care related to sedation and mechanical ventilation are not completely standardized across ICUs in different institutions (or indeed often within the same institution), generalizing these data to other care settings requires inherent assumptions that could be erroneous.

References

1. Shigemitsu O, Hadama T, Miyamoto S, et al (2001) Early and long-term results of cardiovascular surgery in octogenarians. Ann Thorac Cardiovasc Surg 7:223–231
2. Udekwu P, Gurkin B, Oller D, et al (2001) Quality of life and functional level in elderly patients surviving surgical intensive care. J Am Coll Surg 193:245–249
3. Dimopoulou I, Anthi A, Michalis A, et al (2001) Functional status and quality of life in long term survivors of cardiac arrest after cardiac surgery. Crit Care Med 29:1408–1411
4. Heyland DK, Hopman W, Coo H, et al (2000) Long term health related quality of life in survivors of sepsis. Short Form 36: a valid and reliable measure of health-related quality of life. Crit Care Med 28:3755–3756

5. Nelson BJ, Weinert CR, Bury CL, et al (2000) Intensive care unit drug use and subsequent quality of life in acute lung injury patients. Crit Care Med 28:3626–3630

6. Korkeila M, Ruokonen E, Takala J (2000) Costs of care, long term prognosis and quality of life in patients requiring renal replacement therapy during intensive care. Intensive Care Med 26:1824–1831

7. Wehler M, Martus P, Geise A, et al (2001) Changes in quality of life after medical intensive care. Intensive Care Med 27:154–159

8. Jones C, Griffiths RD, Humphris G, et al (2001) Memory, delusions, and the development of acute posttraumatic stress disorder-related symptoms after intensive care. Crit Care Med 29:573–580

9. Scragg P, Jones A, Fauvel N (2001) Psychological problems following ICU treatment. Anaesthesia 56: 9–14

10. Schnyder U, Morgeli H, Nigg C, et al (2000) Early psychological reactions to life threatening injuries. Crit Care Med 28:86–92

11. Schelling G, Stoll C, Haller M, et al (1998) Health related quality of life and posttraumatic stress disorder in survivors of the acute respiratory distress syndrome. Crit Care Med 26:651–659

12. Kress JP, O'Connor MF, Pohlman AS, et al (1996) Sedation of critically ill patients during mechanical ventilation. A comparison of propofol and midazolam. Am J Respir Crit Care Med 153:1012–1018

13. MacIntyre NR (2001) Evidence-based guidelines for weaning and discontinuation ventilatory support: A collective task force. Chest 120:375S–396S

14. Kress JP, Pohlman AS, O'Connor MF, Hall JB (2000) Daily interruption of sedative infusions in critically ill patients undergoing mechanical ventilation. N Engl J Med 342:1471–1477

15. Heffner JE (2000) A wake-up call in the intensive care unit. N Engl J Med 342:1520–1522

16. Puntillo KA (1990) Pain experiences of intensive care unit patients. Heart Lung 19:526–533

17. Turner JS. Briggs SJ. Springhorn HE. Potgieter PD (1990) Patients' recollection of intensive care unit experience. Crit Care Med 18:966–968

18. Griffiths RD, Jones C (1999) Recovery from intensive care. Br Med J 319:427–429

19. Russell S (1999) An exploratory study of patients' perceptions, memories and experiences of an intensive care unit. J Adv Nurs 29:783–791

20. Kress J, Lacy M, Pliskin N, Pohlman A, Hall JB (2001)The long term psychological effects of daily sedative interruption in critically ill patients. Am J Respir Crit Care Med 163:A954 (abst)

21. Stansfeld SA, Roberts R, Foot SP (1997) Assessing the validity of the SF-36 general health survey. Qual Life Res 6:217–224

22. Morrow G, Chiarello R, Derogatis L (1978) A new scale for assessing patients' psychological adjustment to medical illness. Psychol Med 8:605–610

23. Joseph S (2000) Psychometric evaluation of Horowitz's Impact of Event Scale: a review. J Trauma Stress 13:101–113

24. Bieling P, Anthony M, Swinson R (1998) The State-Trait Anxiety Inventory: Trait version structure and content re-examined. Behav Res Ther 36:777–788

25. Spielberger CD (1975) The measurement of state and trait anxiety: conceptual and methodological issues. In: Levi L (ed) Emotions: Their Parameters and Measurement. Raven Press, New York, pp 713–725

26. Lasa L, Ayuso-Mateos JL, Vazquez-Barquero JL, Diez-Manrique FJ, Dowrick CF (2000) The use of the Beck Depression Inventory to screen for depression in the general population: A preliminary anaylsis. J Affect Disord 57:261–265

27. Beck, AT, Steer R A, Brown G K (1980) Beck Depression Inventory, Second Edition Manual. The Psychological Corporation, Harcourt Brace and Company, San Antonio

Improving Methods to Capture Long-term Outcomes in Clinical Studies

Disease-free Survival and Quality of Life as End-points in Clinical Trials

M. Van Glabbeke and A. Bottomley

Introduction

Clinical Research in Oncology

The second half of the 20th century has witnessed an impressive development of clinical research in oncology, motivated by the acute need for effective treatments for most cancers and encouraged by the discovery of the first chemotherapy agents. The availability of computers to store and analyze large quantities of data gave a new dimension to research projects. In parallel, an appropriate methodology was developed for designing, conducting and analyzing the clinical trials that would finally lead to improvement of cancer treatment.

Multicenter Trials and Cooperative Groups

It appeared rather early that medical practice would only be improved on the basis of the results of randomized clinical trials including large number of patients, while single centers were generally unable to recruit patients fast enough in pivotal studies. The oncology community began conducting multicenter, and sometimes multinational clinical trials to accrue patients at a reasonable speed, and optimize the research strategies. The resulting heterogeneity of the patient population included in multicenter trials favored broad generalization of their results. Clinical investigators formed 'clinical cooperative groups' to organize and manage these trials. These networks are still at the origin of most clinical research conducted in oncology today, and also of most methodological developments. Since 1955, the United States National Cancer Institute has supported a large Cooperative Groups Program, and is currently sponsoring projects from 12 different groups. The European Organization for Research of Treatment of Cancer (EORTC), that celebrated its 40th anniversary in 2002, is the largest cancer research organization in Europe, while national and regional groups are growing in number and expanding their activities.

One of the keys of success of cancer cooperative groups is the integration of scientists with different types of expertise, including biology, statistics, and, more recently, psychology and economics.

Statistical Support

Following the model of pioneering US cancer research organizations, such as the Southwest Oncology Group (SWOG) and the Eastern Cooperative Oncology Group (ECOG), one of the early priorities of the EORTC was to create a Data Center that would provide statistical and data management support to the clinical groups. Involvement of biostatisticians in cancer research is not limited to data analysis: on the contrary, they actively participate to the design and set-up of clinical trials. From the beginning, they have underlined the need of objective measurement scales to evaluate the outcome of investigated treatments, and they have contributed to the definition and development of such scales as well as the elaboration of statistical techniques to analyze the collected data.

Quality of Life

In the early eighties, the recognition of quality of life as an important end-point for cancer research lead to the creation of an EORTC Quality of Life Study Group, and, in the early nineties, a Quality of Life Unit was added to the EORTC Data Center to promote quality of life as an end-point for cancer clinical trials, to develop an appropriate methodology and to apply it to EORTC trials.

The Example of oncology

With an experience of more than half a century, oncology is a leading field of clinical research.

The present chapter gives an overview of the different end-points currently used in cancer clinical trials, with a short description of their origin, development, applicability and a discussion of particular problems encountered in their statistical analysis. It underlines the efforts dedicated to develop tools and instruments for assessing the impact of disease and treatments on the quality of life of cancer patients. This can be taken as an example for developing appropriate end-points for evaluating treatment results in other types of disease.

Overall Survival

The most intuitive and commonly used end-point in cancer trials is patient overall survival. This reflects the fact that a large part of cancer research aims at prolonging survival of patients affected by a type of tumor for which no curative therapies are available.

Overall survival is an unbiased end-point, and is easy to assess. Methods are available to use the information that a patient is still alive at a known date and exploit this information in different types of statistical analyses. The date of last follow-up provides a lower limit of the survival estimate for alive patients (censored data). Actuarial methods (the most commonly used is the Kaplan-Meier method

[1]) use censored data for the estimation of survival rates at different time points. Statistical tests have been developed (the most commonly used being the Logrank test [2]) to compare the survival profiles of different groups of patients, using censored data.

Techniques initially developed for survival analysis can be used for any end point defined as 'time to a particular event', like disease free survival or time to treatment failure.

Performance Status

The Karnofsky Index

The first attempt to measure treatment outcome is the Karnofsky index, that classifies patients according to their performance status [3]. David Karnofsky has developed an 11 points ordered scale, varying from 100 (fully normal activities) to 0 (death), reflecting the impact of disease symptoms on the patient's ability to work, care for him/herself, and the level of assistance, medical care and supportive treatment required.

This index was used to demonstrate the palliative effect of chemotherapy. It was the first effort aiming at assessing treatment outcome in an objective way, despite the fact that the scale incorporates some subjective elements.

Simplified Scales

The experience acquired with the Karnofsky index suggested that it could be difficult to apply, the distinctions between the different categories being sometimes too subjective to classify patients in a reliable way. A simplified five points scale was consequently proposed by Zubrod et al. [4] and adopted by most US cancer cooperative groups. This scale has been subsequently adopted by the World Health Organization (WHO) consensus meeting in (see hereunder) [5] and is now often referred as the 'WHO scale for performance status'.

Although presently performance status does not contribute to the assessment of 'palliative affect' or 'response to therapy', it has been demonstrated to be an important prognostic factor in most cancers. Performance status is generally recorded and followed in clinical studies, and often used as a stratification factor for randomization and statistical analysis.

Efficacy of Therapies

In the seventies, the availability of radiological techniques to follow cancer lesions and measure their size with an increased precision opened new perspectives for measuring efficacy of cancer treatments. Objective response to therapy started to be evaluated on the basis of tumor measurements rather than performance status. Radiological evidence was required to document disease progression.

When discussing the methods currently used to assess the efficacy of cancer therapies, two types of trials have to be distinguished:

- Trials on advanced disease, where patients with active tumors are submitted to a treatment aimed at decreasing the tumor burden, as well as the signs and symptoms of disease, and, eventually, cure them from their disease.
- Adjuvant trials, where patients who are free of any sign or symptom of disease, after a radical treatment, are submitted to an additional adjuvant therapy to avoid or delay possible relapses.

Response to Treatment for Advanced Disease

The use of a mixture of subjective (performance status) and objective (imaging) elements to assess the disease response to new treatments underlined the need for standardization, the only way to allow reliable comparisons of published results of cancer clinical trials.

In the late seventies, the WHO organized an international consensus meeting with representatives of major cooperative groups in Europe and the US to standardize the reporting of results of cancer treatment [5]. One of the outcomes of this conference was the definition of a standardized method for response assessment, mainly based on repetitive bi-dimentional measurements of a few 'target' cancer lesions. The aim was to provide an objective method for rapidly screening new agents, and identify biological antitumor activity in specific types of cancer.

The evolution of the size of target lesions was used to classify treatment outcome as "complete response" (CR: complete disappearance of all signs and symptoms of disease), "partial response" (PR: decrease of at last 50% of the total tumor load), "progression" (PD: increase of at least 25% of the total tumor load) or "disease stabilization" (SD: no or small changes in the total tumor load that do not qualify as partial response or progression).

The 'WHO response criteria' were universally used for nearly 30 years in new drug screening.

The RECIST Criteria

The experience acquired with these criteria underlined some problems and ambiguities that progressively lead to different interpretations amongst the different groups. In 1994, the EORTC, the National Cancer Institute of the US, and the National Cancer Institute of Canada Clinical Trials Group set up a task force to review the WHO response criteria on the basis of the experience and knowledge acquired since their original publication. This resulted in the edition of a new set of criteria, the Response Evaluation Criteria In Solid Tumors (RECIST) that have now been adopted worldwide [6]. Principal differences with the WHO criteria lie in the use of single dimensions of tumor lesions, clarification of previously encountered ambiguities, and guidelines for the use of the currently available radiological techniques to measure lesions. When designing these new simplified measurement criteria, the four points scale (CR, PR, SD, PD) was maintained, and major discrepancies in the meaning and concept of partial response were avoided, to retain ability to compare results of future therapies to those already available.

In order to avoid misinterpretation or individual modification of the criteria, the RECIST working party maintains a "RECIST Question and Answers" web site (http://www.eortc.be/recist). Adequate communication between the users and the working party is expected to contribute to keep the system standard and consistent with time.

Other efforts have been made to adapt the WHO response criteria to specific situations, not covered by the RECIST criteria. Cheson and colleagues have developed a set of response criteria to be used for the lymphoma, addressing the specific issue of measuring node lesions, and incorporating the response of liver, bone marrow, and other extra-nodal sites [7].

An important point of the RECIST publication, that is generally applicable to any response criteria, is that it underlines the applicability of 'objective response' as an end-point in clinical trials. Response criteria have been developed to identify new cancer agents and regimen worthy of further investigation in comparative trials. These criteria are not intended to be used alone to guide decision in daily clinical practice, where elements less objective but more relevant to the patients may indicate clinical improvement. They are not intended either to be used as the principal end-point of comparative clinical trials, that are designed to provide an estimate of the therapeutic benefit for the patient: objective response is not necessarily a good surrogate for therapeutic benefit.

Time to Progression for Advanced Disease

Time to disease progression may be used as an end-point in comparative clinical trials. In such case, particular attention has to be paid to the definition of events that will be considered as progression. Both the WHO and RECIST criteria provide a definition of progressive disease, based on the growth of cancer lesions, or appearance of new lesions. Other events can, however, also be considered, like the increase of biological tumor markers, or the deterioration of the performance status. Therefore, time to disease progression should not be considered as a standardized end-point.

Time to progression is sometimes used to document anticancer activity of non-cytotoxic agents that are not expected to induce a reduction in the size of lesions. In such case, it is recommended to use the RECIST definition of progressive disease, and to document all progression by tumor measurements.

Disease Free Survival in Adjuvant Trials

Disease free survival is defined as the period during which a patient is 'free from disease', i.e., not affected by any disease sign or symptoms. This end-point can only be used in trials where the patients are 'disease free' at treatment start, typically in the adjuvant situation. The definition of 'tumor recurrence' in these trials is essential, and therefore needs to be prospectively and objectively defined. The problems encountered here are the same as those encountered when trying to define 'progression' in trials on advanced disease. Special attention has to be paid to patients who die while they are still free of recurrence. There is a distinction here between 'disease free survival', where those deaths are considered as events, and 'disease free interval', where these patients are censored on the date of death. Special attention should be paid to this distinction, as these two end-points are often confused. Analysis of this end-point will, of course, be based on 'time to events' methods.

Side Effects of Cancer Therapies

Acute Side Effects

Most anticancer treatments have side effects, and the choice of an appropriate treatment is often a compromise between treatment efficacy and toxicity. Treatment side effects, during and after treatment, are, of course, important components of the patients quality of life. Quality of life issues are discussed later in this chapter.

Early assessments of anticancer treatment toxicity were based on semi-subjective severity scales, grading adverse treatment reactions as 'absent', 'mild', 'moderate', 'severe', 'life threatening' or 'lethal.

The WHO consensus meeting and resulting WHO Criteria for Reporting Results of Cancer Treatment [5] were also the first attempt to measure treatment toxicity according to objective scales. In these guidelines, all types of adverse events commonly expected from cancer therapies were graded according to a five point scale, according to criteria as objective as possible. Grades were defined to correspond to the previously used 'absent' to 'lethal' scales.

Discovery of new types of anticancer agents with new types of toxicity lead the US National Cancer Institute to review these criteria in 1990, and issue the NCI 'Common Toxicity Criteria'. Uncontrolled adaptation of these criteria by different organizations underlined, again, the need to appoint an international working party to maintain standardization. The International Common Toxicity Criteria' are now submitted to a regular update policy. The successive versions are distributed via the Internet (http://ctep.cancer.gov/reporting/ctc.html).

This working party is also maintaining specific criteria for particular patient population (children) or treatments (bone marrow transplants).

Late Side Effects of Radiotherapy

While acute toxicity (occurring during of shortly after the end of treatment) is a major concern for chemotherapy treatments, the maximum tolerated dose of radiotherapy is rather defined on the basis of late sequellae in long survivors.

The EORTC-RTOG late toxicity scale provides an objective five point grading system for these late sequellae. This scale is published as an appendix of the International Common Toxicity Criteria.

It should be noted that most events occur in the irradiated area, and will therefore depend on the irradiated organ. Consequently, different scales are used for the different sites of cancer (and irradiation).

When estimating the rate of late treatment complications, one should take into account the fact that the risk of developing sequellae increases with the duration of survival, that may largely vary from one patient to the other. Therefore, censored analysis techniques are often used to analyze the proportion of late sequellae observed with a treatment; patients are censored in this analysis on the date of death. The possible confusion of late effects and disease symptoms sometimes suggests restricting the analysis of late side effects to the remission period. In such cases, the patient is censored on the date of relapse or progression.

The SOMA-LENT scale

It is clear that late side effects of radiotherapy may have a large impact on patient quality of life, and, consequently, the US Radiation Therapy Oncology Group (RTOG) and EORTC Radiotherapy Group joined forces in the eighties to replace their previous 'late toxicity scale' by an instrument taking into account Subjective, Objective, Management and Analytical elements to grade Late Effects on Normal Tissues. The resulting grading scales are known as the SOMA/LENT grading system.

The ambitious objective was to develop, for each possible late side effect of radiotherapy, a multidimensional scale that would reflect not only the grading of objective symptoms by the physician (the basis of the previous scale), but also subjective patient perception (quality of life), the medical management of the symptoms, reversibility and treatability, and analytical parameters (laboratory and imaging). A scoring system has been defined for 37 different organs. For each organ, relevant parameters have been identified and graded on a scale varying from 0 to 4, and a summary score of the 4 dimensions is proposed.

This scale was simultaneously published in 1995 in *Radiotherapy and Oncology* [8] and in the *International Journal for Radiation Oncology and Biology Physics*.

This scale is not yet fully validated, but currently piloted in a few studies.

Quality of Life

Introduction

In the early eighties the need to evaluate the impact of cancer treatment on quality of life, as perceived by patients, started to gain recognition. However, it was not until the 1990s that interest in this field became so well accepted that many research organizations and clinical trialists frequently started to measure this as an endpoint in randomized clinical trials (RCTs). Due partly to researchers faced with situations where patients may not gain benefits in terms of traditional endpoints, such as survival, or disease-free survival, this new aspect showed that it is possible to see significant changes in quality of life, or as it is often refered to as health-related quality of life (HRQL) [9]. Other reasons for the rise in interest relates to an increased empathy from professional bodies, including the US Food and Drug Administration (FDA) and the European Agency for the Evaluation of Medicinal products (EMEA); both recognize the possible benefits of HRQL as a basis for the approval of new anticancer drugs. Without doubt, influential cancer organizations, such as the American Society of Clinical Oncology (ASCO) have also played a leading role, influencing many practicing clinicians to consider HRQL as a useful tool not only to help in research, but also daily clinical practice. Finally, another important factor which has pushed HRQL into the forefront of clinical trial research is patient involvement. This comes mainly from the USA. Here, influential cancer groups influence the clinical trial process by ensuring patient HRQL is a key issue for consideration when appropriate.

However, the process of introducing HRQL into research and clinical trials has not always been easy. One of the most difficult challenges is dealing with a multi-dimensional construct and an important concept that has, for many years, proved difficult to define. Many definitions of HRQL exist, for example, "it is the state of well being that is a composite of two components: the ability to perform everyday activities that reflect physical, psychological, and social well-being; and patient satisfaction with levels of functioning and control of the disease [10]; "it is the subjective evaluation of the good and satisfactory character of life as a whole" [11]; "it is the gap between the patient's expectations and achievements. The smaller the gap, the higher the quality of life" [12]. Although in some respects HRQL is poorly defined, after considerable debate, over a decade, it is believed that HRQL is now generally regarded as covering the subjective clinical perceptions of the positive and negative aspects of cancer patient domains, including physical, emotional, social and cognitive functions, and, importantly, disease symptoms and treatments.

Even with an agreed definition, there are a number of barriers to acceptance of HRQL as an outcome in clinical oncology trials. Most frequently these are related to oncologists' and clinicians' attitude problems towards the subjective nature of the data collected, something that is somewhat different from most other aspects of medical management, and collection of patient data. Fortunately, in recent years, clinicians have shown a greater understanding of HRQL not only as a research-based tool, but also its potential use in helping to direct patient care [13–15]. For example, clinicians working with esophageal cancer patients held to the traditional view that dyspnea was one of the most significant patient concerns. However, data from HRQL studies, reveal that fatigue and its effects on HRQL are more of an issue. This has lead some clinicians to address patient management by, for example, treating fatigue, possibly using erythropoietin or other interventions [16].

Challenges of Measuring HRQL

That patients are the best judges of their HRQL is one fundamental lesson learned in oncology over the last decade. Several authors have reported that when HRQL assessment is made, clinicians consistently underestimate the level of patient HRQL problems, particularly related to pain and nausea, when compared to patients rating themselves [17, 18]. Patient preferences for treatment are also known to be different from clinicians and health care providers. For example, it is known that many cancer patients undergoing chemotherapy are prepared to accept a significantly greater degree of toxicity and reduced HRQL and, sometimes, minimal increase in change or survival or cure than health care professionals report. This suggests that patients, as opposed to clinicians, are the only people who should evaluate the life and death decisions they face [19]. Therefore, for a number of years the use of patient-reported questionnaires has become standard practice in the assessment of cancer patient HRQL.

However, developing a robust and valid HRQL measuring instrument, useful in clinical trials, is resource intensive. Presently, there are several types of measuring instruments available; for example, *generic instruments*, intended for general use, and can be used on patients irrespective of the disease of the patient. Indeed, many such tools can be used on healthy patients, tools such as the Short Form (SF)-36, perhaps one of the most widely used tools for measuring HRQL. While such tools are valuable, and cover a wide range of HRQL issues, they lack a focus on disease-specific issues and may lack sensitivity to detect HRQL issues in some patient populations. For example, whilst the SF-36 is useful for a general population, asking questions on general health, activities, etc, it will not detect key issues in cancer patients, such as levels of lymphedema in breast cancer patients, or hair loss for instance. Therefore, *disease specific instruments* were developed for many fields that address such shortfalls. In oncology, hundreds of tools exists at present that claim to measure HRQL. While there are many measures to select from, there are many problems in using such tools appropriately in the clinical setting; if well-validated instruments are not used in the correct manner, there is an inherent issue of concern regarding appropriate interpretation [9]. If an HRQL instrument is not well known it needs to be examined in detail to ensure psychometric properties of reliability and validity are suitable before any interpretation of the results can be undertaken. Kong and Gandhi reviewed 265 articles reporting on HRQL assessment in clinical trials: only 23 % provided reliability data, and only 21 % provided validity data [20]. Therefore, the tools used in this instance are inadequate for the purpose intended.

In the 1980s, the EORTC Quality of Life Group recognized that not only was HRQL a key issue, but that it represented an area where methodological challenges lie; it would need to be addressed if HRQL was to be successfully integrated into cancer clinical trials. The key to success was the formulation of an instrument development and validation system usable across clinical trials and within a number of different populations. After a review of existing instruments, the Quality of Life Group decided that none were fully appropriate, deciding to develop a set of cancer-specific HRQL questionnaires focusing on health-related issues and practical enough to be completed by the patients themselves. A modular approach was adopted, with one core questionnaire applicable to all types of cancers, and a series of specific modules applicable to particular types of cancers. As a result, the EORTC QLQ-C30 core questionnaire is now one of the most widely accepted standardized methods for assessing the HRQL of cancer patients worldwide; several disease-specific modules are now either fully validated, or in their development phase [21, 22].

Developing HRQL Measures in Oncology – the EORTC Approach

The development of an HRQL tool begins with the definition of a questionnaire that would ultimately quantify different aspects of health-related HRQL according to a multidimensional scale. The EORTC instrument incorporates five functional scales (physical, role, cognitive, emotional and social), three symptom scales (fatigue, pain, nausea and vomiting), six single items symptom scales (constipation, diarrhea, appetite, sleep, dyspnea, financial) and a global health and quality of life scale [23]. Answers to the different questions are combined to obtain a score on each scale, varying from 0 to 100. The definition of the questions is based on the knowledge of the disease to be assessed, and the problems frequently encountered by patients.

Developed instruments must be subsequently validated on patients. The questionnaires should avoid upsetting or confusing questions and should be easily completed by the patient with limited assistance. Based on statistical techniques, such as simple factor analysis, or more complex techniques such as item response theory modules, instrument developers will then check that each item (question) of the instrument appropriately contributes to one of the hypothesized scales. The resulting scales should be reliable, i.e., produce reproducible and consistent results, and valid, i.e., measure what they are supposed to measure. The EORTC approach to instrument development has been reported in detail by several authors [24–26].

One of the unique challenges that faces HRQL researchers in the European setting, is having robust, culturally-valid measures. Therefore, the EORTC pays considerable attention to the applicability of its instruments in a wide range of cultural settings. This implies that all questionnaires are translated into a large number of languages, and that the translation is validated by a back translation to the original. A large number of other steps must then be followed to check on the validity of the translation, including pilot-testing with patients and expert review before accepting a final translation. This is extremely resource intensive, following the procedure reported by Cull et al. [27]. It is recognized that not all measures produced in oncology, or for that matter in other diseases, have followed this process. While presently there is no internationally agreed standard for the translation and cultural adaptation of measures, the general procedure adopted by the EORTC is one broadly followed by other international research groups, such as the USA Functional Assessment to Cancer Therapy Measurement Group [28] and groups such as the WHO. (WHO GROUP) [29]. In many respects, when conducting translations and cultural validation, failure to adhere to these general practices and principles of validation can lead to problems in both administering measures; this may ultimately lead to confusing and incorrect assumptions based on patient reported data.

Practical Aspects of Design and Analysis of Quality of Life Studies

The inclusion of HRQL as an endpoint in a clinical trial requires that it must be based on a clear hypothesis, and, as for any other end-points, HRQL hypotheses must be defined, clearly indicated in the clinical trial protocol, and tested in the final analysis. This also serves to inform those clinicians who are perhaps less motivated, into collecting more data to better understand the exact value of this work.

The next step is the selection of the appropriate measurement instrument. This should be a valid and reliable tool, and one that is suitable to detect the HRQL issues of a given population. Assessment time-points are an important component of any study. An initial (pre-study) evaluation is always needed: follow-up evaluations would be useless without any baseline assessment for comparison. Baseline data can help ascertain whether HRQL characteristics of RCTs are equally distributed in both arms; this can also help explain reasons for missing follow-up data, and can be used to help minimize any systematic biases that can develop from data that are not missing at random. The number of assessments should be weighted to the patient burden, and the probability of obtaining an adequate compliance to the completion of the questionnaires. Ideally, to reduce burden on clinical staff who already suffer a considerable workload, consideration should be given to collecting HRQL data at the same time other clinical data are collected. This not only reduces the burden on patients, and clinicians, but can also lead to higher compliance of data collection [30]. The choice between fixed time-points and treatment related time-points should be considered in the interpretation of the results. Of course, the timing of HRQL assessments will relate to the research question being asked. Whilst it might be desirable to measure HRQL after progression of the disease, this has often proven to be difficult, and associated with poor compliance. The frequency of 'off treatment' assessments will be dependent on the purpose and feasibility of assessments.

Compliance with HRQL data in multinational, or even national trials can be a problem at times, one that has plagued the success of many HRQL studies. However, compliance issues are a limited problem when data are collected from single institutions; however, in many clinical trials this is not the case. To obtain good compliance, data collection should be prospectively organized in all centers. Any number of strategies can be considered to improve compliance, a problem faced by many cancer clinical trial organizations; for example, providing training courses for data managers, clinicians, and other health professionals on how to collect, use and implement all aspects of HRQL studies prior to commencing trials. Providing written guidelines for administering HRQL measures can also help [30]. The EORTC recommends handing the questionnaire to the patient during a visit, rather than sending it by mail, as often compliance can be reduced when the postal service is used. In addition, it is possible that bias may be an issue, for example, with the patient's family or relatives helping to complete the HRQL measure. Hopefully, by collecting data in a clinical setting, these biases can be reduced.

The major problems faced by the statistician during the analysis are related to the treatment of missing data. Models for missing data mechanisms are important topics of research; missing data can be an important source of bias in HRQL analysis, and results have therefore to be interpreted with particular care and in line with the formulated analysis plan. Interpretation of HRQL data represents a challenge in many other respects. For example, very few HRQL tools have clear cut-off levels where it is known patients can be classed within a clinically defined group: if patient A scores 50 and patient B scores 60 on a 1–100 scale (1 being worse and 100 being the best) then this does not necessarily mean the patients are clinically worse than each other. Statistical significance does not imply clinical relevance for patients. This is an area where a good deal of research in HRQL is presently being undertaken. In oncology, some success is evident; research by Osoba et al. [31], Juniper et al. [32], and Lydick and Epstein [33] are helping clinicians to understand patient meaning and responses on HRQL instruments.

Finally, it cannot be over stressed that one critical issue to ensure HRQL studies are regarded as valuable, at the research level and to influence practice, is ensuring high standards of reporting and publishing of results. In many respects, the collection, analysis and reporting of HRQL data must be to the same standards as that of other clinical data collected in cancer clinical trials. Lee and Chi [34] provide evidence that much past reporting of HRQL data from clinical trials is not optimal; there is room for improvement. In their review of some 72 articles on HRQL many studies failed to have a defined hypothesis or rationale for including HRQL, and in many cases interpretation is limited by poor descriptions of methodology used or methods to handle missing data are not explained, or adherence to assessment schedules and lack of data on the validity of measures selected. Bottomley et al. [16] report this to be such a major problem that in many cases it has proven difficult to make robust and meaningful conclusions about many HRQL questions in certain disease sites [34]. Minimum standards are proposed by several groups and organizations, such as the International Society of Quality of Life Research or Staquet et al. [35]. Such standards require full explanation of the rationale, instrument selection and validity and other psychometric details, and should include details of clinical significance, as reported above.

Conclusion

Half a century of experience in clinical cancer research has demonstrated the success of the multidisciplinary approach, and the important role of cooperative groups. Standardized instruments to measure treatment outcome are the basis of a common language, an essential tool to compare the experience and results of different research teams. Scoring systems based on objective criteria and measurements and on assessments made by the physicians are the most widely used for evaluating treatment results. They do not, however, necessarily reflect the patient's perception of quality of life. Systems based on patient reported questionnaires are now available to incorporate this new important end-point in trial conclusions.

Worldwide acceptability of measurement and scoring scales is obtained by involving experts from all major groups of potential users in the development of these instruments. All scales have to be validated and appropriate statistical techniques need to be created to analyze the resulting data. Easy communication channels (like web sites, e-mails and forums) can be used for publication and information, user's feed back and discussions; this helps to maintain the scoring systems standard and consistent.

End-points used in clinical research are based on large efforts of conception, validation, and maintenance that should not be underestimated.

References

1. Kaplan EL, Meier P (1958) Nonparametric estimation from incomplete observations. J Am Stat Ass 53:457–481
2. Peto R, Peto J (1972) Asymptotally invariant rank test procedures. J R Stat Soc A135:185–206
3. Karnofsky DA, Abelman WH, Craver LF, Burchenal JH (1948) The use of nitrogen mustards in palliative treatment of carcinoma. Cancer 1:643–656
4. Zubrod CG, Schneiderman SM, Frei E III, et al (1960) Appraisal of methods for the study of chemotherapy of cancer in man: comparative therapeutic trial of nitrogen mustard and thio phosphoamide. J Chron Dis 11:7–33
5. WHO (1979) Handbook for Reporting Results of Cancer Treatment (1979).: World Health Organization Offset Publication No 48, Geneva
6. Therasse P, Arbuck SG, Eisenhauer E, et al (2000) New guidelines to evaluate the response to treatment in solid tumors. J Natl Cancer Inst 92:205–216
7. Cheson BD, Horning SJ, Coiffier B, et al (1999) Report of an international workshop to standardize response criteria for non-Hodgkin's lymphomas. NCI Sponsored International Working Group. J Clin Oncol 17:1244
8. Pavy JJ, Denekamp J, Letschert J, et al (1995) EORTC Late Effects Working Group. Late effects toxicity scoring: the SOMA scale. Radiother Oncol 35:11–15
9. Velikova G, Stark, D, Selby P (1999) Quality of life instruments in oncology. Eur J Cancer 35:1571–1580
10. Cook-Gotay C, Korn EL, McCabe MS, et al (1992) Quality-of-life assessment in cancer treatment protocols: Research issues in protocol development. J Natl Cancer Inst 84:575–577
11. van Knippenberg FC, de Haes JC (1988) Measuring the quality of life of cancer patients: psychometric properties of instruments. J Clin Epidemiol 41:1043–1053
12. Calman KC (1984) Quality of life in cancer patients – an hypothesis. J Med Ethics 24:127
13. Tanaka T, Gotay CC (1998) Physicians' and medical students' perspectives on patients' quality of life. Acad Med 73:1003–1005
14. Morris J, Perez D, McNoe B (1998) The use of quality of life data in clinical practice. Qual Life Res 7:85–91
15. Detmar SB, Aaronson NK (1998) Quality of life assessment in daily clinical oncology practice: a feasibility study. Eur J Cancer 34:1181–1186
16. Bottomley A, Thomas R, Van Steen K, Flechtner H, Djulbegovic B (2002) Human recombinant erythropoietin and quality of life: A wonder drug or something to wonder about? Lancet Oncol 3:145–153
17. Stephens RJ, Hopwood P, Girling DJ, Machin D (1997) Randomized trials with quality of life endpoints: are doctors' ratings of patients' physical symptoms interchangeable with patients' self-ratings? Qual Life Res 6:225–236
18. Titzer S, Christensen O, Manzke O, et al (2000) Vaccination of multiple myeloma patients with idiotype-pulsed dendritic cells: immunological and clinical aspects. Br J Haematol 108:805–816
19. Slevin ML, Stubbs L, Plant HJ, et al (1990) Attitudes to chemotherapy: comparing views of patients with cancer with those of doctors, nurses, and general public. Br Med J 300:1458–1460
20. Kong SX, Gandhi SK (1997) Methodologic assessments of quality of life measures in clinical trials. Ann Pharmacother 31:830–836
21. Gotay CC, Wilson M (1998) Use of quality-of-life outcome assessments in current cancer clinical trials. Eval Health Prof 21:157–178
22. Fayers P, Bottomley A (2002) Quality of Life Research within the EORTC – The EORTC QLQ-C30, on behalf of the EORTC Quality of Life Group. Eur J Cancer 38 (suppl 4):125–133
23. Aaronson NK, Ahmedzai S, Bergman B, et al (1993) The European Organization for Research and Treatment of Cancer QLQ-C30: a quality-of-life instrument for use in international clinical trials in oncology. J Natl Cancer Inst 85:365–376

24. Fayers P, Aaronson N, Bjordal K,Groenvold M, Curran D, Bottomley A (2001) EORTC QLQ-C30 Scoring Manual. 3rd Edition. EORTC Publications, Brussels
25. Blazeby J, Cull A, Groenvold M, Bottomley A (2001) Guidelines for developing Quality of Life Questionnaires, 3rd Edition. EORTC Publications, Brussels
26. Vachalec S, Bjordal K, Bottomley A, Blazeby J, Flechtner H, Ruyskart P (2000) EORTC Item Bank Guidelines. EORTC Publications, Brussels
27. Cull A, Spranger MA, Aaronson N (1998) Translation Guidelines for EORTC Modules. EORTC publications, Brussels
28. Cella D, Davis K, Breitbart W, Curt G. (2001) Cancer-related fatigue: prevalence of proposed diagnostic criteria in a United States sample of cancer survivors. J Clin Oncol 19:3385-3391
29. WHOQOL Group, (1993) "Study Protocol for the World Health Organization Project to Develop a Quality of Life Assessment Instrument," WHOQOL Special Report. Qual Life Res 2:153-159
30. Young T, Maher J (1999) Collecting quality of life data in EORTC clinical trials - what happens in practice? Psychooncology 8:260-263
31. Osoba D, Rodrigues G, Myles J, Zee B, Pater J (1998) Interpreting the significance of changes in health-related quality-of-life scores. J Clin Oncol 16:139-144
32. Juniper EF, Guyatt GH, Willan A (1994) Determining a minimal important change in a disease-specific quality of life questionnaire. J Clin Epidemiol 47:81-87
33. Lydick E, Epstein RS (1993) Interpretation of quality of life changes. Qual Life Res 2:221-226
34. Lee CW, Chi KN (2000) The standard of reporting of health-related quality of life in clinical cancer trials. J Clin Epidemiol 53:451-458
35. Staquet M, Berzon R, Osoba D, Machin D (1996) Guidelines for reporting results of quality of life assessments in clinical trials. Qual Life Res 5:496-502

Surrogate Measures of Patient-centered Outcomes in Critical Care

G. D. Rubenfeld

"... a surrogate endpoint of a clinical trial is a laboratory measurement or a physical sign used as a substitute for a clinically meaningful endpoint that measures directly how a patient feels, functions or survives. Changes induced by a therapy on a surrogate endpoint are expected to reflect changes in a clinically meaningful endpoint." [1]

Introduction

The ultimate goal of medicine is to improve health in ways that matter to patients. A variety of outcomes are important to patients: symptoms, quality of life, duration of life, quality of dying, the effect of their health care on their loved ones, and the cost of medical care. Because of the importance of these outcomes to patients they are referred to as 'patient-centered' outcomes. Ideally, clinicians will offer, insurers will pay for, and patients will have the opportunity to use treatments that have been shown to improve patient-centered outcomes. Patient-centered outcomes are distinct from any number of chemical, physiologic, and radiographic variables that may be measured in clinical research. There are many reasons investigators choose to measure these important *alternate* or *auxiliary* measures. They often provide essential information about how a treatment works, about complications, and about the study population and subgroups. However, when one of these variables is used specifically as a substitute for a patient-centered outcome, it is referred to as a *surrogate* outcome variable. Other synonyms for these variables are *intermediate* or *proxy* outcome variables [2]. Common examples of surrogate outcomes are substituting blood pressure for survival in a study of antihypertensives, left ventricular function for quality of life in a study of therapy for congestive heart failure, and tumor size for survival in a study of cancer therapy.

Surrogate outcomes are usually proximal physiologic or laboratory effects of the treatment and therefore very sensitive to the treatment's effects. The surrogate outcome is a factor that is known (or highly suspected) to be in the causal pathway to the patient-centered outcome [3]. For example, sustained elevations in blood pressure cause atherosclerosis, congestive heart failure and stroke which lead to death and morbidity. The calcium channel blocking drug nifedipine dilates blood vessels and lowers blood pressure. If blood pressure is a valid surrogate for survival, then demonstrating the hypotensive effect of nifedipine is sufficient to prove its benefit in improving patient-centered outcome. A similar argument can be constructed for cholesterol level. Elevated cholesterol causes coronary atherosclerosis leading to myocardial infarction and death. The cholesterol lowering drug clofibrate reduces blood lipid levels. Presumably, a study that demonstrates the effect of clofibrate on lipid levels is sufficient to demonstrate its beneficial effect on survival and quality of life.

There are enormous advantages to studying blood pressure and cholesterol level instead of survival, mortality* or quality of life. Surrogate outcomes hold out the promise of shorter studies of fewer patients to demonstrate the effectiveness of treatments [4, 5]. This is particularly desirable in chronic diseases where a treatment's effect on survival or quality of life may not be observed for years while its effect on a surrogate may be observed over weeks or months. Surrogate outcomes, by definition, are very sensitive to the treatment's direct effect and therefore are more responsive variables than patient-centered outcomes. Since surrogate outcomes are frequently laboratory or physiologic measures they can usually be measured reliably and precisely. By increasing the sensitivity, precision, and reliability of the outcome variable, surrogate outcomes can increase the statistical power of clinical studies requiring smaller numbers of patients to demonstrate a statistically significant effect [6].

Patient-centered Outcomes

While the definition of a patient-centered outcome offered above, 'how a patient feels, functions, or survives', has face validity, it allows for a spectrum of application in practice. At one end of the spectrum, physiologic and laboratory measures are clearly not patient centered since they do not directly measure feeling, function, or survival. Other measures, for example, validated quality of life instruments, are clearly patient-centered. In between these ends of the spectrum, there is room for debate about whether a given outcome is patient-centered or not. Frequently, decisions evolve through regulatory and peer review. When an outcome is measured can affect whether it is patient-centered or a surrogate. For example, mortality differences at 12 hours (if not sustained) are unlikely to matter to patients while differences at 5 years will matter. Questions about the exact timepoint when intensive care mortality should be measured continue. Twenty-eight day mortality has become an accepted standard, however, others have advocated longer timepoints [7]. If we know with confidence that the effect of the treatment or the mortality rate of the disease plateau after a specified timepoint, then this informa-

---

* The terms mortality and survival are used specifically throughout this chapter. Mortality as an outcome is the difference in the probability or odds of death at a specific time point (7 days, 28 days, hospital discharge, 5 years) expressed as a risk ratio, risk difference, or odds ratio. Survival as an outcome is the difference in time until death (truncated at some study observation end point) expressed as a difference in median survival time or as a hazard ratio (a ratio of rates of death). 'Survival' and 'mortality' should not be used interchangeably. Different statistical techniques are used to analyze survival and mortality data and they are subject to different study biases.

tion can help choose a window for observation. It is not unusual for critical care interventions to show a mortality difference at ICU discharge that disappears by hospital discharge [8]. Survival is a patient-centered outcome except when the study observation window is brief. For example, survival analysis of a critical care intervention that truncates patient observation at 28 days can find statistically significant differences in survival rates when the actual differences in survival time is hours or days [8, 9]. It is unlikely that these survival differences reflect meaningful differences to patients.

Restricting the analysis of mortality and survival to deaths from a specific cause can also affect their patient-centeredness. Although some patients may have a strong preference for dying from a specific disease, a treatment that reduces death from a specific cause without affecting overall mortality provides small patient-centered benefits. In fact, well designed studies that show a reduction in cause specific mortality without a similar reduction in total mortality raise the possibility that the treatment actually increases mortality from causes other than the one specified as the outcome.

Are Surrogate Measures Valid?

The utility of surrogate outcomes relies entirely on the validity of the assumption that the surrogate outcome's response to therapy reflects the net effect of the treatment on patient-centered outcomes [3]. If surrogate measures reliably predict patient-centered outcomes, far more efficient clinical studies could be designed. This would lead to less expensive drug development and more rapid identification and distribution of effective treatments. Therefore, it is not surprising that an extensive literature has evolved to examine whether surrogate outcomes are valid predictors of patient-centered outcomes. Not surprisingly, the evaluation of surrogate outcomes is most advanced in the diseases where the causal pathways linking potential surrogate outcomes with patient-centered outcomes are best understood and where a sufficient quantity of studies with both surrogate and patient-centered outcome data exist. These areas of medicine include cardiovascular diseases, oncology, and human immunodeficiency virus (HIV) infection [2]. The literature evaluating the validity of surrogate outcomes speaks with a uniform voice: surrogate outcome measures are not reliable predictors of the effect of treatments on patient-centered outcomes and treatment decisions based solely on data from surrogate outcomes can be misguided [2, 10–13].

Perhaps the most frequently cited example is the Cardiac Arrhythmia Suppression Trial which explored a very reasonable hypothesis [14]. Sudden death after myocardial infarction from cardiac arrhythmia is strongly associated with the presence of premature ventricular contractions and other ventricular dysrhythmias in the post-myocardial infarction period. Suppression of these dysrhythmias should prevent sudden death after myocardial infarction which is presumed to be due to a cardiac rhythm disturbance. Effective drugs exist to suppress these dysrhythmias. However, in a large randomized clinical trial, drug therapy which was effective at suppressing the dysrhythmia was associated with increased mortality.

No hypothesis could make greater sense than the hypothesis that drugs that halt tumor growth would prolong survival in patients with cancer. The causal relation between tumor progression and cancer death is unquestioned. Tumor response as measured by reduction in size is an accepted surrogate endpoint for oncology trials. Again studies that measure both tumor response and survival repeatedly show that reductions in tumor size are not reliably translated into prolonged survival or quality of life [15].

The validity of blood pressure as a surrogate outcome is so entrenched that an abnormality in this surrogate measure is a disease – hypertension. The goal of treating hypertension turned into the goal of blood pressure reduction rather than the goal of preventing strokes, heart failure, and death. Here, too, the literature has shown that not all treatments that affect the surrogate outcome of blood pressure have similar effects on patient-centered outcomes [16, 17]. Specifically, diuretics and beta-blocker medication appear to be more effective at reducing mortality (or at least not increasing mortality) than calcium channel blockers.

The uniform failure of surrogate outcome measures is likely due to the many possible sources of error in extrapolating surrogate outcomes to patient-centered outcomes. The surrogate outcome may not fully capture the negative effects of the treatment on patient-centered outcomes. In this setting negative effects of the treatment on patient-centered outcomes may exceed any benefits of the treatment measured by the surrogate (Table 1). For example, the pro-arrhythmic effects of quinidine in causing ventricular tachycardia may obviate any benefit it provides in keeping patients out of atrial fibrillation [18]. The surrogate outcome may not reflect the long-term effects of the treatment. Short-term benefits may wane for a variety of reasons and long-term patient-centered benefits will be overestimated by the short-term surrogate. For example, the short-term effects of nucleoside analogs on CD4 counts may not reflect long-term effects on survival since HIV develops resistance to single drug therapy [12, 13, 19]. The surrogate outcome may only reflect one pathway the disease has for affecting patient-centered outcome. Measuring the response in the surrogate variable does not reflect the disease's effects via other pathways. For example, inotropic medication and fluids may improve the oxygen delivery problem in septic shock and increase blood pressure, but they do not affect its inflammatory and coagulation derangements. The surrogate outcome may only be associated with, but not part of the causal pathway of the disease. In this situation, surrogate measure response is irrelevant to the overall outcome of the disease. Frequently, more than one of these explain why a persuasive surrogate outcome fails to predict a treatment's effect on patient-centered outcome.

Is Critical Care Different?

A major goal of critical care is to restore and support physiology [20]. If this is true, then perhaps physiologic measures are the best outcome variables to study to decide whether the goal of critical care has been achieved. Given this rationale, it is possible that surrogate outcome variables may show better performance in critical care than their poor performance in other fields of medicine. Unfortunately,

Table 1. Validity of surrogate endpoints

Disease	Treatment	Effect on surrogate outcome	Effect on patient-centered outcome
Sudden death from cardiac arrhythmia	Encainide, flecanide, and moricizine [14]	Reduction in premature ventricular contractions	Increased mortality and suppression of arrhythmias
Atrial fibrillation	Quinidine [18]	Maintenance of sinus	Increased mortality rhythm
Acute myocardial infarction	Lidocaine [39]	Prevention of ventricular	Increased mortality tachycardia
Congestive heart failure	Milrinone [40]	Increased cardiac output,	Increased mortality improved exercise tolerance
Coronary heart disease	Fibrate lipid lowering drugs [41]	Reduced lipid levels, reduced mortality from coronary heart disease	No effect on total mortality, increased mortality from causes other than coronary heart disease
Colon cancer	5-fluorouracil plus leucovorin [15]	Reduced tumor size	No effect on mortality
HIV infection	Nucleoside analogs [19]	Increased CD4 count	No effect or increased mortality

adapted from [2]

experience with clinical research in critical care suggests that surrogate outcomes are no better at predicting patient centered outcomes in critical illness than they have proven to be in other fields (Table 2).

The treatment of acute respiratory distress syndrome (ARDS) provides a typical example. For over 20 years, investigators have explored therapies to reduce mortality from ARDS. Many treatments, including inhaled nitric oxide, inhaled prostacyclin, liposomal prostaglandin E1, prone positioning during mechanical ventilation, partial liquid ventilation, and tracheal gas insufflation have shown improvements in gas exchange in patients with ARDS. To date, none of these treatments have been shown to improve patient-centered outcomes despite, in the cases of inhaled nitric oxide and prone positioning, large multi-center clinical trials [21–23]. Contrary to the beneficial effects on gas exchange noted in these treatments, lung protective ventilation for ARDS, a treatment that uses low tidal volumes and allows carbon dioxide to 'permissively' build up, generally and intentionally worsens the surrogate outcome of gas exchange in patients with ARDS [7]. Despite its negative effect on patient physiology, mortality is significantly improved. Therefore, gas exchange does not appear to be a valid surrogate outcome for mortality in ARDS.

Human growth hormone provides an even more cautionary tale about adopting treatments based on studies using surrogate endpoints. Critical illness is associated with a highly catabolic state reflected by a persistently negative nitrogen balance which is associated with mortality [24]. A number of studies demonstrated that negative nitrogen balance could be reduced or reversed with human growth hormone [25]. The clinical significance of improving nitrogen balance with human growth hormone was unknown. Two studies reported by Takala and colleagues were actually designed to explore the surrogate endpoints of duration of intensive care unit (ICU) stay, muscle strength, and organ failure [26]. Human growth hormone supplementation caused a doubling of mortality even though the patients' nitrogen balance improved. This lead to a "Dear Doctor" letter from the manufacturer warning about the risks of human growth hormone supplementation in critical illness. There are no data to indicate how many intensivists had adopted human growth hormone based on the surrogate outcome studies. If nitrogen balance alone had been used as an outcome measure in these studies, investigators would have concluded that human growth hormone was effective. If the effect on mortality had been smaller or if the study had enrolled fewer patients, the results may have demonstrated a 'benefit' in nitrogen balance and no effect on mortality.

Critical care does not differ from other fields of clinical investigation at least with regard to the performance of surrogate outcomes in predicting patient-centered outcome. In fact, as Table 2 shows, 'beneficial' surrogate outcome data are occasionally associated with increased mortality. Unfortunately, the failure of surrogate outcomes in critical care has been interpreted by some critics as a failure to identify the optimal surrogate outcome for studies of critical illness rather than a reason to reject surrogate outcomes in general [28, 29]. The overwhelming experience from clinical research outside of critical illness suggests that surrogate outcome measures frequently yield misleading information about patient centered treatment effects and reflect a failure of these measures in general rather than problems with their specific application in critical illness. In fact, there are several reasons to believe that surrogate outcome measures have less to offer and greater potential for misinformation than in other fields.

One of the major advantages of surrogate outcomes is to increase the frequency of study outcomes. Investigators studying acute myocardial infarction, congestive heart failure, and even many cancers deal with short-term mortality rates between 0–15 %. Low event rates require large sample sizes to demonstrate statistically significant results. Shifting to an outcome like ejection fraction or tumor size provides significantly more patients with 'poor' outcomes than mortality. This is not a problem for investigators studying critical illness syndromes like ARDS, severe sepsis, and acute respiratory failure where short-term mortality rates of 30–60 % are common. Therefore, surrogate outcomes are unlikely to increase the statistical power of clinical studies by increasing the event rates. Clinical investigators studying chronic diseases like congestive heart failure, diabetes, and hypertension must observe cohorts of patients for years to identify patient-centered outcomes. Although the long-term effects of critical illness are just beginning to be appreciated, most studies indicate that the majority of deaths attributable to critical

Table 2. Validity of surrogate endpoints – examples from critical care

Disease	Treatment	Effect on surrogate outcome	Effect on patient-centered outcome
ARDS	Prone ventilation [23]	Improved oxygenation	No effect on mortality
ARDS	Inhaled nitric oxide [21, 22]	Improved oxygenation	No effect on mortality
ICU anemia	Blood transfusion [42]	Improved hematocrit	Increased mortality
Critical illness	Hemodynamic goal directed therapy [43, 44]	Increased oxygen delivery	No effect or increased mortality
Critical illness	Human growth hormone [26]	Improved nitrogen balance	Increased mortality, prolonged duration of intensive care
Sepsis	Ibuprofen [45]	Reduces levels of prostacyclin and thromboxane, decreases fever and lactic acidosis	No effect on mortality
Sepsis	Recombinant human interleukin-1-receptor antagonist [9, 46]	Improved survival time and reduced short-term mortality	No effect on mortality

illness occur within the first 60 days [30, 31]. Therefore, by chronic disease standards critical care studies already benefit from a brief time horizon. Finally, surrogate outcomes may have worse performance in critical illness because the causal pathways in critical illness syndromes are poorly understood. Current understandings of the body's response to injury, infection, and hypoperfusion stress the complexity of this response and the heterogeneity of the response depending on the age and comorbidity of the patient [32]. If surrogate outcomes fail in single organ diseases like cardiac dysrhythmia and cancer, it is difficult to imagine how they would perform better in the less well characterized critical illness syndromes.

Are Death, Cost, and Quality of Life the only Outcomes that Matter?

Even if surrogate measures are not valid predictors of patient-centered outcomes in studies of critical illness, variables other than death, cost, and quality of life are important in clinical research. Clinical research to understand mechanisms of critical illness requires a broad range of biochemical and physiologic as well as patient-centered variables. Phase II or hypothesis testing studies will continue to use surrogate variables to identify promising treatments to study in larger studies. When a class of treatments, for example beta blocking drugs, have been shown to yield patient-centered benefits, surrogate outcome studies may be used to extend the results to a modified treatment that is a member of the same class without repeating patient-centered studies. Nevertheless, even within a class of drugs, some will confer risks that outweigh benefits and post-marketing surveillance is essential to detect these outcomes when a new treatment is adopted based on extending surrogate outcome data.

However, an important question remains, are there outcome variables besides death, cost, and quality of life that should affect treatment choices? There is no simple answer to this question. As one moves away from the fixed points of death, cost, and quality of life, outcomes are subject to increasingly difficult questions about their clinical relevance. Several important and arguably patient-centered outcomes are missed by studies of death, cost, and quality of life. These include major morbid events, process of care, quality of death and dying, and patient and family experience of intensive care.

Are there some major morbid outcomes in the ICU that are worth preventing as long as their prevention does not worsen patient-centered outcomes? If a treatment reduces ventilator-associated pneumonia (VAP) but has no effect on cost of care, mortality, or quality of life, should it be adopted? Is a treatment that prevents intubation worth adopting even if it offers no improvement in survival? Decubitus ulcers? Gastrointestinal bleeding? Delirium? If the answer is yes, how much information will we need to decide that the treatment is safe and how much would we be willing to pay for 'avoiding a catheter-related bacteremia' that may or may not affect patient-centered outcomes. These decisions will turn on an accurate understanding of the costs of the treatment, the risks of the treatment, the costs imposed by the morbid outcome, and some valuation of the outcome itself, either by patients, their families, or by clinicians. For example, we may think about preventing VAP differently if we can be virtually certain that the intervention is safe and cheap (semirecumbent bed positioning) than if the intervention has even theoretic costs and risk (rotational bed therapy, selective decontamination). We may choose to adopt semirecumbent bed positioning given the evidence of a reduction in VAP yet expect evidence of cost or mortality reduction to initiate selective decontamination.

Process of care variables may be important exceptions to some of the criticisms offered about surrogate outcomes. Investigators studying interventions to improve the quality of care can choose to study the *outcomes* of their quality improvement intervention (mortality, for example) or whether their intervention changes the *process* of care. When a treatment has been shown to improve patient-centered outcomes for a disease, for example, aspirin therapy for acute myocardial infarction, the treatment is known to be in the causal pathway for improving patient-centered outcomes. Studies of interventions to improve quality of care can gain considerable improvements in efficiency by studying process of care as a surrogate outcome rather than outcome [33]. There are three important assumptions in this analysis:

1. The treatment's efficacy regarding patient-centered outcomes is well defined.
2. The treatment's effectiveness in the study setting will be similar to its efficacy.
3. The intervention used to increase use of the treatment will not worsen patient-centered outcomes via other mechanisms.

It is the relative acceptability of this last assumption for quality improvement interventions that make process of care an acceptable surrogate for these studies.

The importance of end of life care in the ICU is increasingly recognized as are its inadequacies [34]. While efforts to identify a measure of the quality of death and dying proceed, it is important to recognize that none of the current patient-centered outcomes capture this important patient-centered outcome. In considering the design of studies that might improve the quality of death and dying in the ICU, it is interesting to consider the possibility that better end-of-life care and communication may actually increase mortality and worsen survival by early identification of patients who do not wish ongoing life sustaining treatments.

While long-term quality of life and functional status after intensive care are clearly patient-centered outcomes, the symptoms of patients in the ICU and the experience of families are also important. Outcome measures to capture these important domains and research into these fields are ongoing. The critical care nursing field has taken an early leadership role in this research. As the focus of weaning from mechanical ventilation shifts from optimizing exercise while weaning to optimizing comfort while evaluating for readiness, the patient's experience on mechanical ventilation takes on a central, and poorly understood, role [35]. Investigators face considerable barriers in studying patients' experiences in the ICU. Endotracheal tubes, delirium, and medication often preclude communication. Many patients have poor recollection of their ICU experiences and most studies of patients' symptoms rely on clinician assessment of level of sedation and discomfort.

Competing Mortality

Whenever an outcome other than mortality is studied, investigators must consider the potential that the outcome is not observed because patients die before developing the outcome. For example, duration of mechanical ventilation may be shorter in a treatment group because the patients have a higher mortality rate and shorter survival than controls rather than any effect from the treatment on the course of mechanical ventilation. This is a problem common to all clinical research and is not unique to critical care [36]. There are a number of solutions to the problem – none is perfect. One can ignore the problem and simply report the difference in the surrogate outcome. This is acceptable if the treatment is known not to affect mortality or if the mortality rate is negligible in both groups. One can compare the outcome in survivors and non-survivors separately but the results of this analysis can be misleading [37]. One can combine the mortality and non-mortality outcome(s) into a single outcome, for example, 'cardiac death, non-lethal myocardial infarction, or hospitalization due to progression of heart failure' is a common outcome in heart failure studies. Another solution is to weight survival by the non-mortality outcome into a single measure of mortality and morbidity [38]. A number of different outcomes use this option including: quality adjusted life year, relapse free survival, symptom-free days, and disability free survival. The 'ventilator-free day' and 'organ failure-free day' outcomes proposed for critical illness studies are versions of these weighted outcomes. These scores assign an arbitrary weight of 1 to a day alive without organ failure and a weight of zero for days when the patient is dead, has the organ failure, or is alive with the organ failure beyond a window date. Finally, there are a number of statistical procedures for sequentially testing the mortality outcome first for evidence of harm followed by a test of the non-fatal outcome for effect [39]. Relatively little theoretic or simulation testing has been performed to explore the implications of competing mortality in surrogate outcome analysis or to identify the optimal solution in studies of critical illness. For example, there have been no empiric studies of the limitations, statistical power, or interpretation of the 'free-day' outcome in studies of critical illness.

Conclusion

Studies of surrogate outcomes have repeatedly provided misleading information about patient-centered treatment effects in many areas of clinical investigation. The appeal of surrogate outcomes, particularly in a physiologically oriented field like critical care, is understandable. Designing studies to address patient-centered outcomes requires larger, longer, and more expensive clinical trials than surrogate outcome studies. Nevertheless, ample evidence exists to make clinicians pause before adopting a therapy based on improvements in surrogate outcomes.

References

1. Temple RJ (1995) A regulatory authority's opinion about surrogate endpoints. In: Nimmo WS, Tucker GT (eds) Clinical Measurement in Drug Evaluation. J. Wiley, New York, p:329
2. Fleming TR, DeMets DL (1996) Surrogate end points in clinical trials: are we being misled? Ann Intern Med 125:605-613
3. Prentice RL (1989) Surrogate endpoints in clinical trials: definition and operational criteria. Stat Med 8:431–440
4. Fleming TR (1994) Surrogate markers in AIDS and cancer trials. Stat Med 13:1423–1435
5. Fleming TR, DeGruttola V, DeMets DL (1997) Surrogate endpoints. AIDS Clin Rev 1997:129–143
6. Hulley SB, Cummings SR (1988) Designing clinical research : an epidemiologic approach. Williams & Wilkins, Baltimore
7. The Acute Respiratory Distress Syndrome Network (2000) Ventilation with lower tidal volumes as compared with traditional tidal volumes for acute lung injury and the acute respiratory distress syndrome.. N Engl J Med 342:1301–1308
8. Amato MB, Barbas CS, Medeiros DM, et al (1998) Effect of a protective-ventilation strategy on mortality in the acute respiratory distress syndrome. N Engl J Med 338:347-354
9. Knaus WA, Harrell FE, Jr., LaBrecque JF, et al (1996) Use of predicted risk of mortality to evaluate the efficacy of anticytokine therapy in sepsis. The rhIL-1ra Phase III Sepsis Syndrome Study Group. Crit Care Med 24:46–56
10. De Gruttola V, Fleming T, Lin DY, Coombs R (1997) Perspective: validating surrogate markers-are we being naive? J Infect Dis 175:237–246
11. Fleming TR (2000) Surrogate end points in cardiovascular disease trials. Am Heart J 139:S193–S196
12. Fleming TR, Prentice RL, Pepe MS, Glidden D (1994) Surrogate and auxiliary endpoints in clinical trials, with potential applications in cancer and AIDS research. Stat Med 13:955–968

13. De Gruttola VG, Clax P, DeMets DL, et al (2001) Considerations in the evaluation of surrogate endpoints in clinical trials. summary of a National Institutes of Health workshop. Control Clin Trials 22:485–502
14. Echt DS, Liebson PR, Mitchell LB, et al (1991) Mortality and morbidity in patients receiving encainide, flecainide, or placebo. The Cardiac Arrhythmia Suppression Trial. N Engl J Med 324:781–788
15. Advanced Colorectal Cancer Meta-Analysis Project (1992) Modulation of fluorouracil by leucovorin in patients with advanced colorectal cancer: evidence in terms of response rate.. J Clin Oncol 10:896–903
16. Psaty BM, Smith NL, Siscovick DS, et al (1997) Health outcomes associated with antihypertensive therapies used as first-line agents. A systematic review and meta-analysis. JAMA 277:739–745
17. Psaty BM, Weiss NS, Furberg CD, et al (1999) Surrogate end points, health outcomes, and the drug-approval process for the treatment of risk factors for cardiovascular disease. JAMA 282:786–790
18. Coplen SE, Antman EM, Berlin JA, Hewitt P, Chalmers TC (1990) Efficacy and safety of quinidine therapy for maintenance of sinus rhythm after cardioversion. A meta-analysis of randomized control trials. Circulation 82:1106–1116
19. Sande MA, Carpenter CC, Cobbs CG, Holmes KK, Sanford JP (1993) Antiretroviral therapy for adult HIV-infected patients. Recommendations from a state-of-the-art conference. National Institute of Allergy and Infectious Diseases State-of-the-Art Panel on Anti-Retroviral Therapy for Adult HIV-Infected Patients. JAMA 270:2583–2589
20. Guidelines Committee, Society of Critical Care Medicine (1992) Guidelines for the definition of an intensivist and the practice of critical care medicine. Crit Care Med 20:540–542
21. Dellinger RP, Zimmerman JL, Taylor RW, et al (1998) Effects of inhaled nitric oxide in patients with acute respiratory distress syndrome: results of a randomized phase II trial. Inhaled Nitric Oxide in ARDS Study Group. Crit Care Med 26:15–23
22. Lundin S, Mang H, Smithies M, Stenqvist O, Frostell C (1999) Inhalation of nitric oxide in acute lung injury: results of a European multicentre study. The European Study Group of Inhaled Nitric Oxide. Intensive Care Med 25:911–919
23. Gattinoni L, Tognoni G, Pesenti A, et al (2001) Effect of prone positioning on the survival of patients with acute respiratory failure. N Engl J Med 345:568–573
24. Rennie M (1985) Muscle protein turnover and the wasting due to injury and disease. Br Med Bull 41:257–264
25. Gore DC, Honeycutt D, Jahoor F, Wolfe RR, Herndon DN (1991) Effect of exogenous growth hormone on whole-body and isolated-limb protein kinetics in burned patients. Arch Surg 126:38–43
26. Takala J, Ruokonen E, Webster NR, et al (1999) Increased mortality associated with growth hormone treatment in critically ill adults N Engl J Med 341:785–792
27. Sibbald WJ, Vincent JL (1995) Clinical Trials for the Treatment of Sepsis. Springer-Verlag, Heidelberg
28. Zapol WM (1998) Nitric oxide inhalation in acute respiratory distress syndrome: it works, but can we prove it? Crit Care Med 26:2–3
29. Angus DC, Musthafa AA, Clermont G, et al (2001) Quality-adjusted survival in the first year after the acute respiratory distress syndrome. Am J Respir Crit Care Med 163:1389–1394
30. Davidson TA, Rubenfeld GD, Caldwell ES, Hudson LD, Steinberg KP (1999) The Effect of Acute respiratory distress syndrome on long-term survival. Am J Respir Crit Care Med 160:1838–1842
31. Marshall JC (2000) Complexity, chaos, and incomprehensibility: parsing the biology of critical illness. Crit Care Med 28:2646–2648
32. Mant J, Hicks N (1995) Detecting differences in quality of care: the sensitivity of measures of process and outcome in treating acute myocardial infarction. Br Med J 311:793–796

33. Curtis JR, Rubenfeld GD (2000) Managing Death in the ICU:The Transition from Cure to Comfort. Oxford University Press, New York
34. Hansen-Flaschen JH (2000) Dyspnea in the ventilated patient: a call for patient-centered mechanical ventilation. Respir Care 45:1460–1464
35. Diehr P, Patrick D, Hedrick S, et al (1995) Including deaths when measuring health status over time. Med Care 33 (Suppl 4):AS164–AS172
36. Heitjan DF (1999) Causal inference in a clinical trial: a comparative example. Control Clin Trials 20:309–318
37. Sullivan DF (1971) A single index of mortality and morbidity. HSMHA Health Rep 86:347–354
38. McMahon RP, Harrell FE Jr (2001) Joint testing of mortality and a non-fatal outcome in clinical trials. Stat Med 20:1165–1172
39. Hine LK, Laird N, Hewitt P, Chalmers TC (1989) Meta-analytic evidence against prophylactic use of lidocaine in acute myocardial infarction. Arch Intern Med 149:2694–2698
40. Packer M, Carver JR, Rodeheffer RJ, et al (1991) Effect of oral milrinone on mortality in severe chronic heart failure. The PROMISE Study Research Group. N Engl J Med 325:1468–1475
41. Law MR, Thompson SG, Wald NJ (1994) Assessing possible hazards of reducing serum cholesterol. Br Med J 308:373–379
42. Hebert PC, Wells G, Blajchman MA, et al (1999) A multicenter, randomized, controlled clinical trial of transfusion requirements in critical care. Transfusion Requirements in Critical Care Investigators, Canadian Critical Care Trials Group. N Engl J Med 340:409–417
43. Gattinoni L, Brazzi L, Pelosi P, et al (1995) A trial of goal-oriented hemodynamic therapy in critically ill patients. SvO2 Collaborative Group. N Engl J Med 333:1025–1032
44. Hayes MA, Timmins AC, Yau EH, Palazzo M, Hinds CJ, Watson D (1994) Elevation of systemic oxygen delivery in the treatment of critically ill patients. N Engl J Med 330:1717–1722
45. Bernard GR, Wheeler AP, Russell JA, et al (1997) The effects of ibuprofen on the physiology and survival of patients with sepsis. The Ibuprofen in Sepsis Study Group. N Engl J Med 336:912–918
46. Fisher CJ, Jr., Dhainaut JF, Opal SM, et al (1994) Recombinant human interleukin 1 receptor antagonist in the treatment of patients with sepsis syndrome. Results from a randomized, double-blind, placebo-controlled trial. Phase III rhIL-1ra Sepsis Syndrome Study Group. JAMA 271:1836–1843

Measuring Health Status After Critical Illness: Where Are We and Where Do We Go From Here?

J. R. Curtis

Introduction

In the past, research concerning the outcomes of critical illness often focused on physiologic endpoints (such as oxygenation, ventilation, and tissue perfusion) and clinical endpoints (such as extubation rates, ICU survival, and hospital survival). Such outcomes are very appropriate for many critical care studies because of the high short-term mortality and life-threatening physiologic abnormalities in these patients. However, there is increasing evidence that mechanical ventilation strategies and critical care treatments such as sedation and restoration of tissue perfusion may have important effects not just on short-term physiology and survival, but also on long-term survival and the quality of that survival. For example, recent studies suggest that survivors of acute respiratory distress syndrome (ARDS) have marked reductions in the quality of their lives compared to other individuals with comparable critical illness but no ARDS [1]. Furthermore, patients with sepsis may survive to hospital discharge but have ongoing decrements in their survival for years that seems to be a result of their critical illness rather than their underlying medical problems [2]. Finally, there is growing evidence that critical care treatment strategies effect long-term cognitive function [3] and influence the prevalence of post-traumatic stress disorder [4–6]. These studies suggest that critical care therapies may influence not just organ function and short-term survival, but also long-term survival and quality of life. These findings imply that critical care clinical research should expand its horizons and look at some of the longer-term outcomes of critical care if we are to maximize the survival and the quality of that survival for our patients.

Survival is, in most situations, the most important outcome for critical care because the mortality is high and the general goal of most critical care therapy is to allow patients to survive a critical illness or injury. However, long-term critical care outcomes must not be limited to survival alone. Other outcomes that are important to patients and their families include quality of life, functional status, and freedom from pain and other symptoms. Much has been written about increasing the focus of medical research on these 'patient-centered' outcomes [7]. Such outcomes became increasingly popular in the assessment of treatments for chronic diseases in the 1980s and early 1990s with improvements in the science of health status and quality of life measurement [8]. The last decade has seen an explosion in the use of these outcomes in critical care research, although the quality of these studies has been variable [9].

Health status outcomes are inherently subjective, since they describe a patient's subjective experience. However, the subjective nature of these outcomes is not a shortcoming, but an essential component: if we are concerned with the patient's perspective on health outcomes, we should measure it directly from the perspective of the patient. The fact that these outcomes are subjective does not mean that they are therefore inherently immeasurable or 'soft' data. The crucial attribute of 'hardness' is the reliability of a measure [10]. Patient-assessed outcome measures are able to provide adequate and often excellent reliability.

Clinical researchers assessing the outcomes of critical care cannot, and should not, measure every outcome in every study for two reasons. First, a study that measured all possible outcomes would be too cumbersome to conduct. Second, not all outcomes are relevant in all studies. The goals of this chapter will be to describe the long-term, patient-centered health outcomes of critical care with particular focus on health status, to identify important issues and pitfalls in measuring these outcomes, and to identify future directions for improving research on these outcomes in critical care.

Terms and Definitions

Health outcomes represent a broad group of end-points used in clinical trials and other clinical research to assess the efficacy or effectiveness of interventions and the outcomes of disease and treatment [11]. Traditional health outcomes in critical care include mortality, physiologic endpoints, and clinical endpoints. More recently, there has been a growing body of research concerning endpoints that are assessed directly by patients and can be termed 'patient-assessed health outcomes'. Patient-assessed health outcomes can be divided into four categories: health status, health utilities, adherence to treatment, and patient satisfaction with health care. A patient's self-reported health status includes health-related quality of life (HRQL) and functional status. Health status can be defined as the impact of a person's health on their ability to perform and derive fulfillment from activities of daily life.

The expression 'quality of life' seems conceptually easy to understand, has great currency and face value in our society, and yet can be difficult to define [12]. One definition of quality of life is the 'holistic, self-determined evaluation of satisfaction with issues important to the individual'. A person's quality of life can be influenced by a number of factors. The degree to which a patient's health status affects a patient's self-determined evaluation of their satisfaction with their life has been defined as HRQL [13]. Individuals with no health problems, in theory, should have a good HRQL. However, this does not preclude them from other experiences, such as poverty or family strife, which may affect their overall quality of life. It is generally agreed that quality of life is considerably more comprehensive than health status and includes aspects of the environment that may or may not be affected by health or treatments. Because the global environment is outside health, the term HRQL is often used to indicate that the outcome measure is focused on the health concept, or aspects of human life and activities that are generally affected by health conditions and/or health services [14].

Functional status refers to a person's ability to perform a variety of activities, including physical, emotional, and social. An individual's functional capacity will be influenced and potentially limited by their overall health. Although there is overlap between functional status and quality of life, they are conceptually distinct from one another and sometimes do not correlate highly [13].

Many health status instruments include items that measure both functional status and HRQL, making it difficult to separate the effect of health on these concepts. Furthermore, for some patients and caregivers, HRQL may affect diverse realms of their overall quality of life not usually considered 'health-related'. Whatever concepts are applied to a health status or quality of life measure in the various applications of the measure, the concepts should be matched as closely as possible to the purpose for each specific application of the measure and, whenever possible, in reference to a theoretical model used in definition of the concept being measured.

Assessment of Health Status Instruments

Before researchers and clinicians use health status instruments, these instruments should have established and published evidence on their reliability, validity, and responsiveness. The instruments themselves are not inherently 'valid' but rather are valid for the specific uses for which the instrument has been evaluated. Without performing the research to document these basic measurement properties of an instrument, it is not possible to determine if this instrument is capable of detecting true signal as opposed to noise.

Reliability

Conceptually, reliability refers to the amount of error found in any form of measurement and can be considered the degree to which an instrument will give the same result when measuring the same phenomenon under different circumstances. Practically, reliability translates into how reproducible the results of an instrument are when applied under various conditions. Reliability can be assessed by a number of methods that include internal consistency, intra- and inter-rater reliability, and stability. An instrument is internally consistent if different components of the instrument administered at the same time yield similar results. The commonly used statistical method to assess internal consistency is Cronbach's alpha. Reliability includes the agreement between different observers (inter-rater reliability) and between the same observer on different occasions (intra-rater reliability). Stability refers to the reproducibility over time and can be described by assessing the same subject on different occasions under circumstances where the concept being measures, such as health status, has not changed (test-retest reliability). Once an instrument has been demonstrated to be reliable, it does not necessarily need to be re-tested for reliability with every use, unless it is to be used in a new, untested population.

Validity

Whereas reliability refers to reproducibility, validity commonly refers to the ability of an instrument to measure what it purports to measure. Classically, validity has been described by the '3 Cs': content, construct, and criterion. Content validity refers to ability of the instrument to reflect the domains of the concepts it purports to measure. The content validity of any patient self-assessed measure can be judged best by the persons or populations being assessed. Ideally, a HRQL instrument should contain questions that cover all domains of HRQL for the population under study.

Criterion validity refers to the ability of an instrument to test a subject in comparison to an accepted 'gold' standard. This can occur in the present (concurrent validity) or can be used to predict the future (predictive validity). Concurrent validity is most commonly tested when comparing a new test to an existing standard with the intent of replacing the existing standard. Predictive validity can only be assessed by applying the instrument and finding out how well it predicts the outcome under study at a later point in time. Few opportunities exist for applying the logic of concurrent criterion or gold standard validity to self-reported health status measures, particularly for the concepts and domains that are inherently subjective and unobservable, since no 'gold standard' exists.

How do we show that an instrument is valid if a gold standard does not exist? This is the situation often faced when measuring relatively new concepts such as HRQL. When there is no gold standard, we must rely on theoretical 'constructs' to infer validity. There are a number of methods that can be used to infer construct validity, but since there is no measure that can unequivocally prove it, construct validity takes the form of on-going hypothesis testing and can rarely be considered 'finished'. The most common methods of assessing construct validity are through convergent and divergent validity. That is, how well does the construct under question correlate with other measures that assess the same or related constructs? The instrument should correlate with both related clinical and health status instruments (convergent) and should not correlate with unrelated or dissimilar ones (divergent).

Responsiveness and the Minimally Important Difference

The responsiveness of a measure refers to the ability of a test to detect change over time. Responsiveness of a health status measure can be viewed as the ability of a particular measure in a particular application to detect change at all or minimally important changes. Determining the responsiveness of an instrument is imperative in trials that test an intervention. In this situation, it is important for the test to be able to detect small, but minimally important differences. Unlike well-known physiologic measures such as forced expiratory volume (FEV_1), where clinicians have a conceptual understanding of how much clinical change occurs with an improvement of 200 ml, health status values often do not have the same shared meaning.

It is important for investigators to report not only the degree of change, but whenever possible, to determine and explicitly state what defines a clinically-relevant change. This is true whether it is positive change (such as would define the success of a treatment) or a negative change (reflecting significant deterioration in health). The best method to determine the 'minimally important difference' (MID) is a matter of some contention [15–17]. Some authors have used patients' or clinicians' judgments of whether the patient had improved since the prior measurement period (often after treatment) and divided patients into groups with significant change and those without significant change. Using this method, the MID is estimated as the change seen in the group identified as slightly or mildly improved. Redelmeier and colleagues used a different approach of defining the MID in which patients are asked to judge themselves relevant to others currently rather than relevant to the way they were at a prior assessment [17]. These authors found that both methods seemed to define the same MID on a chronic obstructive pulmonary disease (COPD)-specific instrument, the Chronic Respiratory Questionnaire. Although all of these methods have been criticized, they remain the most commonly used and best-accepted methods. The MID will be discussed further below in the section on 'future directions'.

Generic versus Disease-Specific Measures

Health status instruments range from generic to disease-specific measures. Generic instruments assess many facets of health status, including such diverse realms as emotional functioning (mood changes and other psychological symptoms), social role functioning (employment, home management, and social/family relationships), activities of daily living (self-care skills and mobility) and the ability to engage in enjoyable activities (hobbies and recreation) [18, 19]. Pulmonary disease-specific measures focus often on particular pulmonary diseases, such as asthma [20] or COPD [21] and the effect that these diseases have on a patient's life. One pulmonary-disease specific measure originally designed for patients with COPD [22] has been found to be reliable and valid in a number of lung-related illnesses including ARDS [1].

Critical care is not used in the treatment of one specific disease with specific symptoms and functional impairments and, therefore, it is unlikely that a 'critical care' disease-specific health status instrument will be more sensitive to change than a generic health status instrument. Nonetheless, the unique features of critical illnesses make it important that instruments be chosen based on the specific disease and the impairment that disease causes. Further research is needed to fully define the diverse realms of impairment experienced by survivors of critical illness. It is also important that the instruments have been used in studies of survivors of critical care and been validated in this setting before they are used in clinical studies.

Utilities and Cost-Effectiveness

Cost-effectiveness analyses are a common approach to evaluate the economic impact of medical care technologies [23]. A cost effectiveness analysis produces a ratio, such as the cost per year of life gained, where the denominator reflects the gain in health from a specific intervention and the numerator reflects the cost in dollars of obtaining that gain [23]. Cost utility is a type of cost-effectiveness where effects are expressed as utilities, such as quality-adjusted survival, facilitating comparisons across different diseases and interventions (e.g., quality-adjusted life years [QALYs)). The core purpose of these analyses is to determine the value or trade-off of a therapy or program. In other words, for a therapy known to be effective, cost-effectiveness analyses ask "what is the cost to achieve that effect (gain in survival)?" This is expressed as the ratio of the incremental, or additional, costs divided by the incremental effects. Measuring the denominator, QALY, requires information about quality of life that permits the investigator to adjust survival for the quality of that survival. The QALY is a measure of health outcome that assigns to each period of time a weight ranging from 0 to 1, corresponding to the quality of life during that period, where a weight of 1 corresponds to perfect health and a weight of 0 corresponds to a health state judged equivalent to death. The number of QALYs represents the number of 'healthy years of life' that are valued equivalently to the actual outcome [23]. This numeric value for a given health state is a utility. There are several approaches and methodologies for assessing utilities. Utilities can be measured either by comparing one health outcome state to another with techniques such as the standard gamble [23] or time trade-off [12, 24] or by administering a health status instrument for which standard utility weights have been determined, such as the Quality of Well Being scale [25, 26], EuroQOL [27], or the Health Utilities Index [28]. Economic analyses of critical care interventions are an important area of research in this cost-conscious era. The unique features of these analyses in the critical care setting are the subject of a recent workshop report from the American Thoracic Society [29].

Additional Measurement Issues for Survivors of Critical Illness

There are a number of unique features of critical care that effect the assessment of these outcomes. First, many critically ill patients are too ill to complete questionnaires or interviews even after discharge from the hospital. Excluding such patients from studies of health status after critical care would obviously introduce a bias in the assessment of the health status of this population of patients. This raises the issue of whether family members can complete these instruments by proxy. A number of studies have used family members to assess a patient's health status or quality of life after ICU care [30–32]. Research in this area suggests that the information obtained from proxies is not as useful as that obtained directly from the competent patient, but nonetheless can be a reliable and valid assessment of the patient's health status [33]. Information from proxies is likely to be more reliable when it relates to observable phenomenon such as ability to perform the

Table 1. Common outcomes for observational outcomes research and the most appropriate point in time for measuring these outcomes.

Outcomes	Site of Measurement		
	ICU	Hospital	Long-term
Patient/Family assessed			
Quality of life & health-relatedquality of life			X
Functional status			X
Symptoms	X	X	X
Satisfaction with care	X	X	X
Process of care			
Processes known to improve outcomes (e.g., DVT prophylaxis)	X		
Reintubation/ICU readmission	X		
Economic outcomes			
ICU/hospital costs	X	X	
TISS	X		
Post-ICU health care costs		X	X
Loss of employment			X
Quality of death			
Satisfaction with end-of-life care	X	X	
Concordance between care and patient's wishes	X	X	X
Support for family	X	X	X
Pain/suffering/anxiety	X	X	X

DVT: deep vein thrombosis; TISS: therapeutic intervention severity score

activities of daily living and much less reliable when it relates to less observable phenomenon such as symptoms of pain or dyspnea or feelings of depression [34].

A second important issue about patient-assessed outcomes in the critical care setting is when they should and should not be measured. In some settings, mortality is the most important outcome and quality of life or other patient-assessed outcomes are much less important. This would be the case in the treatment of an acute illness with a high mortality affecting healthy people, for which survivors generally return to their pre-morbid health status. However, there are also circumstances when quality of life would be a primary outcome of equal or more import than mortality. For example, in a study of the outcomes of respiratory failure for patients with malignant cancer, many patients might judge the quality of life after an episode of critical illness to be more important than the quantity of life. As patients' life expectancy decreases and the burden of disease increases, the importance of quality of life as an outcome of critical care will likely increase.

A final important issue about patient-assessed outcomes involves the timing of the measurement. For research that focuses on the ICU stay, outcomes such as symptoms and patient or family satisfaction with care may be very important, but functional status or quality of life in the ICU are generally not relevant. For research focusing on outcomes after the ICU stay, quality of life and functional status are very important to patients and their families. Table 1 summarizes the appropriate timeframe for measurement of long-term and patient-assessed outcomes in most critical care studies.

Health Status and Related Concepts After Critical Care

Health Status

There are an increasing number of studies that have examined the long-term effect of ARDS or other critical illnesses on the quality of life and health status of survivors. McHugh and colleagues, using the Sickness Impact Profile, demonstrated a significant decrement in health status among survivors of ARDS and showed that health status improved during the first 3 months after discharge from the hospital but remained relatively stable thereafter [35]. Davidson and colleagues [1], using the Medical Outcomes Study Short Form-36 (SF-36) and the Saint Georges Respiratory Questionnaire, showed that there were significant decrements in most domains of health status among survivors of ARDS and that these decrements were significantly worse for patients with ARDS compared to patients with a comparable severity of illness from sepsis or trauma, but who did not meet criteria for ARDS. This study suggested that decrements in physical function might be the most severe. Weinert and colleagues [36] studied 24 survivors of acute lung injury with the SF-36, also showing reductions in many domains of health status and particularly severe reductions in social functioning and mental health domains. Finally, Angus and colleagues [37] used the Quality of Well Being to assess health status in a cohort of 200 previously healthy patients who developed ARDS and showed marked decrements in many domains of health status at 6 months and no significant change from 6 to 12 months.

In addition to ARDS, there have been a number of studies demonstrating reductions in health status for patients with other critical illnesses including sepsis [38], multiple organ dysfunction [39], and general ICU patients [40–42]. Although results vary, these studies also suggest decrements in a wide range of the domains of health status.

There have been a number of studies that have attempted to define the predictors of decreased health status among survivors of ARDS or other critical illness. Several studies suggest that the health status prior to admission to the ICU is a strong predictor of the health status after discharge [43, 44]. A study by Wehler and colleagues [43] showed that patients with the best health status prior to critical illness were more likely to have reductions in their health status while those patients with the lowest health status prior to admission to an ICU were actually more likely to improve from their baseline health status. Similarly, Konopad and colleagues [45] showed that among the very elderly, health status may actually increase from baseline after an ICU admission. Severity of illness is also a significant predictor of health status after discharge from the ICU [35, 43, 44]. Increasing age predicts decreased health status after critical illness in some studies [43, 44], but other studies did not find age to be an important independent predictor of health status

[40] and suggest that even those over the age of 70 who receive more than 30 days of intensive care are often satisfied with their health status and would choose to receive ICU care again if needed [41]. Schelling and colleagues [6] showed that pulmonary function impairment predicted worse health status suggesting that treatment strategies designed to minimize lung injury may have diverse effects improving health status in ARDS survivors.

Symptoms

Symptoms can be viewed as an additional patient-assessed outcome of import and interest to patients and their families and studies of symptoms may shed light on health status after critical illness. There have been a few studies documenting significant symptom burden for critically ill patients while in the ICU [46–48], but relatively few studies explicitly examining the symptoms of survivors of critical illness. Studies of health status among survivors of critical illness incorporate the effect that these symptoms have on individuals' lives, but it may also be important for investigators to explicitly examine the specific symptoms that are troubling to patients after critical illness as one way to understand the potential ways to decrease the symptom burden and the effect these symptoms have on patients' quality of life. For example, in the study by Angus and colleagues [37], the symptom domain of the QWB accounted for a larger decrement in quality of life than other domains including physical activity, social activity, and mobility. Symptoms accounted for approximately 70% of the reduction in health status seen in this study. The types of symptoms that were most bothersome to these patients included lower respiratory tract symptoms, but also depression and anxiety, constitutional symptoms, and cognitive symptoms. These data provide some direction for investigators interested in decreasing the diverse symptom burden experienced by survivors of ARDS.

Psychological Outcomes

There has been increasing interest in examining the effect of critical illness, and especially ARDS, on the emotional, and psychological functioning of survivors. For example, there has been recent research looking at the prevalence and predictors of post-traumatic stress disorder after ARDS. Schelling and colleagues [49] used a questionnaire called the Post Traumatic Stress Syndrome 10-Questions Inventory (PTSS-10) with 80 survivors of ARDS with a median time since ARDS of 4 years and excluded patients with head trauma or pre-existing neurological or psychiatric diseases. These authors found that 28 % of the ARDS survivors had a PTSS-10 score above the cut-off for post-traumatic stress disorder, a significantly higher proportion than two control groups: patients who had undergone maxillofacial surgery and German United Nations soldiers who had prolonged service in Cambodia [49]. They showed that if patients reported memories of traumatic experiences during their ICU stay, including memories of respiratory distress, feelings of anxiety, pain, or nightmares, they were more likely to have symptoms of post-traumatic stress disorder.

It remains unclear exactly what aspects of critical illness or acute lung injury predispose patients to long-term cognitive or psychological effects. Hopkins and colleagues provide some data suggesting it may correlate with desaturations [3]. Nelson and colleagues [50] performed a cross-sectional study of 24 survivors of acute lung injury that showed significant correlations between both symptoms of depression and symptoms of post-traumatic stress disorder and a number of variables including days in the ICU, days on mechanical ventilation, and days of sedation. Interestingly, these authors did not show a correlation between symptoms of either depression or post-traumatic stress disorder and APACHE III score. In an interesting preliminary study, Schelling and colleagues [5] performed a small retrospective case-control study comparing patients who received corticosteroids for treatment of septic shock to similar patients who did not receive corticosteroids. These authors found that the patients who received corticosteroids had a significantly lower incidence of post-traumatic stress disorder (5 of 27 compared to 16 of 27) and significantly higher scores on the mental health index of the SF-36. Although all of these studies are limited by their small numbers and their observational designs, they provide intriguing preliminary data to suggest that the way patients are managed in the ICU may have important effects on their long-term mental health and cognitive function. Further studies are needed to attempt to identify the components of critical illness or critical care treatments that predispose patients to neuropsychological deficits. Furthermore, randomized controlled trials of different mechanical ventilation and sedation strategies should also examine the potential effects on these neuropsychological outcomes.

Quality of Care at the End-of-life and Quality of Death

Because of the severity of illness in critical care medicine, the mortality among critically ill patients is relatively high compared with other areas of medicine. There is a growing interest in assessing the quality of care for patients who are dying [51, 52]. This interest in improving quality of care is coincident with increasing evidence of significant shortcomings in the provision of end-of-life care in hospitals and ICUs [48]. Furthermore, data from one study suggests that patients cared for by intensivists have increased symptoms and worse quality of end-of-life care compared to other seriously ill, hospitalized patients [53]. There is also some evidence that increased aggressiveness of care results in decreased quality of dying experience, at least as assessed by the patient's family [54]. However, this same study also suggests that death following ICU care is not necessarily a worse quality death than those deaths for which patients do not receive care in an ICU during the last month of their lives [54]. Because the ICU is a setting where mortality is high, further research is needed to find ways to improve the experience of patients who die in or shortly after a stay in the ICU setting as well as improve the experience of their families and of the health care providers [51].

The goals of medicine and the measures of quality of care may change dramatically in patients with terminal illness as compared to patients for whom death is not imminent. Survival time may not be a relevant outcome in patients with an imminently terminal disease. In fact, high quality end-of-life care might actually decrease survival time in some settings. In order to provide high quality of care at the end-of-life, we must find better ways to identify patients' preferences for treatment and improve the quality of communication between health care providers and patients or families [51]. If we can reliably measure the quality of end-of-life communication, it may become another important outcome of critical care [55].

Choosing the 'Best' Health Status Instrument for an Individual Study

The choice of an individual instrument for an individual study must depend on the research questions, the conceptual model and definition for the concept to be measured, and the ability of the candidate instruments to meet these specific needs. In addition, investigators must examine the measurement properties of each of the available instruments including reliability, validity, responsiveness, interpretability as well as administration mode and time and respondent burden. Table 2 shows a checklist for these characteristics and their relative importance in three different kinds of studies. This checklist is based on the criteria defined by the Scientific Advisory Committee of the Medical Outcomes Trust [56]. A recent review assessed the reliability, validity, and responsiveness of a number of the measures that have been used in survivors of critical illness and is a useful resource for the information that was available as of 1998 [57].

Future Directions

Despite the exponential rise in the use of health status instruments in observational and experimental studies in the critical care setting, there remain many areas of improvement that could advance the use and interpretability of these instruments. A consensus group convened by the American Thoracic Society concerning use of health status measure in Pulmonary and Critical Care Medicine identified three specific recommendations for the future [13]. First, to establish standards for evaluating, using, and interpreting health status instruments in clinical research concerning lung disease and critical illness. Second, to facilitate funding for research on health status measurement in lung disease and critical illness. Third, to promote education and training concerning the measurement of health status.

In addition to these recommendations, there are specific areas of research needed to improve the use and interpretability of these instruments. These areas include head-to-head comparisons of existing instruments, increased research concerning the best methods to assess responsiveness and to identify the minimally important differences, and methods to increase the interpretability of these instruments for clinicians and policy makers.

Table 2. Checklist for assessing health status instruments to be used in studies of patients with COPD (based in part on the criteria defined by the Medical Outcomes Trust [56]).

Quality to Be Assessed	Importance for Some of the Potential Use of Health Status Measures		
	Outcome in a Randomized, Controlled Trial	Discriminate Between Groups	Predict Future Outcomes
Measurement Model			
Conceptual model specified	++	++	++
Model verified empirically	+	+	+
Reliability			
Internal consistency	+	++	++
Stability (test-retest reliability)	++	++	++
Inter-rater/intra-rater reliability	++	++	++
Validity			
Content validity	++	++	++
Construct validity	++	++	++
Predictive validity	+/–	+/–	++
Responsiveness			
Detection of change	++	+/–	++
Identification of MID	++	+	+/–
Interpretability	++	++	++
Alternative Modes of Administration			
Testing for comparison	++	+/–	+/–
Cultural and Language Adaptations			
Conceptual and semantic equivalence	+/–	+/–	+/–
Validity testing in different cultures	+/–	+/–	+/–

++: Important in all studies of this type; +: Important in most studies of this type; +/-: May be important depending on the specific study

Head-to-head Comparisons of Health Status Instruments in Survivors of Critical Illness

There are dozens of health status instruments that have been used in the assessment of survivors of critical illness. There have been few head-to-head comparisons to evaluate these instruments in the same population, making it difficult to determine which instrument may perform best in a given setting. Head-to-head comparisons, although important, can be difficult to publish in the clinical literature unless the study has clinical implications that extend beyond measurement issues. However, studies designed to compare health status instruments can usually be simultaneously designed to address other research questions of clinical importance.

Responsiveness and the Minimally Important Difference

There is currently no standard or accepted method to assess what constitutes a MID or to compare the responsiveness of different instruments. As described above, two main methods have been used to assess the MID [15–17]. More research is needed to compare methods of assessing the MID. Responsiveness involves hypothesis testing about the direction of the change (i.e., worse, same, better) and interpretation of the results as to the magnitude of the change (i.e., small, medium, or large). A burgeoning literature focuses on responsiveness because all stakeholders in the evaluation of treatments want to be able to judge if the treatment is effective, how effective it is, under what conditions, and in what populations. Statistical reporting of effect sizes has long been the focus of clinical trial methodologies, with consensus around the definition of effect size and standardization of effect sizes [58, 59]. Alternative measures of responsiveness have been proposed, essentially changing what is in the denominator or the measure of variability or noise [60]. Which statistical measure of change should be calculated and reported across treatment effectiveness evaluations remains an important question for scientific inquiry and consensus development.

Interpretability

The field of health status measurement is in need of the development of specific methods to translate instrument scores into clinically interpretable results. This process of increasing interpretability begins with selecting and justifying the external measure used to define the importance of the change, the same process needed to identify the MID. Interpretability also requires that we examine the relationship between the self-reported health status measure and the most relevant external measures. The external measures used could be widely variable, including groups of patients with different severity of illness or events such as re-hospitalization. This work needs to be done before we can expect to see greater acceptance of these instruments outside the academic research community.

Conclusion

Critical care medicine entails the provision of technologic, aggressive, and expensive medical care to individuals with serious illness. An outcome of major importance for this care is survival. However, the diseases that predispose many patients to critical illness, and in some circumstances, the critical care therapies themselves, can have profound residual effect on the health status, quality of life, and functional capacity of patients who receive critical care. Therefore, we must consider these other outcomes of critical care in our efforts to identify care that is effective and cost-effective. Measurement of these other outcomes presents important theoretical and practical problems. However, in an era when we are expected to demonstrate the effectiveness and value of the care we provide, we must confront these challenges.

Acknowledgement

Dr. Curtis is support by an RO1 from the National Institute of Nursing Research (NR-05226-01).

References

1. Davidson TA, Caldwell ES, Curtis JR, Hudson LD , Steinberg KP (1999) Reduced quality of life in survivors of acute respiratory distress syndrome compared to critically ill controls. JAMA 281:354–360
2. Quartin AA, Schein RM, Kett DH , Peduzzi PN (1997) Magnitude and duration of the effect of sepsis on survival. JAMA 227:1058–1063
3. Hopkins RO, Weaver LK, Pope D, Orme J, Bigler ED, Larson-Lohr V (1999) Neuropsychological sequelae and impaired health status in survivors of severe acute respiratory distress syndrome. Am J Respir Crit Care Med 160:50–56
4. Schelling G, Stoll C, Hallar M, et al (1998) Health-related quality of life and posttraumatic stress disorder in survivors of acute respiratory distress Syndrome. Crit Care Med 26:651–659
5. Schelling G, Stoll C, Kapfhammer HP, et al (1999) The effect of stress doses of hydrocortisone during septic shock on posttraumatic stress disorder and health-related quality of life in survivors. Crit Care Med 27: 2678–2683
6. Schelling G, Stoll C, Vogelmeier C, et al (2000) Pulmonary function and health-related quality of life in a sample of long-term survivors of the acute respiratory distress syndrome. Intensive Care Med 26:1304–1311
7. Laine C, Davidoff F (1996) Patient-centered medicine. A professional evolution. JAMA 275:152–156
8. Deyo RA (1991) The quality of life, research, and care. Ann Intern Med 114:695–697
9. Heyland DK, Guyatt G, Cook DJ, et al (1998) Frequency and methodologic rigor of quality of life assessments in the critical care literature. Crit Care Med 26:591–598
10. Feinstein AR (1977) Clinical biostatistics: Hard science, soft data, and the challenges of choosing clinical variables in research. Clin Pharmacol Therapeutics 22:485–498
11. Clancy CM, Eisenberg JM (1998) Outcomes research: measuring the end results of health care. Science 282:245–246
12. Patrick DL, Erickson P (1993) Health Status and Health Policy: Quality of Life in Health Care Evaluation and Resource Allocation. Oxford University Press, New York City
13. Curtis JR, Martin DP, Martin TM (1997) Patient-assessed health outcomes in chronic lung disease: What are they, how do they help us, and where do we go from here? Am J Respir Crit Care Med 156:1032–1039
14. Patrick DL, Chiang YP (2000) Measurement of health outcomes in treatment effectiveness evaluations: Conceptual and methodological challenges. Med Care 9:II14–II27
15. Jones PW, Quick FH, Baveystock CM (1991) The St. George's respiratory questionnaire. Respir Med 85 (Suppl B):25-31

16. Juniper EF, Gordon GH, Willan A, Griffith LE (1994) Determining a minimal important change in a disease-specific quality of life questionaire. J Clin Epidem 47:8–87
17. Redelmeier DA, Guyatt GH, Goldstein RS (1996) Assessing the minimal important difference in symptoms: a comparison of two techniques. J Clin Epi 49:1215–1219
18. Stewart AL, Greenfield S, Hays RD, et al (1989) Functional status and well-being of patients with chronic conditions: results from the medical outcomes study. JAMA 262:907–913
19. Bergner M, Bobbitt RA, Carter WB, Gilson BS (1981) The sickness impact profile: Development and final revision of a health status measure. Med Care 19:787–805
20. Juniper EF, Guyatt GH, Epstein RS, Ferrie PJ, Jaeschke R, Hiller TK (1992) Evaluation of impairment of health-related quality of life in asthma: development of a questionnaire for use in clinical trials. Thorax 47:76–83
21. Guyatt G, Townsend M, Berman L, Pugsley S (1987) Quality of life in patients with chronic airflow limitation. Br J Dis Chest 81:45–54
22. Jones P, Quirk FH, Baveystock CM, Littlejohns P (1992) A self- complete measure of health status for chronic airflow limitation. The St. George's Respiratory Questionnaire. Am Rev Respir Dis 145:1321–1327
23. Gold MR, Siegel JE, Russell LB, Weinstein MC (1996) Cost-Effectiveness in Health and Medicine. Oxford University Press, New York
24. Froberg DG, Kane RL (1989) Methodology for measuring health-state preferences, III: population and context effects. J Clin Epi 42:585–592
25. Kaplan RM, Atkins CJ, Timms R (1984) Validity of a quality of well- being scale as an outcome measure in chronic obstructive pulmonary disease. J Chron Dis 37:85–95
26. Kaplan RM, Feeny D, Revicki DA (1993) Methods for assessing relative importance in preference based. Qual Life Res 2:467–475
27. The EuroQol Group (1990) EuroQol - a new facility for the measurement of health-related quality of life. Health Policy 16:199–208
28. Drummond MF, Stoddart GL, Torrance GW (1987) Methods for the Economic Evaluation of Health Care Programmes. Oxford University Press, New York
29. Angus DC, Rubenfeld GD, Roberts MS, et al (2002) Understanding costs and cost-effectiveness in the ICU: Report from the Second American Thoracic Society Workshop on Outcomes Research. Am J Respir Crit Care Med (in press)
30. Patrick DL, Danis ML, Southerland LI, Hong G (1988) Quality of life following intensive care. J Gen Intern Med 3:218–223
31. Mata GV, Fernandez RR, Carmona AG, et al (1992) Factors related to quality of life 12 months after discharge from an intensive care unit. Crit Care Med 20:1257–1262
32. Mundt DJ, Gage RW, Lemeshow S, Pastides H, Teres D, Avrunin JS (1989) Intensive care unit patient follow up: Mortality, functional status, and return to work at six months. Arch Intern Med 149:68–72
33. Sprangers MA, Aaronson NK (1992) The role of health care providers and significant others in evaluating the quality of life of patients with chronic disease: a review. J Clin Epidemiol 45:743–760
34. Hinton J (1996) How reliable are relatives' retrospective reports of terminal illness? Patients' and relatives' accounts compared. Soc Sci Med 43:1229–1236
35. McHugh LG, Milberg JA, Whitcomb ME, Schoene RB, Maunder RJ, Hudson LD (1994) Recovery of function in survivors of the acute respiratory distress syndrome. Am J Respir Crit Care Med 150:90–94
36. Weinert CR, Gross CR, Kangas JR, Bury CL, Marinelli WA (1997) Health-related quality of life after acute lung injury. Am J Respir Crit Care Med 156:1120–1128
37. Angus DC, Musthafa AA, Clermont G, et al (2001) Quality-adjusted survival in the first year after the acute respiratory distress syndrome. Am J Respir Crit Care Med 163:1389–1394
38. Heyland DK, Hopman W, Coo H, Tranmar J, McColl MA (2000) Long-term health-related quality of life in survivors of sepsis. Crit Care Med 28:3599–3605

39. Pettila V, Kaarlola A, Makelainen A (2000) Health-related quality of life of multiple organ dysfunction patients one year after intensive care. Intensive Care Med 26:1473–1479
40. Chelluri L, Grenvik A, Silverman M (1995) Intensive care for critically ill elderly: mortality, costs,. Arch Intern Med 155:1013–1022
41. Montuclard L, Garrouste-Orgeas M, Timsit J, Misset B, De Jonghe B, Carlet J (2000) Outcome, functional autonomy, and quality of life of elderly patients with a long term intensive care unit stay. Crit Care Med 28:3389–3395
42. Welsh CH, Thompson K, Long-Krug S (1999) Evaluation of patient-perceived health status using the Medical Outcomes Survey Short Form 36 in an intensive care unit population. Crit Care Med 27:1466–1471
43. Wehler M, Martus P, Geise A, et al (2001) Changes in quality of life after medical intensive care. Intensive Care Med 27:154–159
44. Mata GV, Fernandez RR, Carmona AG, et al (1992) Factors related to quality of life 12 months after discharge from an intensive care unit. Crit Care Med 20:1257–1262
45. Konopad E, Noseworthy TW, Johnston R, Shustack A, Grace M (1995) Quality of life measures before and one year after admission to an intensive care unit. Crit Care Med 23:1653–1659
46. Nelson JE, Meier D, Oei EJ, et al (2001) Self-reported symptom experience of critically ill cancer patients receiving intensive care. Crit Care Med 29:277–282
47. Puntillo KA (1990) Pain experience of intensive care unit patients. Heart Lung 19:525–533
48. The SUPPORT Principal Investigators (1996) A controlled trial to improve care for seriously ill hospitalized patients: the study to understand prognoses and preferences for outcomes and risks of treatments (SUPPORT). JAMA 274:1591–1598
49. Schelling G, Stoll C, Haller M, et al (1998) Health-related quality of life and posttraumatic stress disorder in survivors of the acute respiratory distress syndrome. Crit Care Med 26:651–659
50. Nelson BJ, Weinert CR, Bury CL, Marinelli WA, Gross CR (2000) Intensive care unit drug use and subsequent quality of life in acute lung injury patients. Crit Care Med 28:3626–3630
51. Rubenfeld GD, Curtis JR , for the End-of-Life Care in the ICU Working Group (2001) End of life care in the intensive care: A research agenda. Crit Care Med 29:2001–2006
52. Levy MM (2001) Paying attention to death. Crit Care Med 29:2037–2038
53. Desbiens NA, Wu AW (2000) Pain and suffering in seriously ill hospitalized patients. J Am Geriatrics Soc 48:S183–S186
54. Curtis JR, Patrick DL, Engelberg RA, Norris KE, Asp CH , Byock IR (2002) A measure of the quality of dying and death: Initial validation using after-death interviews with family members. J Pain Symptom Manage (in press)
55. Curtis JR, Patrick DL, Shannon SE, Treece PD, Engelberg RA, Rubenfeld GD (2001) The family conference as a focus to improve communication about end-of-life care in the intensive care unit: Opportunities for improvement. Crit Care Med 29:N26–N33
56. Scientific Advisory Committee of the Medical Outcomes Trust (1995) Instrument Review Criteria. Medical Outcomes Trust Bulletin 3:1–4
57. Black NA, Jenkinson C, Hayes JA, et al (2001) Review of outcome measures used in adult critical care. Crit Care Med 29:2119–2124
58. Armitage P, Colton T (1998) Encyclopedia of Biostatistics. J. Wiley, Chichester
59. Cohen J (1988) Statistical Power Analyses for the Behavioral Sciences, 2nd Edition edn. Erlbaum, Hillsdale
60. Liang MH (1995) Evaluating measurement responsiveness. J Rheum 22:1191–1192.

How Should We Assess Neuropsychological Sequelae of Critical Illness?

R. O. Hopkins

Introduction

Critically ill, mechanically ventilated patients in the intensive care unit (ICU) consume a considerable proportion of our medical resources [1]. Patients admitted to an ICU with life-threatening critical illness require invasive procedures, mechanical ventilation, and sedative and analgesic drugs. Sedative and analgesic drugs in conjunction with mechanical ventilation and pain may adversely affect patients' cognitive and emotional outcome following ICU care [2]. The patient's distressing memories of the ICU experience may lead to psychotic symptoms such as hallucinations and delirium [3]. Most outcome studies have focused on survival as the major ICU outcome variable. More recent studies have found large proportions of ICU patients experience impaired health-related quality of life (HRQL) and psychosocial impairments [1, 4]. Forty percent of ICU survivors were unable to return to work due to impaired physical and psychosocial problems [5]. Although medical outcomes research has studied critically ill patients, relatively few studies have assessed neuropsychological function. For example, outcomes research following acute respiratory distress syndrome (ARDS) has been ongoing for a number of years, however, only limited information exists concerning ultimate outcomes. Initial outcome studies assessed survival [6] and pulmonary function [7, 8]. Subsequent studies have found impaired health status [8] and symptoms of posttraumatic stress disorder following ARDS [9]. Only in the past several years have a few studies assessed neuropsychological outcome following ARDS [10–12]. The limited studies of neuropsychological outcome following critical illness may be due in part to the belief held by many physicians that most medical disorders have little effect on the brain and cognitive function [13].

In the past few years, research that assessed the relationship between medical disorders and cognitive function has increased. Recent studies have found neurocognitive impairments in a variety of medical disorders including diabetes mellitus, pulmonary disorders, liver disease, hypertension, cancer, cardiac disorders, thyroid disease, and renal dysfunction (for a review see [14]). Less information is available regarding neurocognitive outcome following critical illness. In order to understand the association between brain function and cognition in critically ill patients, it is necessary to understand the interaction between disease and cognitive capacities [14]. Neurocognitive impairments following a critical illness may occur as a consequence of the pathophysiological disturbances and resulting organ and system pathology such as hypoxia [10]. Alternatively, neurocognitive impairments may be associated with various medical treatments, such as microemboli that occur during cardiac surgery as a result of the cardio-pulmonary bypass machine [15]. Thus it is important to identify the neurocognitive consequences of a critical illness, the correlates of the disease and associated treatments, and differentiate them from individual variables (e.g., age, education, gender, psychiatric history, etc.).

Research in neuropsychological outcomes following critical illness offers new areas of research that will be able to link neuropsychology and neuroscience with medicine through empirical investigation that will help to elucidate pathological and treatment effects with cognitive function. Assessment of neurocognitive function following a critical illness requires measures that are sensitive to cognitive abilities that are reliable, valid, repeatable, and free of (or reduce) measurement error. Neuropsychological tests provide potential advantages to the assessment of cognitive function [16] including:

1. Neuropsychological tests are developed for a wide range of specific neurocognitive domains (e.g., attention, memory, mental processing speed, etc.).
2. Neuropsychological tests are administered and scored using standardized procedures that contribute to their reliability.
3. Neuropsychological tests are objective and require less subjective judgment than other behavioral measures of brain function, such as impairment rating scales (i.e. mild, moderate, and severe).
4. Neuropsychological tests yield continuous ranges of numerical scores, which reflect levels of performance and allow for comparisons across subjects. The continuous scores reflect different levels of performance and are amenable to statistical analyses.
5. Neuropsychological tests measure a wide range of cognitive domains such as attention, memory, executive function, and motor skills to name a few. These measurements have been psychometrically developed and carefully validated in normal control subjects and samples of patients with a variety of medical and neurological disorders.
6. Neuropsychological tests have been shown to have reliability over time and some tests offer equivalent forms in order to reduce the potential for practice effects.

In summary, neuropsychological tests are objective, reliable, and repeatable standardized measures that assess performance in a variety of cognitive domains [16]. In addition, neuropsychological tests may provide information that has ecological relevance to the patient. Ecological validity is the degree to which neurological assessment provides information about the patient that will be useful to their environment. Information regarding the individual's cognitive function can be used to formulate a plan of care, predict problems the individual will have at work, and evaluate the ability of the individual to live independently.

Neurocognitive Domains

The brain is not a unitary organ and is comprised of multiple nuclei, structures, and neural systems, each that subserve different neurocognitive domains. Integration of cognitive domains and function occurs in polymodal association cortices. Neurocognitive domains include sensory, motor, intelligence, attention, memory, mental processing speed, language, executive abilities, emotional components of cognition, etc. For each neurocognitive domain, such as memory, there are multiple types of memory and multiple memory systems in the brain (Table 1). In addition to the types of memory listed in Table 1, memory can be characterized as verbal memory that is predominately dependent on the left hippocampus and visuo-spatial memory that is predominately dependent on the right hippocampus.

The assessment of memory, like most cognitive functions is complex. Given that most standardized neuropsychological tests measure only one or two types of memory; several tests may be necessary in order to determine the effects of critical illness on memory.

Assessment of Premorbid Function

In measuring neuropsychological function following critical illness, a common question regards the interpretation of whether the observed cognitive impairments are due to the critical illness or are simply a measure of an individual's premorbid level of cognitive function. Since premorbid neuropsychological test data are rarely

Table 1. Types of memory

Type of Memory	Definition	Neural Structure(s)
Short term memory	Memory that lasts seconds to minutes	Frontal lobes/hippocampus
Declarative memory	Memory for new facts and events, requires conscious recollection	Hippocampus/medial temporal lobe structures
Long term memory	Memory that lasts minutes to years	Cortex
Motor skills	The ability to learn and remember new motor skills	Basal ganglia
Temporal order memory	Memory for the order of events in time (temporal markers)	Frontal lobes/hippocampus
Working memory	Information held in memory in order to complete a task	Frontal lobes
Emotional memory	Emotional content of memory	Amygdala
Classical conditioning	Stimulus response associations	Cerebellum

available, estimates of the individual's premorbid abilities may help determine if the cognitive performance is a change from the normal pre-illness level. Neurocognitive deficit can be assessed either in comparison to normative standards or compared to the individual's pre-illness level of cognitive function. If a test has normative data available, the extent of the discrepancy between the post-illness ability level and normative standards (standardized data from adults with the same age, gender, and education) for the behavior in question, will allow for the determination of the cognitive decline. Alternatively, the present performance can be compared to an estimate of the patient's original (pre-illness) ability level. A number of methods for inferring premorbid abilities have been used with varying degrees of success. Personal historical (e.g., education level) and observational data have been used for comparison to post-illness or post-injury neuropsychological test performance. The best performance method consists of identifying the highest test score or level of function in every day tasks, which is used as a standard against which all other aspects of the current performance are compared [17]. Alternatively, premorbid abilities can be assessed by tests that measure over-learned skills such as vocabulary and reading, which are highly correlated with intelligence and are more resistant to brain injury [17–20]. Examples of tests that measure these over-learned skills include the Vocabulary subtest of the Wechsler Adult Intelligence Scale (WAIS), the National Adult Reading Test (NART), and the Wide Range Achievement Test.

Demographic data formulas for estimating premorbid ability have also been used, and include education, ethnicity, and occupation as the best predictors. A number of investigators have developed equations to calculate premorbid intelligence. For example, the Barona Index [21] incorporates the above demographic variables with measured intelligence quotient (IQ), geographic region, urban-rural residence, and handedness into the regression formula. Barona and colleagues did not state the rate of misclassification, but other studies have shown that the index misclassifies approximately one-half of the patients [22]. The Oklahoma Premorbid Intelligence Estimate (OPIE) uses a linear prediction algorithm based on the WAIS-R standardization samples and combines the best performance of either Vocabulary or Picture Completion with demographic information [23]. The OPIE provides reasonable estimates of IQ accounting for approximately 75% of individuals. One limitation of the demographic based estimates of premorbid intelligence is the tendency to underestimate ability at the high end and overestimate ability at the low end.

Neuropsychological Test Batteries

A variety of factors must be considered when choosing a neuropsychological test battery to assess outcome following a critical illness. The length of the test battery and areas cognitive function to be assessed must be considered, as well as the endurance and emotional stability of the patients must be incorporated into decisions regarding the neuropsychological test battery. For detailed reviews of neuropsychological tests, administration and scoring see [17–20].

There are a number of different types of neuropsychological test batteries that include brief neurocognitive screening tests, comprehensive test batteries, computerized test batteries, and test batteries designed to assess select domains of cognitive function based on specific hypotheses of brain injury. The four types of neuropsychological test batteries will be discussed below.

Neurocognitive Screening Tests

Neurocognitive screening tests were designed to be brief measures for use in acute-care settings. Professionals who practice in medical/surgical hospital settings are often faced with a limited amount of time to evaluate patients who have a critical illness. The reduced length of stay in many health care systems increases the demand for a brief and rapid assessment of neurocognitive function. Neurocognitive screening tests, like the Mini Mental State Examination (MMSE) [24], Neurobehavioral Cognitive Status Examination (NCSE) [25], and the Cognitive Capacity Screening Exam [26] were designed as diagnostic screening tools for severe neurological disorders like dementia. For a detailed review of the strengths and weakness of cognitive screening tests see [27]. Neurocognitive screening tests are brief, are easy to administer, and can be completed in 3 to 30 minutes. Although the screening tests are easy and quick to administer, they have several significant limitations. Neuropsychological screening tests assess only limited domains of cognitive function and provide limited information regarding the cognitive areas that they assess. Most screening tests were not designed to target specific diseases or cognitive impairments. Some screening tests like the MMSE have a strong language component but provide little information for visual spatial and memory abilities. The neurocognitive screening tests are often insensitive to mild or moderate cognitive impairments, thus they often do not identify individuals with cognitive impairments (i.e., have a high rate of false-negative identification). A number of studies have reported that the above neuropsychological screening tests are not sensitive to cognitive impairments following carbon monoxide poisoning [28], dementia of multiple sclerosis [29], and mild cognitive dysfunction [30]. The Repeatable Battery for the Assessment of Neuropsychological Status (RBANS) is a brief test that measures attention, language, visuospatial/constructional abilities, and memory [31]. The RBANS takes 20–30 minutes to administer and has two comparable alternate forms. Although the RBANS was standardized using a sample of individuals from 20–89, it underestimates mild cognitive impairment and underestimates cognitive impairments in very bright individuals. Given the limitations of neuropsychological screening batteries, the use of screening batteries in the evaluation of neuropsychological function following a critical illness may result in a high false negative rate, that is, not identify individuals in whom neuropsychological function is impaired.

Comprehensive Neuropsychological Test Batteries

There are a few comprehensive neuropsychological test batteries that are in wide use at the present time. There include the Halstead-Reitan Battery (HRB) [32] and the Luria-Nebraska Battery (LNB) [33]. The comprehensive neuropsychological test batteries assess in depth a broad range of cognitive domains, and take two to six hours to administer. The length of the testing session can be prohibitive in patients who have been in the ICU, as they require a significant amount of time for administration and scoring, which often results in patient fatigue or inability to complete the testing. One way to reduce the length of the standardized neuropsychological test battery is to shorten the test battery by administering only some of the tests thereby omitting or inadequately assessing some domain(s) of cognitive function. Another limitation of the standardized neuropsychological test batteries are that some areas of cognitive function, such as memory, are not well assessed by the HRB or LNB [34].

An alternative to pre-selected test batteries, are individualized comprehensive neuropsychological test batteries. For example in assessing traumatic brain injury [35] we formulated a test battery for use at LDS Hospital in Salt Lake City, Utah, USA. The current neuropsychological test battery in use at LDS Hospital is shown below (Table 2) by domain of cognitive function assessed. All tests are fully standardized, normed and are administered according to standardized protocols. However, because of individual patient needs, some aspects of the battery may be abbreviated. Whenever test battery abbreviation occurs, we try to obtain some measure within each domain. These neuropsychological tests, their standardized administration procedures and implications for lateralized functions have been fully discussed elsewhere [17].

One major limitation of the comprehensive neuropsychological test batteries is the length of the battery that requires two to six hours to administer with resultant patient fatigue and possible loss of subjects. In a study that assessed neuropsychological outcome following ARDS [10] we shortened the test battery to 1.5 hours in order to measure cognitive function at the time of hospital discharge and one year post hospital discharge. The neuropsychological tests were selected based on an *a priori* hypothesis regarding effects of hypoxia on the brain. For example, the ARDS patients were administered only select tests from the memory, executive function, language, and attention domains and no motor tests were administered. In addition most questionnaires regarding affect were only administered at the one-year follow-up session. Even with the shortened neuropsychological test battery, the tests administered prior to hospital discharged were carried out in three to four separate sessions of approximately 30 minutes due to patient fatigue [10].

Computerized Test Batteries

Computerized neuropsychological test batteries are more recent developments in neuropsychological assessment. Some computerized tests are standard tests that have been transferred to the computer [47] whereas other tests have been specifically designed for the computer in order to test a cognitive function such as

Table 2. Standardized neuropsychological assessment battery used at LDS hospital

Function assessed	Neuropsychological Test [Reference]
Motor	Finger Oscillation Test [36]
	Strength of Grip Test [36]
	Purdue Peg Board [17]
	Grooved Peg Board [17]
Memory	Wechsler Memory Scale-III [37]
	Recognition Memory Test [38]
	Rey-Osterrieth Complex Figure Design [39]
	Rey Auditory Verbal Learning Test [17]
Visual-Spatial	Trail Making Test [36]
	Block Design from WASI [40]
Language	Controlled Oral Word Association [17]
	Wide Range Achievement Test - R [41]
	Boston Naming Test
	Verbal IQ - Selected subtests from the WASI [40]
Attention	Stroop Test
	Digit span from the Wechsler Memory Scale-III [37]
General Cognition	Wechsler Abbreviated Scale of Intelligence (WASI) [40]
Executive Function	Category Test [36]
	Wisconsin Card Sorting Test [42]
	Trail Making Test [36]
Affect	Beck Depression Inventory [43]
	Beck Anxiety Inventory [44]
	Symptom Checklist 90-Revised [45]
	Davidson Trauma Scale [46]

memory. Advantages of computerized neuropsychological tests are decreased administrator error, speed or data capture, immediate data analyses, and response times can be measured in milliseconds. Several of the computerized neuropsychological test batteries will be discussed below. Computerized versions of previous neuropsychological tests, such as the Wisconsin Card Sorting Test, and computerized tests that only assess one cognitive domain such as memory will not be discussed.

MicroCog is a computerized screening test that assesses nine areas of cognitive function including attention, memory, reasoning, accuracy, and cognitive processing speed [48]. In addition MicroCog was designed with test-retest ability, to monitor cognitive status over time. The Cognitive Evaluation Protocol (CEP) assesses cognitive function and has three versions: the CEP-Short for basic screening (18–22 minutes); CEP-Complex for advanced evaluation of persons with limited capacities (15–22 minutes); and the CEP-Extended which combines the other two versions (45 minutes) [49]. One major limitation of the CEP software is that it requires a touch screen to administer the tests. CogState is a computer-based test to be delivered and scored via the Internet [50]. CogState tests a variety of cognitive domains including alertness, attention, working memory, spatial awareness, memory, and executive function. CogState takes 15 to 20 minutes to administer and is automatically scored. An almost infinite number of forms are available due to randomization, making it ideal to situations in which test-retest is advantageous [50]. Computerized testing requires a compatible computer, and if you want to see inpatients, then a laptop computer is required. One major limitation of all computerized neuropsychological test batteries is that most of the companies charge a fee for the administration of one test (approximately $100 US). In addition, computerized tests are inappropriate for certain populations, such as dementia, where the requisite memory and executive function capabilities needed to perform the task are impaired [33].

Hypothesis Driven Neuropsychological Test Batteries

Given the limitations of comprehensive neuropsychological test batteries for assessing neuropsychological sequelae of a critical illness, it would seem reasonable to design test batteries that are hypothesis driven. That is, what components of an illness and/or treatments are likely to result in brain injury? In order to understand the association between brain function and cognition following critical illness, the relationships between the disease and cognitive function must be determined. Brain injury following a critical illness may result from a number of factors including hypoxia, decreased cerebral perfusion, and toxic and metabolic effects. Previous research has shown that hypoxia may result in neurocognitive sequelae and brain injury. The severity of the brain injury depends on the length and severity of the hypoxic episode; although nonspecific degenerative neuropathologic changes can ensue, the hippocampus appears to be more selectively vulnerable than other brain structures. Several recent studies using quantitative magnetic resonance imaging (MRI) analyses showed significant hippocampal atrophy and concomitant memory impairments in select hypoxic subjects [51–53]. Alternatively, hypoxic brain injury may result in diffuse damage throughout the brain in some cases [54]. Hypoxia-induced cognitive impairments occur in a variety of pulmonary disorders including ARDS [10], chronic obstructive pulmonary disease (COPD) [55, 56], following cardiac or respiratory arrest [51, 52], and obstructive sleep apnea syndrome [57].

In a study that assessed neuropsychological outcome following ARDS the neuropsychological tests were selected based on *a priori* hypothesis regarding effects of hypoxia on the brain [10]. The study hypothesized that ARDS-induced hypoxia would result in hippocampal damage and subsequent memory impairments. Neurocognitive outcome was assessed in 55 ARDS survivors using a prospective within subjects design. At the time of hospital discharge, 100 % of the patients experienced cognitive impairments, including problems with memory, attention, concentration, and global loss of cognitive function. At one-year follow-up, 30 % of the patients experienced impaired general intelligence and 78 % had at least one of the following; impaired memory, attention, concentration and/or mental processing speed (48 %). At one year only 19 % had impaired intellectual function, 40 % had impaired executive function, and 42 % had decreased mental processing speed. Continuous oxygen saturation data were automatically collected and hypoxemia significantly correlated with impaired attention, memory, intelligence, speed of processing, visual-spatial skills (block design) and executive function at one year [10].

Although the hypoxemia was related to impaired memory in the ARDS patients, it was also related to slow mental processing speed, and impaired intellectual function, visual-spatial skills, and attention. Thus it appears that ARDS-induced hypoxemia results in diffuse brain injury rather than selective injury to memory systems such as the hippocampus. The severity of the brain injury was related to the duration and severity of the hypoxic episode as measured by pulse oximetry. These results support previous data which showed that the degree of cognitive impairment appears to parallel the degree of morphologic abnormality as demonstrated by quantitative MRI analysis [53].

Other factors in addition to hypoxia may contribute to the cognitive impairments and concomitant brain injury following ARDS. Other possible causes of brain injury include ischemia and metabolic effects such as cytokines and inflammation, and associated sepsis. For example severe sepsis results in acute organ dysfunction due to generalized inflammatory and procoagulant response to infection [58]. Memory impairments are commonly associated with infectious diseases [59]. A study that induced cytokine activation in healthy male volunteers using intravenous injection of *Salmonella abortus equi* endodotoxin, found impaired verbal and nonverbal memory that were correlated with endotoxin-induced cytokine secretion [60]. Patients with chronic fatigue syndrome and elevated cytokine levels exhibit impaired attention, concentration, and memory [61]. Finally a study of sepsis and multiple organ failure found that three out of five patients experienced cognitive impairments [62].

Another example of a hypothesis driven study is one that assesses the effects of a treatment on brain integrity such as cardio-pulmonary bypass during open-heart surgery. Clinical studies indicate that 30–80 % of patients who undergo open-heart surgery experience a decline in cognitive function [63]. Possible causes of neurological damage include bypass equipment leading to fat emboli [64], air bubbles [65], and platelet aggregates [66]. The appearance of emboli has been reported to correlate with various events during the surgical protocols [67], such as during aortic cannulation, cardioplegia, placement and removal of the cross clamp, cross clamp time, side clamp placement and removal, side clamp bypass, initial ejection, and aortic decannulation. An alternate source of emboli is suggested by previous reports of hypothermia-induced platelet aggregation (HIPA) in whole blood exposed to biomaterials and hypothermia, with a maximum response at 24 centigrade. HIPA was found in 34 % of volunteers and produced platelet aggregates with sufficient strength to occlude micropores at 50 mmHg [68]. A study was conducted to determine if HIPA may contribute to the cerebral injury (expressed as cognitive impairment) associated with hypothermic coronary artery bypass graft (CABG) surgery (Hall et al., unpublished data). Patients (n=45) undergoing hypothermic (32–28 °C) CABG surgery had pre- and post-operative (4–6 days) neuropsychological testing. The CABG with HIPA patients experienced a significant ($p < 0.05$)

decline in cognitive function in the mental processing speed, memory and executive function compared to those CABG patients that did not have HIPA (Hall et al., unpublished data). These results support the idea that medical intervention may cause or increase the severity of the neuropsychological impairments. Specific hypothesis driven research has the potential to significantly increase our understanding of the neuropsychological effects following a critical illness.

Conclusion

Critically ill, mechanically ventilated patients in the ICU consume a considerable proportion of the medical resources and require multiple interventions including invasive procedures, mechanical ventilation, and numerous medications. The nature of a critical illness and the life saving treatments may result in brain injury and neuropsychological sequelae following ICU care. Assessment of neuropsychological sequelae in critically ill patients will help to determine if cognitive function may be impaired due to the pathophysiology of the illness or subsequent treatments. Future research should be directed at understanding the effects of critical illness on neurological integrity and neuropsychological outcome. In addition, research should be directed at investigating the effectiveness of new and existing treatments that influence the course of a critical illness, which may indirectly influence cognitive outcome, and treatments specifically aimed at improving cognitive dysfunction.

References

1. Spicher JE, White DP (1987) Outcome and function following prolonged mechanical ventilation. Arch Intern Med 147:421–425
2. Jones C, Griffiths RD, Humphrys G (2000) Disturbed memory and amnesia related to intensive care. Memory 8:79–94
3. Jones J, Griffiths RD, Macmillian RR, Palmer TEA (1994) Psychological problems occurring after intensive care. Br J Intensive Care Feb:46–53
4. Konopad E, Noseworthy TW, Johnston R, Shustack A, Grace M (1995) Quality of life measured before and one year after admission to an intensive care unit. Crit Care Med 23:1653–1659
5. Goldstein RL, Campion EW, Thibault GE, Mulley AG, Skinner E (1986) Functional outcomes following medical intensive care. Crit Care Med 14:783–788
6. Lee J, Turner S, Morgan CJ, Keogh BF, Evans TW (1994) Adult respiratory distress syndrome: has there been a change in outcome predictive measures? Thorax 49:596–597
7. Suchyta M, Clemmer T, Elliott CG, Orme JJ, Weaver L (1993) The adult respiratory distress syndrome. A report of survival and modifying factors. Chest 104:647–648
8. McHugh LG, Milberg JA, Whitcomb ME, Schoene RB, Maunder RJ, Hudson LD (1994) Recovery of function in survivors of the acute respiratory distress syndrome. Am J Respir Crit Care Med 150:90–94
9. Schelling G, Stoll C, Haller M, et al (1998) Health-related quality of life and posttraumatic stress disorder in survivors of the acute respiratory distress syndrome. Crit Care Med 26:651–658
10. Hopkins RO, Weaver LK, Pope D, Orme JF, Jr, Bigler ED, Larson-Lohr V (1999) Neuropsychological sequelae and impaired health status in survivors of severe acute respiratory distress syndrome. Am J Respir Crit Care Med 160:50–56

11. Rothenhausler HB, Ehrentraut S, Stoll C, Schelling G, Kapfhammer HP (2001) The relationship between cognitive performance and employment and health status in long-term survivors of the acute respiratory distress syndrome: results of an exploratory study. Gen Hosp Psychiatry 23:90–96

12. Marquis KA, Curtis JR, Caldwell ES, et al (2000) Neuropsychologic sequelae in survivors of ARDS compared with critically ill control patients. Am J Respir Crit Care Med 16:A383 (abst)

13. Ryan CM, Adams KM, Heaton RK, Grant I, Jacobson AM, DCCT Research Group (1991) Neurobehavioral assessment of medical patients in clinical trials: The DCCT experience. In: Mohr E, Brouwers P, (eds) Handbook of Clinical Trials: The Neurobehavioral Approach. Swets & Zeitlinger, Amsterdam, pp 215–241

14. Butters MA, Beers SR, Tarter RE (2001) Perspective for research on neuropsychological assessment of medical disease. In: Tarter RE, Butters MA, Beers SR (eds) Medical Neuropsychology, 2nd edn. Kluwer Academic/Plenum Publishers, New York, pp 1–3

15. Jacobs A, Neveling M, Horst M, et al (1998) Alterations of neuropsychological function and cerebral glucose metabolism after cardiac surgery are not related only to intraoperative microembolic events. Stroke 29:660–667

16. Borhstein RA (1991) The role of neuropsychological assessment in clinical trials. In: Mohr E, Brouwers P (eds) Handbook of Clinical Trials. Swets and Zeitlinger, Amsterdam, pp 11–28

17. Lezak M (1995) Neuropsychological Assessment, 3rd edn. Oxford University Press, New York

18. Bigler ED, Clement PF (1997) Diagnostic Clinical Neuropsychology, 3rd edn. University of Texas Press, Austin

19. Grant I, Adams KM (1996) Neuropsychological Assessment of Neuropsychiatric Disorders, 2nd edn. Oxford University Press, New York

20. Spreen O, Struss E (1998) A Compendium of Neuropsychological tests: Administration, Norms and Commentary, 2nd edn. Oxford University Press, New York

21. Barona AC, Reynolds C, Chastain R (1984) A demographically based index of premorbid intelligence for the WAIS-R. J Consult Clin Psychol 52:885–887.

22. Sweet J, Moberg P, Tovain S (1990) Evaluation of Wechsler Adult Intelligence Scale-Revised premorbid IQ clinical formulas in clinical populations. Psychol Assessment 2:41–44

23. Krull KR, Scott JG, Sherer M (1995) Estimation of premorbid intelligence from combined performance and demographic variables. Clin Neuropsychologist 9:83–88

24. Folstein MF, Folstein SE, McHugh PR (1975) "Mini-Mental State": A practical method of grading the cognitive state of patients for the clinician. J Psychiatr Res 12:189–198

25. Kiernan RJ, Mueller J, Langston JW, Van Dyke C (1987) The neurobehavioral cognitive status examination: A brief but differentiated approach to cognitive assessment. Ann Intern Med 107:481–485

26. Jacobs JW, Bernhard MR, Degado A, Strain JJ (1977) Screening for organic mental syndromes in the medically ill. Ann Intern Med 86:40–46

27. Mitrushina M, Fuld PA (1996) Cognitive screening methods. In: Grant I, Adams KM (eds) Neuropsychological Assessment of Neuropsychiatric Disorders, 2nd edn. Oxford University Press, New York, pp 118–138

28. Weaver LK, Hopkins RO, Larson-Lohr V (1996) Neuropsychologic and functional recovery from severe carbon monoxide poisoning without hyperbaric oxygen therapy. Ann Emerg Med 27:736–740

29. Beatty WE, Goodkin DE (1990) Screening for cognitive impairment in multiple sclerosis. Arch Neurol 47:297–301

30. Filey CM (1998) The behavioral neurology of cerebral white matter. Neurology 50:1535–1540

31. Randolph C (1998) Repeatable Battery for the Assessment of Neuropsychological Status. The Psychological Corporation, Harcourt Brace and Company, San Antonio

32. Reitan RM, Davidson LA (1974) Clinical neuropsychology: Current status and applications. Hemisphere, New York

33. Golden CJ (1981) A standardized version of Luria's neuropsychological tests: A quantitative and qualitative approach to neuropsychological evaluation. In: Filskov S, Boll TJ (eds) Handbook of Clinical Neuropsychology. Wiley, New York, pp 608–648

34. Albert MS (1991) Criteria for the choice of neuropsychological tests in clinical trials. In : Mohr E, Brouwers P (eds) Handbook of Clinical Trails: The Neurobehavioral Approach. Swets and Zeitlinger, Amsterdam, pp 131–139

35. Bigler, ED, Blatter DD, Andersen CV, et al. (1997) Hippocampal volume in normal aging and traumatic brain injury. Am J Neuroradiology 18:11–23

36. Reitan RM, Wolfson D (1985) The Halstead-Reitan Neuropsychological Test Battery. Neuropsychology Press, Tucson

37. The Psychological Corporation (1999) Wechsler Memory Scale-III. Harcourt Brace and Company, San Antonio

38. Warrington EK (1984) Recognition Memory Test. Western Psychological Services, Los Angeles

39. Osterrieth R (1944) Le teste de copie d'une figure complexe: Contribution a l'etude de la perception et la memoire. Archives de Psychologie 30:286–356

40. The Psychological Corporation (1999) Wechsler Abbreviated Scale of Intelligence. Harcourt Brace and Company, San Antonio

41. Systems JA (1984) Wide Range Achievement Test. JASTAK Associates, Wilmington

42. Nelson HE (1976) A modified card sorting test sensitive to frontal lobe deficits. Cortex 12:313–324

43. Beck AT (1987) Beck Depression Inventory. The Psychological Corporation, San Antonio

44. Beck AT, Steer RA (1993) Beck Anxiety Inventory. The Psychological Corporation, San Antonio

45. Derogatis LR, Lipman RS, Covi L (1973) SCL-90: An outpatients psychiatric rating scale, preliminary report. Psychopharmacol Bull 9:13–27

46. Davidson J, (1996) Davidson Trauma Scale. Multi-Health Systems Inc., North Tonawanda

47. Randt CT, Brown ER (1983) Randt Memory Test. Life Science Associates, Bayport

48. Powell D, Kaplan E, Whitla D, Weintraub S, Catlin R, Funkenstein H (1996) MicroCog™: Assessment of Cognitive Function Version 2.4. The Psychological Corporation, San Antonio

49. Anonymous (1998) Cognitive Evaluation Protocol. Eval-Flex Inc., Sherman Oaks

50. Westerman R, Darby DG, Maruff P, Collie A (2001) Computer-assisted cognitive function assessment of pilots. ADF Health 2:29–36

51. Hopkins RO, Kesner RP, Goldstein M (1995) Memory for novel and familiar spatial and linguistic temporal distance information in hypoxic subjects. J Int Neuropsychological Soc 1:454–468

52. Kesner RP, Hopkins RO (2001) Short-term memory for duration and distance in humans : Role of the hippocampus. Neuropsychology 15:58–68

53. Hopkins RO, Gale SD, Johnson SC, Anderson CV, Bigler ED, Blatter DD (1995) Severe anoxia with and without concomitant brain atrophy and neuropsychological impairments. J Int Neuropsychol Soc 1:501–509

54. Gale SD, Hopkins RO, Weaver LK, Bigler ED, Booth EJ, Blatter DD (1999) MRI, quantitative MRI, SPECT, and neuropsychological findings following carbon monoxide poisoning. Brain Inj 13:229–243

55. Heaton RK, Grant I, McSweeny AJ, Adams KM, Petty TL (1983) Psychologic effects of continuous and nocturnal oxygen therapy in hypoxemic chronic obstructive pulmonary disease. Arch Intern Med 143:1941–1947

56. Grant I, Heaton R, McSweeny A, Adams K, Timms R (1982) Neuropsychological findings in hypoxemic chronic obstructive pulmonary disease. Arch Intern Med 142:1470–1476

57. Bedard M, Montplaisir J, Richer F, Roulea I, Malo J (1991) Obstructive sleep apnea syndrome: Pathogenesis of neuropsychological deficits. J Clin Exp Neuropsychol 13:950–964

58. Bone RC, Grodzin CJ, Balk RA (1997) Sepsis: a new hypothesis for pathogenesis of the disease process. Chest 112:235–243

59. Capuron L, Lamarque D, Dantzer R, Goodall G (1999) Attentional and mnemonic deficit associated with infectious disease in humans. Psychol Med 29:291–297
60. Reichenberg A, Yirmiya R, Schuld A et al (2001) Cytokine-associated emotional and cognitive disturbances in humans. Arch Gen Psychiatry 58:445–452
61. Patarca-Montero R, Antoni M, Fletcher MA, Klimas NG (2001) Cytokine and other immunologic markers in chronic fatigue syndrome and their relation to neuropsychological factors. Appl Neuropsychol 8:51–64
62. Sieser A, Schwarx S, Brainin M (1992) Critical illness polyneuropathy: clinical aspects and long-term outcome. Wien Klin Wochenschr 104:294–300
63. Newman S, Stygall J, Kong R (2001) Neuropsychological consequences of coronary artery bypass surgery: In: Waldstein SR, Elias MF (eds) Neuropsychology of Cardiovascular Disease. Lawrence Erlbaum Associates, Mahwah, pp 189–218
64. Caguin F, Carter MG (1963) Fat embolism with cardiotomy with use of cardiopulmonary bypass. J Thorac Cardiovasc Surg 46:665–672
65. Deklunder G, Roussel M, Lecroart JL, Prat A, Gautier C (1998) Microemboli in cerebral circulation and alteration of cognitive abilities in patients with mechanical prosthetic heart valves. Stroke 29:1821–1826
66. del Zoppo GJ (1998) The role of platelets in ischemic stroke. Neurology 51 (Suppl 3):S9–14 (abst)
67. Stump DA, Kon NA, Rogers AT, Hammon JW (1996) Emboli and neuropsychological outcome following cardiopulmonary bypass. Echocardiography 13:555–558
68. Hall MW, Goodman PD, Alston SM, Solen KA (2002) Hypothermia-induced platelet aggregation in human blood in an in-vitro model: identification of a high responder subpopulation. Am J Hematology 69:45–55

How Can We Evaluate Information Provided to Family Members in the ICU?

E. Azoulay, D. Moreau, and F. Pochard

Introduction

Admission to the intensive care unit (ICU) signals the eruption of an acute disease process that puts, or may put, the patient's life in danger by compromising one or more vital functions. To stay alive, the patient must rely on sophisticated machines and highly skilled caregivers. This dependency indicates a condition so critical that many ICU patients are unable to understand their prognosis, diagnosis, or treatment; to draw conclusions by logical thinking; or to communicate their wishes about their own care [1–3].

Because ICU caregivers cannot inform their patients, they naturally turn towards the families. Family members are not viewed as simple visitors to the ICU but as people fully involved in what is happening and capable of bearing testimony to the patient's history and wishes [4].

Clearly, informing patients in the ICU raises specific issues. Recommendations on patient information are evolving in a way that challenges the 'paternalistic' nature of the patient-physician relationship. ICU admission does not involve any loss of the rights guaranteed to every individual by law. Implementing laws and regulations about patient information may not be feasible in the ICU. Yet, this neither relieves intensivists of their obligation to inform their patients nor severs the patient-physician relationship [5].

In the ICU, patients are so ill that they are often unable to make decisions. Thus, a specific characteristic of the ICU is that the traditional patient-physician relationship expands into a caregiver team-patient and family relationship. This expansion requires a profound and appropriate change in communication: in most cases, information of the patient is mediated by communication with family members and friends. In 1994, the quality of information given to families was added to the accreditation criteria used for ICUs affiliated to the Society of Critical Care Medicine (SCCM) [6]. Nevertheless, the goals pursued by informing ICU patients or their family remains intensely debated. The deontological and ethical principles on which the patient-physician relationship is built (beneficence, non-maleficence, autonomy, and justice) [7] require that the patient and family receive high-quality information on the diagnosis, prognosis, and management: this is the *first level* of family involvement in the ICU. The *second level* consists of asking family members to speak for the patient; their role here is to assist the caregivers in providing the type of care that the patient would choose if he or she were capable of expressing their wishes. This level of involvement implies optimal information that makes the family members aware of the crucial role they are being asked to play in an extraordinarily sensitive situation. At the *third level*, the ICU caregivers invite family members to participate in making decisions about the patient and in providing selected components of patient care [3, 4]. In the United Kingdom and North America, where patient autonomy is theoretically the rule, involvement of families in medical decision-making is supposedly routine, particularly as it is often the family members who pay at least part of the ICU bill. Sharing in care and decisions has recently been included in a family satisfaction scale [8]. Yet, shared decision-making raises many questions: Do the families have the knowledge needed to share in patient care and decision-making? Should the sharing be confined to issues related to personal values or should it extend to technical problems? Should the source of funds affects doctors choices of legitimate goals?

In France, decisions about ICU patients are usually made by physicians. Family members are usually informed, sometimes asked to give advice, and only rarely involved in decision-making. One factor that may contribute to this pattern is the limited financial cost to the families, as the cost of care is paid for by the national health insurance system.

Numerous studies have evaluated the quality of information delivered to the families of ICU patients. They have identified several factors that are central to fostering effective interactions among all the individuals affected by admission of a patient to the ICU.

Results of Family Information Studies

Three criteria have been suggested as appropriate for evaluating the effectiveness of information supplied to family members: comprehension of the information given by intensivists; satisfaction with both the quality of care and the interactions with caregivers; and severity of symptoms denoting anxiety and depression in family members [8-12].

If the patient or family does not understand, they cannot interact appropriately with the caregivers, and the family members cannot speak for the patient [9]. To be successful in sharing their knowledge, caregivers must deliver information in a manner that is adapted to each patient or family. When the disease process and treatment are extremely complex and change rapidly over time, the caregivers must lead the family to accept that gaps exist in their understanding of the diagnosis, optimal treatment, or prognosis in the patient. The family members and friends are viewed as the patient's natural protectors. They must understand what is at stake so that they can make the changes in family dynamics needed to adjust to the acute event. They can defend the patient's best interests only if they comprehend the diagnosis, become aware of the seriousness of the disease, and receive information on the main treatments used [13].

The satisfaction of family members indirectly reflects the extent to which their expectations are met. These expectations can be measured using the criteria suggested by Molter in 1979 [14] and used by the SCCM in 1994 to develop a family needs assessment tool [6, 15]. The 14 items in this tool were modified in 1998 by

Johnson et al. [11], who explored four domains: whether the family felt welcome at their first visit to the ICU; whether effective communication was established between caregivers and family members; whether the caregivers expressed empathy to the families; and whether the families felt alone during visits to the ICU or time spent in the waiting room. This tool has been evaluated in France and in Canada [10, 11]. A high degree of family satisfaction seems essential to a good interaction with the caregivers. In turn, this good interaction is needed to ensure optimal tailoring of medical decisions to the patient's wishes and to collect consent (or refusal to consent) to suggested treatments. Studies of the expectations of family members have highlighted an ethical aspect of information that is related to the principles of beneficence and autonomy; family members want honest information that is easy to understand, and they expect the ICU physicians to tell them of any changes that occur during the ICU stay.

Admission of a patient to the ICU usually plunges the family into a state of acute distress. Several studies have found that symptoms of anxiety and depression are extraordinarily common among family members of ICU patients [12, 16]. The impact of these symptoms on the decision-making capacity of family members deserves consideration and should be addressed by specific studies. A reasonable assumption is that symptoms of anxiety or depression impair the ability of family members to understand, to draw conclusions from logical thinking, and to communicate. Studies of such effects are urgently needed given the current trend towards increased involvement of families in medical decision-making.

Investigations conducted in Europe and North America have measured comprehension, satisfaction, symptoms of anxiety and depression, and the determinants of these characteristics in family members of ICU patients. They have identified several factors that can be acted on to better meet the informational needs of families [9–13, 16–18]. French studies have pinpointed the determinants of incomprehension, dissatisfaction, and symptoms of anxiety and depression. Here, we will focus on determinants that are dependent on the attitude of caregivers. These determinants are potential targets for efforts designed to improve the quality of information delivered to families.

In a study of 102 families, half the families did not understand the information they received from ICU physicians [9]. Comprehension was evaluated by asking family members to say in their own words what they had been told. Poor comprehension was more common among families who were allowed less time to receive information and who were not given a family information booklet. The results underlined the difficulty in providing understandable information to patients and families whose cultural background is different from that of the physician. Similarly, Ip et al. [19] pointed out that cross-cultural differences are an obstacle to sharing decision-making with the families of ICU patients.

The FAMIREA study measured satisfaction and symptoms of anxiety and depression in 920 family members of 637 patients enrolled by 43 French ICUs. The Critical Care Family Needs Inventory was used to measure satisfaction and the Hospital Anxiety depression scale (HADS) to measure anxiety and depression [12]. Caregiver-related factors associated with dissatisfaction included perceived contradictions in the information given, information delivered by more than one physician, and absence of knowledge by the families of the role of each caregiver.

Similarly, shorter time spent receiving information and absence of help from the family's own physician were independently associated with dissatisfaction. The perception by the family members that they were not allowed enough time to meet with physicians was a major determinant of dissatisfaction.

Determinants of symptoms of anxiety among family members included absence of regular physician-nurse meetings and absence of a room specifically set aside for informing families. Family members with symptoms of anxiety were more likely to ask for help from their own physician. Half the family members requested an interview with a psychologist, and family members who made such a request were twice as likely to have symptoms of anxiety than those who did not. Determinants of symptoms of depression were absence of a waiting room and perception by the family that they were receiving contradictory information.

In another study, 204 families received either a standardized family information leaflet or a blank sheet of paper, according to a random allocation scheme. Of the 175 evaluable family members, 87 received the leaflet and 88 did not. Symptoms of anxiety and depression occurred with similar prevalence in the two groups. In contrast, poor comprehension occurred in 40 % of family members who did not receive the leaflet as compared to only 12 % of those who did. Furthermore, in the subgroup with good comprehension, satisfaction was significantly better with the leaflet [20].

Three lessons can be drawn from these studies:
1) Family members of ICU patients want individualized information provided by a single physician. When a single physician is in charge of delivering information to the family, there is no risk of contradictory information. The leaflet used in the above-mentioned study was given to the family members by the informing physician, who wrote his or her name on the leaflet, thus becoming that family's own ICU physician.
2) Family members want help from their own physician (if they have one, whether a general practitioner or a specialist), who is usually aware of the family dynamics and can provide an independent point of view, promote communication and, if needed, explain recommendations made by the intensivists. Some families ask their own physician to help them speak for the patient. This is sparking interest into the possible benefits of enlisting the help of someone from outside the ICU to inform family members [21] and, if that person is a physician, to act as a mediator in ethical conflicts encountered in the ICU (including during end-of-life decisions). The French Consultative Committee of Ethics has recently recommended that patients designate representatives of their choice. A study conducted by Roupie et al. in an emergency department [22] suggests that family doctors, if they accept this role, may have a key part to play as patient representatives; nearly one-third of the study individuals designated not one but two representatives, ascribing to each a specific role. One representative was to receive information about the patient's condition and the other to participate in decisions should the patient become unable to do so. This model, in which one person receives information and another participates in decisions, may apply to many situations.

Table 1. Ten recommendations to intensivists about information in the ICU [23]

I. *Global information given orally, with adjunctive written information in three documents:*
   the patients medical chart
   the nurses log
   a family information booklet

II. *Information given to the families of the ICU patients*

III. *Information provided by a structured and accessible team*
   knowledge by the families of the role of each caregiver
   information provided by an intensivist-nurse dyad
   regular intensivist-nurse meetings at least once a week
   waiting room and room for providing information to families of the ICU patients

IV. *Family information leaflet*
   Standardized leaflet developed by the SRLF
   (Société de Réanimation de Langue Française)

V. *Modalities for providing information to families*
   reach out to the family without waiting for them to request information
   allow enough time
   provide information in a room set aside for that purpose
   give information on diagnosis, prognosis, and treatment
   give information in a setting-appropriate and timely manner

VI. *Attention to the specific issues raised by informing families from other cultures*

VII. *Accessibility of the ICU*
   visiting hours
   involvement of the family's usual physician
   involvement of a person from outside the ICU

VIII. *Interview with the patient before ICU discharge*

IX. *Clinical research and training specifically designed to improve information*

X. *Information and accreditation*

3) Finally, the place of choice given to spouses as recipients of information and as representatives raises a number of problems. In the FAMIREA study, which included all family members of each patient, spouses accounted for 25 % of family members. The spouse is acutely aware of the absence of the patient from home. Because the relationship in a couple is intimate, caregivers tend to feel particularly sympathetic toward spouses. However, in the FAMIREA study, 81 % of spouses had symptoms of anxiety and 47 % of depression, as compared to figures of 69 % and 35 %, respectively, for family members overall. This

difference invites an evaluation of the decision-making capacity of spouses of ICU patients.

Conclusion

Informing ICU patients and their families is central to improving the quality of care. Studies have evaluated the quality of information delivered to families of ICU patients. The results have been used by the Société de Réanimation de Langue Française to establish ten recommendations aimed at assisting caregivers in delivering information that is easy to understand, perceived as satisfactory, and designed to minimize anxiety and depression [23]. These recommendations are summarized in Table 1. Further evaluations are needed to build on the impetus propelling ICUs towards ever better procedures and caregiver skills.

References

1. Cohen LM, McCue JD, Green GM (1993) Do clinical and formal assessments of the capacity of patients in the intensive care unit to make decisions agree? Arch Intern Med 153:2481–2485
2. Ferrand E, Bachoud-Levi AC, Rodrigues M, Maggiore S, Brun-Buisson C, Lemaire F (2001) Decision-making capacity and surrogate designation in French ICU patients. Intensive Care Med 27:1360–1364
3. Jacob DA (1998) Family members' experiences with decision making for incompetent patients in the ICU: a qualitative study. Am J Crit Care 7:30–6
4. Molter NC (1994) Families are not visitors in the critical care unit. Dimens Crit Care Nurs 13:2–3
5. Cook D (2001) Patient autonomy versus parentalism. Crit Care Med 29:N24–N25
6. Harvey MA, Ninos NP, Adler DC, Goodnough-Hanneman SK, Kaye WE, Nikas DL (1993) Results of the consensus conference on fostering more humane critical care: creating a healing environment. Society of Critical Care Medicine. AACN Clin Issues Crit Care Nurs 4:484–549
7. Pochard F, Grassin M, Azoulay E (2001) Ethical principles for everyone. Ann Intern Med 134:1152
8. Wasser T, Pasquale MA, Matchett SC, Bryan Y, Pasquale M (2001) Establishing reliability and validity of the critical care family satisfaction survey. Crit Care Med 29:192–196
9. Azoulay E, Chevret S, Leleu G, et al (2000) Half the families of intensive care unit patients experience inadequate communication with physicians. Crit Care Med 28:3044–3049
10. Azoulay E, Pochard F, Chevret S, et al (2001) Meeting the needs of intensive care unit patient families: a multicenter study. Am J Respir Crit Care Med 163:135–139
11. Johnson D, Wilson M, Cavanaugh B, Bryden C, Gudmundson D, Moodley O (1998) Measuring the ability to meet family needs in an intensive care unit. Crit Care Med 26:266–271
12. Pochard F, Azoulay E, Chevret S, et al (2001) Symptoms of anxiety and depression in family members of intensive care unit patients: ethical hypothesis regarding decision-making capacity. Crit Care Med 29:1893–1897
13. Azoulay E, Pochard F (2002) Information provided to family members of ICU patients: beyond satisfaction. Crit Care Med (in press)
14. Molter NC (1979) Needs of relatives of critically ill patients: a descriptive study. Heart Lung 8:332–339
15. Harvey MA (1998) Evolving toward—but not to—meeting family needs. Crit Care Med 26:206–207

16. Perez-San Gregorio MA, Blanco-Picabia A, Murillo-Cabezas F, Dominguez-Roldan JM, Sanchez B, Nunez-Roldan A (1992) Psychological problems in the family members of gravely traumatised patients admitted into an intensive care unit. Intensive Care Med 18:278–281
17. McGaughey J, Harrison S (1994) Developing an information booklet to meet the needs of intensive care patients and relatives. Intensive Crit Care Nurs 10:271–277
18. Medland JJ, Ferrans CE (1998) Effectiveness of a structured communication program for family members of patients in an ICU. Am J Crit Care 7:24–29
19. Ip M, Gilligan T, Koenig B, Raffin TA (1998) Ethical decision-making in critical care in Hong Kong. Crit Care Med 26:447–451
20. Azoulay E, Pochard F, Chevret S, al (2002) Impact of a family information leaflet on the quality of the information provided to family members of intensive care unit patients. Am J Respir Crit Care Med 165:438–442
21. Pochard F, Azoulay E, Chevret S, Zittoun R (2001) Toward an ethical consultation in the ICU? Crit Care Med 29:1489–1490
22. Roupie E, Santin A, Boulme R, et al (2000) Patients' preferences concerning medical information and surrogacy: results of a prospective study in a French emergency department. Intensive Care Med 26:52–56
23. Azoulay E, Cattaneo I, Ferrand E, Pochard F (2001) L'Information au patient de Réanimation et à ses proches: le point de vue de la SRLF. Réanimation 10:571–581

Approaches to Improve Long-term Outcomes

How should we Measure the Economic Consequences of Critical Illness?

B. A. van Hout and D. C. Angus

Introduction

Florence Nightingale, surrounded by wounded soldiers, had only limited time, and choices had to be made about who to treat, how intensely to treat them, and for how long. It was a war, she was with few, and she became a hero. Health care in western societies is much more sophisticated, there are no domestic wars, doctors and nurses are with many, and they rarely become heroes. However, the need to make choices has not changed. Choices are made at all levels of health care; they are made at the governmental level when considering, for example, vaccination programs, and they are made at the level of doctor and patient when considering the best treatment.

Florence Nightingale could not do all she wanted. She was budgeted in terms of time, materials, and in the number of colleagues. Health care budgets – or limited resources – span across time, and intensive care, an area in health care that is associated with high costs, is not without its budgets. Costs of intensive care per day are often above $1,500 and an average admission costs over $10,000. Though costly, results are often heroic. Lives are saved and there can be little discussion about the value of intensive care unit (ICU) treatment. Within western society, it is hard to think of any person who would argue that $10,000 for a life saved is not offering value for money. But what if a new therapy comes available that increases the cost by $10,000 and for which the number needed to treat is around 100? In this case, the costs to save one additional life are $1,000,000. Does that still offer good value for money? The answer may be positive when imagining a young adult with a prognosis of 30 years after being discharged. But what if this concerns a cancer patient with a prognosis of one year or less? In this case one may argue that the same money might also be allocated to other types of medication or towards hiring more nurses. One might also argue that the money could be spend outside health care, for example for safety measures or to improve education, and naturally, that it may be used as free disposable income.

Without answering the questions of what is worthwhile and what is not, choices about the allocation of scarce resources in health care are best based on complete information about the consequences. Moreover, these consequences are best expressed in a structured way. This may facilitate comparisons, for example between buying a modern sepsis medication and hiring more nurses. Structuring the required information is an area of research labeled as 'medical technology assessment'. Within this area, therapies are assessed, in terms of costs, benefits, ethical aspects and legal considerations [1]. In this chapter, emphasis is placed on the economic consequences. In doing so, we will not be complete and we will concentrate on those aspects that are typical for critical illness. Over the last decade, excellent books have been published about assessing costs and effects [2, 3]. Moreover, guidelines have been published about how to make such assessments, for example, in Canada [4] and Australia [5]. We refer the reader to these books for a more extensive review.

Critical Illness

An economist, expressing himself in lay terms, may define critical illness as a certain stage within a disease process, say cancer or heart failure, where organ systems fail and where support is needed to help the human body to recover. Correspondingly, an economist may look at an ICU as a place where doctors are equipped with a number of measures to support failing organ systems, in such a way that natural recovery is catalyzed. For example, when the lung fails, there are lung-machines, when the kidney fails there is dialysis. There are medications to help the circulation of the blood and medications to support the functions of the heart and the liver.

So, the economist may look at the ICU as a production unit in which services are offered by intensive care doctors and ICU nurses who have access to a number of instruments in and outside the ICU. In all cases, fine-tuning is important. All organ functions depend on each other, many treatments are associated with serious side effects and all treatments are surrounded with uncertainty. The patient's health state may change per day and this may not always happen in a predictable way. Choosing the most appropriate diagnostics and the best treatment may be as much an art as a science. However, without exception, usage is made of scarce resources and they may be used in an alternative way. This implies costs and – even in the world of Scrooge McDuck – there comes a moment in which one may want to assess the various options in comparison with their effects.

The Health Care Costs

Thinking about costs is meaningless without thinking about effects. One does not spend $2,000 for an ICU day when one just wants a place to sleep. That would be rather expensive! However, it may be a bargain when one is critically ill. Thinking about costs is also meaningless without the possibility of using the same resources otherwise. Without a choice one does not have to think. So, costs always have to be seen in perspective of effects and in comparison to another strategy. It is therefore preferable to express the results of an economic evaluation in a two-dimensional plane such as in Figure 1. In this so-called cost effectiveness plane [6], four quadrants are found. When a therapy is associated with increased costs and increased effectiveness, it ends up in the northeast quadrant. When the therapy combines additional effectiveness with cost savings it ends up in the southeast

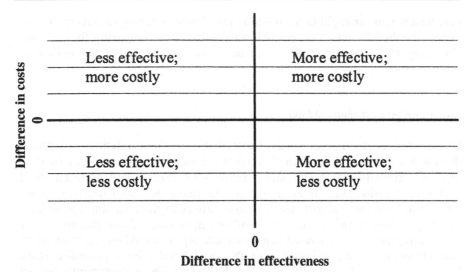

Fig. 1. The cost effectiveness plane

quadrant. If it is cost saving but less effective, it ends in the southwest quadrant, when it is increasing costs and less effective, it ends in the northwest.

Perspectives

The costs of a treatment may be assessed from various perspectives. From the perspective of a well-insured patient, costs may be limited to the costs of travelling to and from the hospital and to the costs associated with a decrease in income while ill. From the perspective of an insurance company the costs may be limited to the costs of the charges they need to reimburse. What perspective is taken is of crucial importance [7]. Imagine, for example, a new therapy with cost-offsets due to a decrease in the number of ICU days. As long as this does not have any financial consequences for the hospital, for example due to long term contracts, these savings may not be seen and the costs from the hospital perspective may just be the costs of the new therapy. Sure, one might treat more patients or one might treat patients longer with better effectiveness. But in that case, the question has to be raised what the value is of these changes, and again this has to be done from the perspective of the hospital.

The appropriate perspective depends on the question asked and on who asks the question. Here, it will be assumed that the question is posed from a societal point of view. This means that all consequences of critical illness should be included, monetary or non-monetary. Taking this perspective, it is usual to categorize costs as medical and non-medical costs and as direct and indirect costs. Additionally, taking this perspective, the outcomes of interest are 'life years gained' and 'quality adjusted life years (QALYs) gained'. The additional number of survivors may be a very meaningful outcome measure when comparing various treatment options on the ICU. It is, however, of limited value when comparing, for example, allocating more money to ICUs versus more money to the prevention of osteoporosis.

Direct and Indirect Medical Costs

Direct medical costs are those medical costs that have a direct relationship with the disease being treated. Indirect medical costs are the costs associated with treating other, non related diseases. The categorization between direct and indirect medical costs is often easily made. For example, when assessing the costs of heart transplantation, the direct medical costs are those associated with the screening, the surgery, the hospital admission, the costs of rehabilitation, the costs of immunosuppressive medication and the costs of re-admissions due to rejections. When heart transplant patients incur costs due to lung-cancer, they are labeled as indirect medical costs. Whether the indirect medical costs need to be included in an assessment is subject to debate. According to the Canadian and US guidelines they should be included. According to the Dutch and the Australian guidelines they should not.

With heart transplantation, the costs on the ICU are part of the direct medical costs and the division direct/indirect poses no problem. This is different for treatments that are started on the ICU. Patients are treated here for a variety of reasons, often in relation to surgery or to a complication occurring during the course of treating a disease. And so, whether the costs on the ward, and the costs after discharge are related to the costs of the critical illness is not as straightforward. The following argument will show that, whatever label the costs are given, they should be included.

Imagine a society in which families have to pay for their own health care. Additionally, imagine a large – say Dutch – family in which a family council takes the decisions about health care. Imagine further that the council consists of two lawyers, two accountants, and a grandmother. And further, imagine that a 90-year-old grandfather needs treatment on an ICU. The family council may come together and may want to assess the options. They are informed that treatment will cost $10,000 and that there will be a 75 % change that grandfather will survive. If grandfather is not admitted, he will die. Depending on the family's wealth, they may think this is worthwhile and may immediately decide on admission. Probably – remember this is a Dutch family – this decision will not be taken that fast. One of the accountants will realize that the information is not complete.

He will realize that the costs of critical illness may not be limited to the ICU. If grandfather survives, he will need to recover on a ward, at a cost of $5,000. Moreover, grandfather was already ill and after discharge he will need life long medication at $1,000 a year. Additionally, in relationship to the same underlying illness, it can be expected that grandfather will be hospitalized once a year at a cost of $9,000 per admission. So, when his life expectancy after discharge is estimated at 3.5 years, the expected costs are estimated at $40,000 = ($10,000 + 0.75 × 5,000 + 0.75 × 3.5 × ($1,000 + $9,000). Finally, the accountant may realize that (neglecting the time in the ICU) the expected number of life years is 2.625 years (0.75 [the probability of survival] times 3.5). And, being an accountant, he may want to express these costs in relationship to the effects. Calculating the costs per life year gained, here being equal to $15,238, may do this. Now, the family council may accept this or not. Probably, the lawyers will realize that whatever decision is taken, it may work as a precedent. They may think that if we are spending this money on grandfather, we also have to spend it on the other family members in case they need health care. Therefore, they decide to put a limit on what is acceptable or not. After ample discussion this limit is put at $30,000 per life year gained and grandfather is sent to the ICU.

Now, imagine that after grandfather has been admitted to the ICU, the family council is informed that grandfather has a diagnosis for which a new treatment is available. The costs are $5,000 and it will increase his probability of survival from 75 to 80 %. Will the family fund this? The family council may come together again and may again calculate the costs per life year gained. Following the same strategy as before, it will be estimated that the additional costs after ICU discharge are $2,000 and that treatment will increase his life expectancy by 0.175 years. So, including the $5,000 for the treatment, the costs per life year gained are estimated at exactly $40,000. Cruel, but they regard this as unacceptable. Grandfather will be treated on the ICU, but he will not get the new treatment.

Now, grandmother, who loves her husband, may suggest that the other members are biased by inclusion of the costs after discharge. She may suggest that the decision should be taken on the basis of the costs limited to the choice at that moment: whether grandfather should be treated on the ICU or not. And so, she may argue that the costs per life year gained are only $5,000/0.175: less than $30,000. It can be expected that the council's accountants will not agree. They will explain that the life expectancy that grandmother is using in her calculation depends on the costs in later years. In doing so, they may estimate that, when grandfather is not treated on the ward and if grandfather is not given the medication, that his life expectancy will only be 2 years. So, when no account is taken of the additional costs after being treated on the ICU, one should choose the corresponding life expectancy, which is then equal to 2 years. In that case the costs per life years gained are $5,000/0.05*2 = $50,000, which is again unacceptable.

The Short-term Costs on the ICU

When comparing the costs of two new therapies, costs are best calculated as the product of volumes of resource utilization and unit costs. How to calculate these most efficiently depends on the question asked and the way the data are most easily collected. Here, two approaches are distinguished. The first is labeled as a 'resource-data-driven' approach. The second is labeled as a 'disease-data-driven' approach.

The 'ressource-data-driven' approach. The 'ressource-data-driven' approach refers to situations where data about resource utilization can be collected per patient together with data about effects, typically alongside randomized clinical trials [8, 9]. The main question is what to collect. When the assessment concerns a therapy that is expected to decrease length of stay without changing the average resource use per day, one may limit oneself to registering the length of stay and to calculating the average costs per day. When one assumes that the new therapy also changes resource utilization during the time on the ICU, one may want to collect more detailed costs. Sometimes, this can be done very precisely, for example when the study is carried out in only one center and usage can be made of automated billing systems (or when several centers use the same type of billing system). When this is not possible, collecting information may best be limited to the big-ticket items and to these items where differences are expected. In any case, a distinction between the hotel costs, the time spent by doctors and nurses, the costs of medication, and a distinction between the costs of diagnostic and therapeutic interventions may be helpful in understanding the effects of the treatment on the costs.

Ideally, unit costs reflect the real costs associated with the unit of resource utilization. Often, such estimates are not available and tariffs can be used as a first approximation. However, this may bias the results and corrections may be needed. For example when applying US tariffs, one may apply 'cost-to-charge ratios'. Another example may concern the cost of nursing. Nursing time may differ per day and assuming no differences may not reflect the real differences in cost related to the compared therapies. A potential solution is found in the registration of therapeutic intervention scoring system (TISS) points. If one knows the total number of TISS-points on a department, one might calculate the costs of nursing per TISS point per day and calculate the costs of nursing per patient. This is the product of the patient's total TISS points (during the whole admission) and the cost per TISS point per day. In all cases cost-calculations can be laborious, and the resources that are needed to collect the relevant data have to be weighed against the value of the added information.

The 'disease-data-driven' approach. When weighing the value of the added information about costs, the decision is often that only limited data will be collected. And this is often in contrast with data about effectiveness. In those cases it may be worthwhile to establish a relationship between effectiveness data and costs. For example, it may happen that there are no detailed data about costs but that there are detailed data about organ failure as measured by the sequential organ failure assessment (SOFA) score [10]. Estimating a relationship between the costs of treatment and the SOFA score may then be very helpful. Such a relationship may, for example, be estimated using data that were not necessarily collected during the study comparing the new therapy. For this purpose, data might be used from one's own hospital or country. When this relationship is identified one may predict the costs of treatment by using this relationship in combination with the collected SOFA score data. Such an approach might be labeled a 'disease-data-driven' approach; it may also be very helpful when the effectiveness data are collected in an international study. While data about efficacy are often assumed to be universal, data about costs are not allowed to cross borders knowing that treatment patterns may differ considerably. Additionally, given the variability of cost data, data from international trials may be insufficient to identify country differences in treatment patterns. This may be relevant particularly when considering rare events. Additional data, collected outside the study, focusing on the treatment patterns and costs per country may be most appropriate [11].

The Long-term Costs after Discharge from the ICU

As indicated before, the costs of treatment are not limited to the costs on the ICU and data collection should not be limited to the ICU-treatment or to 28 days after starting the treatment. Nevertheless, at a certain moment data collection has to end. When – at that moment – there are still differences in survival, extrapolations are needed to calculate the differences in costs and effects [12]. The average expected costs are best extrapolated using a rule, or a model, that predicts costs as a function of each patient's characteristics at the end of the observation period. As such, the precise estimate may depend on the age/gender distribution of the surviving group as well as the presence/absence of co-morbidities. Such predictions are always surrounded with uncertainties. This is even the case in cardiology where data can be used from cohort studies such as the Framingham database. There, the uncertainties arise due to fact that the Framingham population may not represent the average patient, due to changes in treatment patterns, changes in survival after myocardial infarction, increases in the incidence of heart failure, etc. However, despite the uncertainties, cardiologists may consider themselves extremely wealthy in terms of data in comparison to critical care doctors in search of similar data about what happens with patients after an ICU admission. While waiting for better data from large – long term – cohort studies, alternative approaches have to be followed. An example of such an alternative is found in the analysis plan of the Prowess database assessing the life long benefits of activated drotrecogin alfa in severe sepsis [13]. The approach starts with calculating the number of life-years by first generating an age- and gender-specific life expectancy for each 28-day survivor from life table data. Subsequently, this life expectancy is corrected using the relative risk of death for sepsis survivors (0.51) determined from Quartin et al. [14]. By doing do, each patient is assigned a corrected life expectancy. One might interpret this as if each patient is assigned a new age. Someone of 60 years of age suddenly becomes 75 years of age. Now, given each patient's new age (gender remains the same) one may predict each patient's remaining health care costs by combining age specific life tables with estimates of age-specific annual health care costs such as obtained from National Medical Expenditure Surveys.

Direct and Indirect Non-medical Costs

When considering what costs should be included in the economic assessment we imagined a large Dutch family with no health insurance considering the ICU treatment of grandfather. Again taking the perspective of this family, one may easily come to the conclusion that a distinction between medical and non-medical costs is not relevant. All costs need to be included in the assessment, including those related to traveling from and to the hospital and including the costs related to the help of the partner, for example in the case of treatment with home dialysis. These latter costs are traditionally labeled as direct non-medical costs.

Another category of costs, traditionally distinguished in economic assessments, concerns the indirect non-medical costs. To illustrate these, let us assume that it is not the grandfather in need of ICU treatment but a nephew, 35 years of age and working in the family factory. The difference with grandfather is that the nephew, in relationship to his work, earns money for the family. If he dies, that money is lost and the accountants may want to take these losses into account. It is estimated that he would have worked for another 30 years, implying a decreased family-income of 30 times his annual salary. This approach is called the human capital approach. Now, it may be that one of the accountants notes that another nephew is unemployed and that he might take the job of the one who needs the ICU treatment. He may calculate that it will take a couple of months to get him to the same level and he may argue that, in this case, the only relevant cost is that part of the family-income that is lost due to the replacement. Taking account of this substitution process is called the friction-cost approach [15]. What method to choose depends on the potential for substitution.

Grandmother may now note that these rude calculations will discriminate against the elderly and that they may discriminate against the housewives in the family (often having two children). She will be told that it may indeed be possible that the elderly will be discriminated against but she may be given the option to correct for this by assigning some additional value to the lives of the elderly. While telling her this, it may be pointed out to her that savings lives irrespective of age implies that life years gained by the elderly are given a higher weight than those gained by younger patients. While pointing this out, the question can be raised whether we really value life years gained by the elderly higher than life years gained by younger individuals. With respect to the housewives, grandmother will be told that when replacement is needed with financial consequences, that these have to be taken into account. Additionally, one might assign an added value to the fact that their own mother raises the children. In theory, ethical norms may be incorporated in the evaluation process. How to do this in practice may be very difficult and the family council may choose not to do this in an explicit way. Other considerations may be taken into account and it may be a wise idea not to limit decision making on the basis of cost effectiveness calculations alone.

The Health Care Benefits

It is commonly acknowledged that health care does not only aim at increasing survival but also aims at improving quality of life. And when assessing the effectiveness of a therapy, it is becoming more and more common to assess this. Currently, measuring quality of life is a flourishing line of research throughout Western health care [16]. Every disease seems to have its own disease specific questionnaire and already in 1995 Bowling assessed the use of 69 measures of health and of over 200 disease specific measures [17]. Such disease specific measures are especially helpful when assessing the effectiveness of a therapy as they focus on those items that are typically affected by the disease under investigation. For an economist, trying to value the effects of one therapy versus another, disease specific measures are not very useful.

Let us get back to our imaginary Dutch family. The family council has decided to limit what is acceptable at $30,000 per life year gained. Now one nephew may need bypass surgery. It is noted that the survival benefits are limited and the costs per life years gained are estimated at $100,000. According to the decision-rule that is based on costs per life year gained, this would not be acceptable. However, surgery is expected to completely relieve the angina and the decision rule that is based on life years only may nor reflect the preferences of the family. Large gains in quality of life may be valued higher than small gains in length of life. So, a new decision rule is needed, including not only survival but also quality of life. One way to do this is by weighing the various life years with an index reflecting the quality of those life years: by calculating 'QALYs' gained. This implies that life years are multiplied with an index that takes the value 0 for a life year that is valued equal to not being alive. Temporarily, the value may be under zero, reflecting a health state worse than death.

Making choices between quality of life improvements and gains in survival may be a difficult task and family members may state that such is impossible. However, it is not that such choices are never made. Bypass surgery may lead to permanent relief of angina. However, surgery is not without risk and this risk, including the potential of death, has to be weighed against the potential gains. In the case of bypass surgery, most people will decide in favor of surgery. However, there are more risky types of surgery, or leading to smaller benefits, where the choice is not made so easily. Additionally, improvements in one aspect of quality of life may also be weighed against another aspect. For example, people with hernia may weigh the benefits of an operation against the risk of drop-foot as a consequence. And so, tradeoffs are being made between length of life and quality of life and between various aspects of quality of life. This is not impossible, it is daily practice.

The difference here is that the decision is not an individual one, but one of a family council faced with balancing the benefits of various therapies for various family members. The one therapy may have effects on pain, the other on anxiety, a third on mobility and so on. Moreover, gains from one person are weighed against the gains of another, gains in one disease area are weighed against gains in another disease area. Knowing that resources are not unlimited, decisions will be made. And now the main question is how to obtain the weights that will be assigned to the various health states to obtain the QALY estimates.

Since the late eighties economist have been involved with the question of how to obtain weights reflecting the value of quality of life. The most prevalent solution is by using measurement instruments that lead to health state descriptions for which valuations are available. The EQ-5D (Euro Quality of Life – 5 Dimensions) is one of these instruments, the HUI-3 (Health Utilities Index) is another, both developed aimed at measuring as well as valuing differences in quality of life [18, 19]. Recently, algorithms have been published to calculate valuations using measurements obtained with the Short-Form (SF)-36 another well-known generic-measurement instrument [20]. For all instruments, values are obtained that reflect valuations of the general public as if the whole family is included in the way the various weights are defined (and not only those who are ill).

The assessment and valuation of quality of life is still an area of research where a lot of work may be needed in terms of methodology. However, decisions about scarce resources are being taken and when research is aimed to support such decisions it is advised to always add one of the three before mentioned instruments. When considering intensive care treatment, with a variety of underlying diseases, each with its own disease specific questionnaire, using these instruments may even have the additional benefits of enabling straightforward comparisons.

Assessing the Uncertainties

Although the word 'evidence' in evidence-based medicine may suggest some kind of certainty, health care is loaded with uncertainties. In the case of the grandfather being treated on the ICU there is a 30 % probability that he will survive. This is a first type of uncertainty. Additionally, this 30 % is an estimate and this estimate is also surrounded with uncertainty. That is a second type of uncertainty. The same is true for costs, they may be estimated at $10,000, but again, this is an estimate that is surrounded with uncertainty. The magnitude of the uncertainty may have consequences for the decision. Our family council was prepared to have grandfather treated when the costs per additional survivor are under $30,000. However, searching for some certainty, they might change their decision rule for example into the demand that the costs per life year gained have to be under $30,000 with 95 % certainty.

Over the last decade, economists have been very active in developing ways to express the uncertainties surrounding the outcomes of economic assessments. When presenting the results from a randomized clinical trial, uncertainties may be expressed within the cost effectiveness (CE)-plane (Fig. 1) using probability ellipses [21]. Figure 2 presents such an ellipse for the case of a new treatment in which – based on data from a trial with 2,500 patients the additional costs after 28 days are estimated at $5,000 and the additional number of survivors at 5 %. The right-angled shape of the ellipse illustrates the correlation between costs and effects. Patients who die have lower costs and, as a consequence, the higher the difference in the

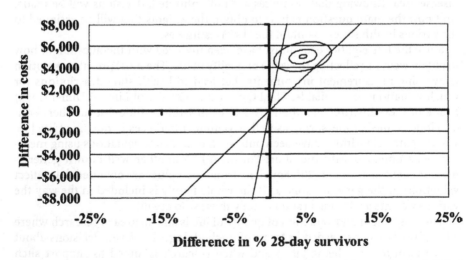

Fig. 2. Uncertainty surrounding costs and effects as measured alongside a randomized clinical trial, expressed by probability ellipses

number of survivors, the higher the differences in costs. The central estimate of the costs per additional survivor is $100,000, the 95 % confidence intervals, illustrated by the straight lines is estimated at ($ 62,000 and $245,000). Suppose that one assumes that $200,000 is the limit of what is acceptable, then the probability that this therapy fulfills this criterion is estimated at 91 %. The latter probability may be estimated for each limit. Figure 3 presents the curve that results after calculating this probability for each imaginable limit; a so-called acceptability curve.

It is noted that the approach chosen here is parametric. The uncertainties may also be addressed by bootstrapping [22]. This means that a number of new trials, say 1,000 are simulated by drawing at random – with replacement – from the data of the original trial. Each new simulated trial (of similar size) leads to a new estimate of both costs and effects and the results may again be pictured in the CE-plane. Figure 4, shows the results of 250 draws, corresponding to the results from Figures 2 and 3.

The results in the figures are illustrative of an assessment of costs and effects based on data from a randomized clinical trial with a short-term horizon. As indicated before, costs per additional survivor may be informative from the ICU point of view but not from a societal perspective. In that case, estimates of costs per life year gained are better suited. For the purpose of calculating these, extrapolations are needed, and this extrapolation is again surrounded with uncertainty. One way to express this is by multivariate sensitivity analysis. In case of a modeling study, such an analysis starts with defining distributions that reflect the uncertainties surrounding all variables that determine the outcomes. Subsequently, one calculates the main outcomes (expected costs and effects), say 10,000 times while drawing at random from all distributions. The main outcomes differ per simulation. This leads to a distribution of outcomes that reflects the uncertainty surrounding these outcomes. When data are available from a randomized clinical trail with data up till day 28, one may link the model to each patient to predict each patient's

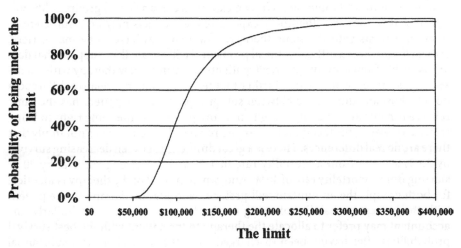

Fig. 3. The acceptability curve

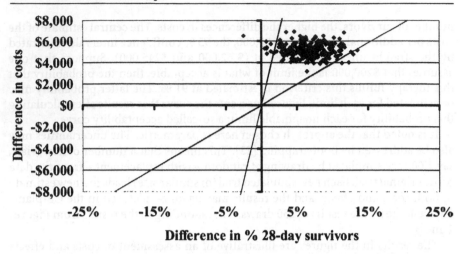

Fig. 4. Uncertainty surrounding costs and effects as measured alongside a randomized clinical trial, resulting from bootstrapping

future costs and effects. Now, new trials can be simulated using bootstrapping and within each bootstrap one may draw at random from the uncertainty distribution. When picturing the results concerning costs and life years gained, similar results are seen as in figure 4 but now with the additional number of life years gained on the vertical axis.

Sub-group Analysis

Often, when introducing new therapies, results are interpreted with skepticism and doctors want to start building their own experience in a selected group. Additionally, new therapies are often more expensive and budgets may be insufficient to treat all patients with the same therapy. Again choices have to be made. Here, critical illness faces a difficult, ethical problem. To illustrate this, suppose that data are available from a study with 2,500 patients assessing a new therapy with a net 5 % increase in survival. Assume further that tests assessing the relative differences do not show any differences between sub-groups. So, every patient has the same relative benefits and one might argue that any person has the same right to being treated. However, the fact that there are no relative differences does not imply that there are no real differences. There is a great difference between decreasing survival by 20 % starting from a mortality rate of 1 % and decreasing survival by 20 % starting from a mortality rate of 40 %. And, when the cost of the therapy is identical for both groups, the accountant will prefer to allocate the therapy to the patient with the highest probability of dying on the ICU. Moreover, and similarly, the accountant may prefer to allocate the therapy to the patient with the best survival probabilities after having been discharged from the ICU. There is a substantial difference in expected gains when confronted with two patients, both with a 30 %

probability of dying on the ICU, but one with a life expectancy of one year and another with a life expectancy of 20 years. So, from a cost effectiveness point of view it will often be most beneficial to limit treatment – when needed – to those patients who benefit the most while being critically ill and with a long life expectation after having been critically ill: patients with bad APACHE scores without co-morbidity.

Naturally, one may also study the data from the trials to find patients for whom the therapy is most beneficial. Unfortunately, these data are often of limited value. Trials are typically powered to find a certain difference in a group of patients and after the trial has confirmed effectiveness, this is mostly for the whole group. Testing for differences of pre-defined sub-groups may be informative but the power of these tests is rather limited. Moreover, the probability that one finds a negative effect in a sub-group, while the real effect is not different than that from the whole is substantial. For example, suppose that the real effect is an increase in survival from 75 to 80 % and that this has been confirmed in a trial with 2,500 patients. Assume further that the trial only includes 200 patients under the age of 45 for whom the same difference applies. The probability of finding a negative result in this subgroup is over 15 %. So, be aware.

Conclusion

Cost effectiveness aims at informing decision makers about the balance between the costs and effects of alternative therapies. In this chapter, a brief introduction is given, concentrating on the problems when doing this type of research in critical illness. We imagined an uninsured Dutch family, where decisions are taken about who to treat. It is hard to imagine that any decision in health care will ever be taken in such a cold, deterministic way as happens in this imaginary family. However, decisions are being taken, hidden or explicit. Moreover, if resources are limited and there are unused possibilities to treat people effectively, there will always be someone who will be treated in a sub-optimal way. That person has a right to know why. Making choices in health care will never be easy and cost effectiveness analysis is no panacea. However, it will make decision making more transparent, more predictable, and it will allow for better-defined criticism. That may be worth a lot.

References

1. Glasser JH, Chrzanowski RS (1988) Medical Technology Assessment, appropriate methods, valuable answers, Health Policy 3:267–276
2. Drummond, B O'Brien, GL Stoddart, GW Torrance (1997) Methods for the Economic Evaluation of Health Care Programmes, 2nd Edition. Oxford Medical Publications, Oxford
3. Gold MR, Siegel JE, Russell LB, Weinstein MC (1996) Cost-effectiveness in Health and Medicine. Oxford University Press, New York
4. Ontario Ministry of Health (1994) Ontario Guidelines for Economic Analysis of Pharmaceutical Products. Ontario Ministry of Health, Toronto
5. Commonwealth department of human services and health (1995) Guidelines for the Pharmaceutical industry on Preparation of Submissions to the Pharmaceutical Benefits Advisory

Committee including major submissions involving economic analyses. Australian Government Publishing Service, Canberra

6. Black WC (1990) The CE plane – A graphic representation of cost-effectiveness, Med Decis Making 10:212–214
7. Mansley EC, McKenna MT (2001) Importance of perspective in economic analyses of cancer screening decisions, Lancet 358:1169–1173
8. Serruys PW, Unger F, Sousa JE, et al (2001) Comparison of coronary-artery bypass surgery and stenting for the treatment of multivessel disease. N Engl J Med 344:1117–1124
9. Serruys PW, Van Hout B, Bonnier B, et al (1998) Randomised comparison of implantation of heparin-coated stent with balloon angioplasty in selected patients with coronary artery disease (Benestent II). The Lancet 352:673–681
10. Vincent JL, Moreno R, Takala J et al (1996) The SOFA (sepsis-related organ failure assessment) score to describe organ dysfunction/failure. Intensive Care Med 7:707–710
11. Zwart-van Rijkom JEF, van Hout BA (2001) Cost-efficacy in interventional cardiology; results from the EPISTENT study. Eur Heart J 22:1476–1484
12. Buxton, MJ, Drummond MF, Van Hout BA, et al (1997) Modeling in economic evaluation: an unavoidable fact of life. Health Econ 6:217–227
13. Bernard GR, Vincent JL, Laterre PF, et al (2001) Efficacy and safety of recombinant human activated protein C for severe sepsis. N Engl J Med 344:699–709
14. Quartin AA, Schein RM, Kett DH, et al (1997) Magnitude and duration of the effect of sepsis on survival. JAMA 277:1058–1063
15. Koopmanschap MA, Rutten FFH, Van Ineveld BM, Van Roijen L (1995) The friction cost method for measuring indirect costs of disease. J Health Econ 14:171–189
16. Fayers PM, Machn D (2000) Quality of Life, Assessment, Analysis and Interpretation. John Wiley and Sons, Chichester
17. Bowling A (1995) Measuring Disease, a Review of Life Measurement Scales. Open University Press, Philadelphia
18. Dolan P (1997) Modeling valuations for EuroQol health states. Med Care 35:1095–1108
19 Feeny D, Furlong W, Torrance GW, et al (2002) Multiattribute and single-attribute utility functions for the health utilities index mark 3 system. Med Care 40:113–128
20. Brazier J, Roberts J, Deverill M (2002) The estimation of a preference-based measure of health from the SF-36. J Health Econ 21:271–292
21. Van Hout BA, Al M ,Gordon GS, Rutten FFH (1994) Costs, effects and C/E-ratio's alongside a clinical trial. Health Econ 3:309–319
22. Briggs AH, Wonderling DE, Mooney CZ (1997) Pulling cost-effectiveness analysis up by its bootstraps: A non-parametric approach to confidence interval estimation. Health Econ 6:327–340

Modifying Triage Decisions to Optimize Long-term Outcomes

C. L. Sprung and P. D. Levin

Introduction

The triage decision determines whether a patient is admitted into an intensive care unit (ICU) and for some patients, this decision will determine whether the patient lives or dies. When standing next to a patient's bed and deciding whether or not to admit the patient, or alternatively, when forced to refuse a patient who could benefit from ICU care due to lack of space, triage decisions may become heart wrenching dilemmas.

Unfortunately, little definitive evidence is available to assist the physician in deciding which patient to admit for medical reasons and sparse data are available for the 'system' to determine strategies to optimize capacity, efficiency and the use of ICUs.

This chapter will describe the background to the triage dilemma, the problems, existing studies in the field, suggestions for future work, and recommendations based on current knowledge.

Background

Deciding which patient will be admitted to ICU is a medical and ethical problem facing intensivists on a daily basis. The demand for medical services such as critical care often exceeds supply [1] and rationing of ICU beds is common [2, 3]. Despite the expense and importance of the issue of triage of ICU beds, few studies have been performed [3–13]. The utilization of intensive care beds is not efficient. The majority of patients and families are willing to undergo intensive care to achieve a one month survival [14] and most ICU doctors admit patients with no hope of surviving more than a few weeks [2, 15].

Spending for intensive care is a significant proportion of health care charges. American health care spending has increased over the last several years to $800 billion, more than 14 % of the gross national product [16]. Since the introduction of ICUs in the 1960s, their number has increased in hospitals throughout the world. Although critical care beds account for approximately 8 % of hospital beds in the United States, 28 % of charges for acute hospital care come from ICUs and comprise more than 1 % of the gross national product [17]. The percentage of ICU beds in

Europe is lower (5 %) but still consumes approximately 20% of the hospital budget [18].

Unfortunately, the indications for ICU admission and discharge remain poorly defined and the identification of patients who can benefit from ICU is extremely difficult. A detrimental mismatch between provision and demands of resources was demonstrated in approximately 75 % of the 89 ICUs studied in 12 European countries [18]. Tremendous and unpredictable diversity was found in the use and costs of different ICUs [18]. Waste of resources occurred in as many as 50 % of ICUs [18]. This was due to the lack of appropriate guidelines for the provision of ICU resources and the dominant use of ICUs for surgical patients who could be cared for in a less expensive unit [18]. None of the ICUs had written admission and discharge policies [18]. Several authors have stressed an urgent need for more appropriate ICU admission criteria [6, 11, 12].

It is likely that with the advent of more complex medical procedures and with increasing patient expectations, ICU costs will increase further and the demand will exceed the available health care budget. As a result, it is imperative that the available resources are used effectively. This will require the appraisal of not only traditional endpoints such as ICU and hospital survival, but also long term survival, quality of life and cost effective analyses.

Present Recommendations

The demand for intensive care exceeds its availability [1, 19]. Demand has increased due to physician and family requests, an aging, more chronically ill population, new technologies, and more difficult operations, whereas capacity is limited by inadequate reimbursements, facilities and staff [1]. When the demand for ICU beds exceeds their supply, how should physicians decide who to admit? In theoretical discussions of the micro allocation (selection between individual patients) of scarce resources, several criteria have been proposed.

Beauchamp and Childress described the need for two sets of substantive and procedural rules [20]. Their first rule is to determine the relevant pool of potential recipients or those eligible for the scarce resource and the second for final selection or the definitive decision who to admit. Various criteria for the final selection are shown in Table 1 [20, 21].

The Society of Critical Care Medicine's (SCCM) Consensus Statement on triage stated that priority for admission should be given to patients who are more likely to benefit from ICU care when compared with non-ICU care [1]. The American Thoracic Society (ATS) statement on triage did not recommend ICU triage based on grounds of relative benefit if two patients were competing for the same ICU bed [19]. They stated that these decisions are too morally problematic to define and ranking relative degrees of potential benefit without ambiguity, bias or subjectivity is extremely difficult [19]. The ATS recommendation was that all patients who exceed the threshold for minimal benefit and needs should be treated the same on a first-come, first-served basis [19]. But how should this be determined? Is it the patient who arrives in the Emergency Department first, the patient who the intensivist is first called about, or who is examined first? Intensivists do not believe age

Table 1. Criteria for Selection of ICU patients

– Medical benefit	– Social worth
– Life expectancy	– Societal contribution and status
– Medical need or urgency	– Age
– Prospect of successful treatment	– Mental functioning
– Need	– Self created health risks
– Merit	– Compensatory justice
– Committee	– Iatrogenic injuries
– The market	– Chance or queuing

should be used as a criteria to exclude patients from the ICU [15] but several studies demonstrate that the elderly are less likely to be admitted [12, 13]. In practice, some seemingly medically ineligible patients who do not meet the first set of rules are admitted to ICUs; most patients are admitted on a first come, first served basis or as a result of a substantive assessment of greater benefit [1, 19].

The Problem

Triage decisions are extremely complex. There have been few studies of ICU triage and of criteria for ICU admission and discharge. It is important to evaluate the wide context of triage. The triage process is extremely complex and made up of several elements. The classical triage decision relates to whether a patient should be admitted to an ICU but the chain starts before and ends after the ICU [22]. Patients who require ICU admission have to be referred to the hospital (self-triage), the severity of their disease has to be recognized (pre-triage), the ICU physician has to admit the patient (ICU triage), and a place in the ICU may have to be made available (post-triage) (Fig. 1) [22]. Many patients requiring ICU care remain hospitalized on general wards without the ICU triage officer even knowing about their presence in the hospital.

What outcome should be used to define benefit? A National Institute of Health (NIH) consensus conference studying intensive care concluded that ICUs decrease mortality and morbidity for a sub select group of patients but that in a majority of patients the evidence was equivocal [23]. ICUs may prolong life but they can also prolong the dying process [24]. An SCCM Task Force on guidelines concluded that ICUs should be reserved for patients with reversible medical conditions who have "a reasonable prospect of substantial recovery" [25]. If ICU admission should be reserved for those patients that benefit and recover, patients who are 'too well' or 'too sick' should be excluded. But how is benefit and recovery to be defined and by whom? Is benefit ICU, hospital, or one year survival, or is it a good quality of life? Is benefit to be determined by the health care professional, the patient, family, judge or society? Even if physicians evaluate benefit in terms of mortality, is it based on the total risk of death or the difference in the risk between medical treatment in and out of the ICU?

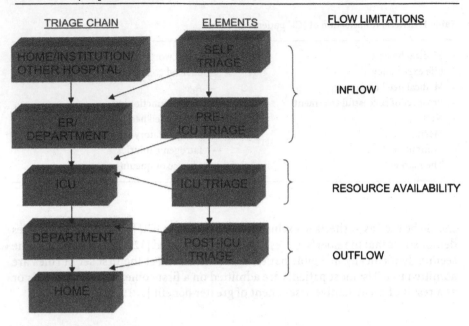

Fig. 1. The spectrum of triage. Adapted from [22] with permission

Factors that have been considered important in determining benefit for triage in a consensus statement include: likelihood of a successful outcome, the patient's life expectancy due to disease(s), anticipated quality of life of the patient, wishes of the patient and/or surrogate, burdens for those affected, health and other needs of the community, and individual and institutional moral and religious values [1].

Is it valid to have exclusion criteria for ICU admission rather than to define patients to be admitted? At times it is easier to define which patients should be excluded rather than included. Conditions have been defined with limited medical suitability, low priority, or for exclusion from the ICU. These include: terminal, irreversible illness; persistent vegetative or permanently unconscious state; irreversible multiorgan failure; unresponsive metastatic carcinoma; brain dead non-organ donors; and patients declining intensive care and/or invasive monitoring [1, 25, 26]. Unfortunately, non-objective factors not related to a patient's illness are sometimes used for triage decisions. These include: doctor or family pressure and persistence; age; difficulty in caring for the patient (patient receiving mechanical ventilation or vasopressors); ICU census; elective surgery; location in hospital; seniority of requesting and triaging physician; socioeconomic status; interpersonal relationships; and hospital priorities [7, 12, 13, 22, 24].

Are there any guidelines presently available to help physicians make these difficult triage decisions? Several guidelines and criteria for ICU and intermediate care admission and discharge have been published [25, 27–29]. These are based on models of prioritization, diagnosis, objective parameters and/or therapies [25, 27–29]. Unfortunately, they have been developed by consensus opinion with few

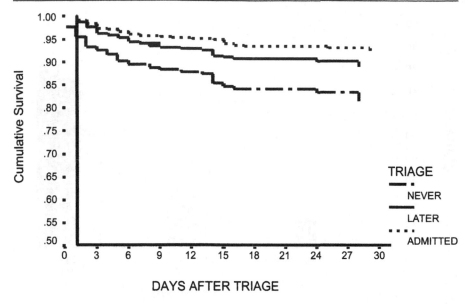

Fig. 2. Cox model comparing the cumulative survival estimates during a 28-day period of triaged patients who were admitted later (solid line; n= 30; relative risk = 1.4; p = 0.40), never admitted (dashed line; n = 43; relative risk = 2.5; p 0.01), and admitted (dotted line; n = 276; relative risk = 1), controlling for APACHE II scores. Adapted from [2] with permission.

or no scientifically rigorous data. There are no prospective studies of patients admitted or not or discharged or not, based on predefined admission or discharge criteria. In addition, the guidelines provide little help for clinicians at the bedside having to make triage decisions on several patients when insufficient beds are available [30].

Why can available outcome measures such as severity scores not be used for triage? Although sophisticated severity scoring systems including APACHE II and III [30, 31], Simplified Acute Physiology Score (SAPS I and II) [32], and Mortality Probability Models (MPM$_0$, I and II) [33] have been developed for prognosticating intensive care mortality, none have been produced for intensive care triage [34]. Current criteria used for intensive care admission and refusal are not based on scientific data and may vary from institution to institution or within the same institution depending on the triaging doctor. At times these decisions are arbitrary.

Previous Studies

Many of the past studies of ICU triage were general studies of patients usually in ICUs but not studies of individual decisions to accept or reject a patient [3–7]. Some evaluated seriously ill patients found in and out of the ICU for effect of ICU care [5, 8, 9]. Recent studies have prospectively examined patients admitted or refused ICU care [11–13] or all patients requiring ICU care within a hospital (Sprung et al.,

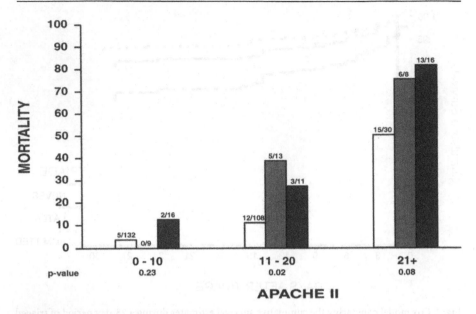

Fig. 3. Hospital mortality of patients initially accepted (white), later accepted (gray), or never accepted (black) to intensive care as a function of APACHE II scores.

unpublished data). None of these studies evaluated long term survival, quality of life or economic issues. In these studies of all triaged patients, non-admitted patients had a significantly higher mortality than admitted patients [11–13] as did patients with a delayed ICU admission [12] (Fig. 2). Triage to intensive care correlated with the number of available beds, diagnosis, age, and severity of illness [12, 13]. The greatest benefit of ICU care appeared to be in the mid range of severity of illness [12, 13] (Fig. 3).

Even the studies examining triaged patients to the ICU, do not recognize actual ICU needs as many doctors do not request ICU beds especially when they are repeatedly told there are no available ICU beds. An accurate estimation of ICU bed requirements would require an evaluation of all hospitalized patients meeting ICU admission criteria. Such a study was recently performed (Sprung et al., unpublished data). During four random days, all hospitalized patients in five Israeli hospitals were screened for ICU admission criteria (Sprung et al., unpublished data). In this prevalence study, 5.5 % of patients met ICU admission criteria and half the patients were treated in regular wards and not ICUs (Sprung et al., unpublished data). Survival was advantageous for ICU patients during the first days but not thereafter (Sprung et al., unpublished data).

When less ICU beds are available for admission, fewer patients are admitted to the ICU and those patients admitted are more severely ill [3, 4]. ICU resources were denied to patients who were to be monitored rather than patients with little likelihood of surviving [3, 4]. Many studies have shown that ICUs are not used correctly. Patients are admitted to the ICU for non-intensive monitoring [35–39].

The number of intermediate care patients in ICUs range from 23–78 % [35–39]. An evaluation of the clinical information available on admission and for the first seven ICU days in 17,440 ICU admissions in 42 US ICUs revealed that current day therapy, APACHE III score, diagnosis, age, chronic health status, emergency surgery, previous day Acute Physiologic Score, and hospital stay and location before ICU admission determined the next day risk for life support [36]. Survival, ICU readmission rate, and the number and type of therapies could predict a < 10 % risk for active treatment suggesting that these patients could be discharged earlier without compromising their safety [36]. Up to 78 % of the neurosurgical patients who underwent monitoring in an ICU were at low risk for subsequent active therapy and may not have required ICU care at all [39]. In addition, up to 25 % of patients die after discharge from the ICU, many with a low predicted mortality, perhaps secondary to premature ICU discharge [40].

Post-ICU triage and outflow have received little if any investigation. This includes ICU discharge criteria and problems moving patients out of the ICU because of lack of intermediate or ward beds or because of physician or family pressure to keep a patient in the ICU [22]. Hopeless patients in ICUs are rarely discharged and do not undergo more rapid withdrawal [3, 4]. Patients often stay in the ICU because wards are incapable of caring for critically ill, dying patients. One study demonstrated that 27 % of total ICU bed days were used for patients who did not benefit as opposed to 4 % for patients who did not require ICU care [41]. The authors concluded that an acute terminal care unit for dying patients was more appropriate than an intermediate care unit [41].

No studies have been performed comparing outcomes of low risk patients treated in ICUs versus those treated in intermediate units or wards, or intermediate units versus wards after treatment in an ICU [42, 43]. The circumstances under which an intermediate care unit is a cost-effective alternative to the traditional ICU or general ward beds have not been determined [42].

Future Research for Triage

- **Prospective study to define which patients are benefited by ICU admission.** Patients should be evaluated by admission or rejection to the ICU and prevalence and incidence studies of all critically ill patients admitted to the hospital. This should include different diagnoses and perhaps other variables such as age, treatments, physiological and/or other parameters. Surgical, medical and cardiac patients should be evaluated separately. Concurrent controls are required. This should lead to more exact admission criteria. End points should include ICU and hospital survival, 6 and 12 month survival, quality of life and cost analyses for patients in ICUs, intermediate units or general wards. Subsequently, borderline patient groups in whom it is not clear whether ICUs benefit or harm them should be randomized to ICU or other care. This will be extremely difficult. Our attempts to set up such a study failed. In addition to ethical constraints, most doctors are unwilling to admit such a patient outside the ICU if there is a bed in the ICU.

- Prospective study to define when patients should be discharged from the ICU and to what location. Patient groups, end points and subsequent studies should follow ICU admission studies above.
- A triage score should be developed. Just as ICU severity scores such as APACHE II and III, SAPS II and III and MPM II have been developed for patients in the ICU, physicians should have more objective scoring systems based on data available at the time of triage and not after the patient has been admitted. Such a study is presently being developed in Europe. Just as severity scores cannot be used in an individual patient, so too this score might not be able to be used to exclude a specific patient but the information might make triage decisions more objective.
- Define for specific diagnoses, patients requiring ICU or intermediate care. Studies on high risk patients with acute gastrointestinal hemorrhage and diabetic ketoacidosis have shown which patients may be more likely or not to benefit from ICU care [44, 45]. These types of studies should be performed for the common ICU admissions. Most importantly, postoperative patients who require ICU versus prolonged or routine post operative recovery unit care should be identified as many of these patients currently consume ICU resources.
- Cost effectiveness study of ICU, intermediate care or regular ward for various diagnoses.
- Define the extent of outflow problems and its effect on inflow.
- Criteria used by triage officers in making decisions.

The above studies are important for the practice of intensive care yet they will be extremely difficult to perform. Problems include funding, multidisciplinary cooperation, ethical issues and methodological difficulties. Some difficulties which we have confronted regarding a triage score recently may be helpful. One must compare patient severity in the different groups studied. How should this be done? What score should be used? Studies have used APACHE II scores [6, 7, 10–12] but this score was developed and validated for patients after 24 hours in the ICU and not for patients not admitted to an ICU [34]. One study [13] utilized the MPM_0 which is performed at the baseline period as opposed to 24 hours later but it too was developed for ICU patients and does not have as many acute physiological parameters as the APACHE II and SAPS II score. What time should be used? Should it be the triage time or the ICU admission time for which APACHE and SAPS were developed? How should missing data be evaluated? Patients admitted to departments often have less tests performed than in the ICU and many values are missing. Should the values be considered normal or should abnormal values found several days before or after the triage be used? Patients on wards may 'appear' less severely ill, merely because they are not monitored closely and have fewer collected data. Clearly, a triage score for potential ICU patients is required but will be difficult to develop.

Recommendations for Current Care

Despite the need for much research in the triage area, several problems have been identified and present knowledge can be used to formulate more optimal care for ICU patients, hopefully with improved long term outcomes. We have previously examined a business model of flow processes to help make the triage process more efficient [22]. The most important recommendations include:

- **Increase resource availability.** There is a lack of ICU beds in many countries. This relates to an actual shortage of beds and/or a lack of trained critical care nurses.
- **Improve resource pooling of ICU beds within a hospital and community.** Greater cooperation must be developed between ICUs in a given institution and between hospitals in a given city. Such cooperation exists in certain cities such as Paris. Turf battles are not uncommon. Medical ICUs may refuse to care for surgical patients and surgical units may refuse to care for medical and particularly coronary patients. Critical care physicians and nurses must be trained and certified to work in all types of units. Resources should be pooled. Specialty units should not keep patients no longer requiring ICU care in a bed so an elective patient can use the bed the next day. Perhaps a triage officer responsible for all ICU beds in an institution is needed despite the seemingly impossible workload [1].
- **Explicit admission and discharge criteria must be developed and exhibited for health care workers and for families. These criteria should be followed.** This should help avoid the admission of patients with no hope of survival and the discharge of patients with little or no anticipated benefit [1]. The SCCM consensus statement declared that such patients could be excluded or discharged from the ICU despite the anticipation of an untoward outcome [1].
- **Appropriate areas outside of ICUs should be developed for the care of terminal patients and patients requiring monitoring and not ICU care.** It should be acknowledged that if these are not available, ICUs will be used for these patients; this may prevent the admission of patients who can truly benefit from ICU care.
- **Mechanisms should be developed to streamline the admission and discharge of patients without delay.**
- **Develop admission and discharge criteria that take into account the probability and length of a successful outcome, quality of life and cost.** Such a model was termed an ICU treatment entitlement index (ICU-EI) and suggested by Engelhardt and Rie many years ago [46]. The equation was:

ICU-EI = P Q L / C

where P indicates the probability of the successful outcome; Q, quality of success; L, length of life remaining; and C, costs required to achieve therapeutic success [46]. As the costs increase and the quantity and quality of the success decrease, the reasonableness of the investment diminishes [46]. The significance of the costs can be appreciated by comparing them to non-ICU costs so as to see the incremental value of ICU care [46]. There may be a score level above which it may be agreed that all patients should be treated [46]. The score would lead to a bias against the elderly which already exists. Although the score might not be able to be used for individual patients much as a severity score is not, objective information concerning all the variables in the equation might be helpful.

A more complete listing of recommendations can be found in a recent editorial [22].

References

1. Society of Critical Care Medicine (1994) Ethics Committee Consensus statement on the triage of critically ill patients. JAMA 271:1200–1203
2. Vincent JL (1999) Forgoing life support in western European intensive care units: The results of an ethical questionnaire. Crit Care Med 27:1626–1633
3. Strauss MJ, LoGerfo JP, Yeltatzie JA, Temkin N, Hudson LD (1986) Rationing of intensive care unit services. JAMA 255:1143–1146
4. Singer DE, Carr PL, Mulley AG, et al (1983) Rationing intensive care Physician responses to a resource shortage. N Engl J Med 309:1155–1160
5. Sax FL, Charlson ME (1987) Utilization of physician triage and patient outcome. Arch Intern Med 147:929–934
6. Franklin C, Rackow EC, Mamdani B, Burke G, Weil MH (1990) Triage considerations in medical intensive care. Arch Intern Med 150:1455–1459
7. Marshall MF, Schwenzer KJ, Orsina M, Fletcher JC, Durbin CG (1992) Influence of political power, medical provincialism, and economic incentives on the rationing of surgical intensive care unit beds. Crit Care Med 20:387–394
8. Charlson ME, Sax FL (1987) The therapeutic efficacy of critical care units from two perspectives: a traditional cohort approach vs a new case-control methodology. J Chron Dis 40:31–39
9. Ron A, Aronne LJ, Kalb PE Dantini D, Charlson ME (1989) The therapeutic efficacy of critical care units. Arch Intern Med 149:338–341
10. Frisho-Lima P, Gurman G, Schapira A, Porath A (1994) Rationing critical care – what happens to patients who are not admitted? Theor Surg 9:208–211
11. Metcalfe MA, Sloggett A, McPherson K (1997) Mortality among appropriately referred patients refused admission to intensive care units. Lancet 350:7–12
12. Sprung CL, Geber D, Eidelman LA, et al (1999) Evaluation of triage decisions for intensive care admission. Crit Care Med 27:1073–1079
13. Joynt GM, Gomersall CD, Tan P, Lee A, Ai Yu Cheng, Lai Yi Wong E (2001) Prospective Evaluation of patients refused admission to an intensive care unit – triage, futility and outcome. Intensive Care Med 27:1459–1465
14. Danis M, Patrick DL, Southerland LI, Green ML (1988). Patients' and families' preferences for medical intensive care. JAMA 260:797–802
15. The Society of Critical Care Medicine Ethics Committee (1994) Attitudes of critical care medicine professionals concerning distribution of intensive care resources. Crit Care Med 22:358–362
16. Chalfin DB, Fein AM (1994) Critical care medicine in managed competition and a managed care environment. New Horiz 2:275–282
17. Berenson RA (1984) Intensive care units (ICU's): clinical outcomes, costs and decision-making. Office of Technology Assessment; Health Technology Case Study 28
18. Miranda DR, Ryan DW, Schaufeli WB, Fidler V (1998) Organisation and management of intensive care. A prospective study in 12 European countries. Springer, Berlin
19. American Thoracic Society Bioethics Task Force (1997) Fair allocation of intensive care unit resources. Am J Respir Crit Care Med 156:1282–1301
20. Beauchamp TL, Childress JF (1983) Principles of Biomedical Ethics, 2nd Edition. Oxford University Press, New York, pp, 183–220
21. Childress JF (1970) Who shall live when not all can live. Soundings 53:339–355

22. Levin PD, Sprung CL (2001) The process of intensive care triage. Intensive Care Med 27:1441–1445
23. NIH consensus conference (1983) Critical Care Medicine. JAMA 250:798–804
24. Strosberg MA (1993) Intensive care units in the triage mode. Crit Care Clin 9:415–424
25. Task Force of the American College of Critical Care Medicine (1999) Guidelines for intensive care unit admission, discharge and triage. Crit Care Med 27:633–638
26. Teres D (1993) Civilian triage in the intensive care unit: The ritual of the last bed. Crit Care Med 21:598–606
27. Nasraway SA, Cohen IL, Dennis RC, et al (1998) Guidelines on admission and discharge for adult intermediate care units. Crit Care Med 26:607–610
28. Donnelly P, Sandifer QD, O'Brien D, Thomas EA (1995) A pilot study of the use of clinical guidelines to determine appropriateness of patient placement on intensive and high dependency care units. J Pub Health Med 17:305–310
29. Dawson JA (1993) Admission, discharge and triage in critical care. Crit Care Clin 9:555–574
30. Knaus WP, Draper EA, Wagner DP, Zimmerman JE (1985) APACHE II: A severity of disease classification system. Crit Care Med 13:818–828
31. Knaus WP, Wagner DP, Draper EA, et al (1991) The APACHE III Prognostic System. Risk prediction of hospital mortality for critically ill hospitalized adults. Chest 100:1619–1636
32. Le Gall JR, Lemeshow S, Saulnier F (1993) A new simplified acute physiology score (SAPS II) based on a European/North American multicenter study. JAMA 270:2957–2963
33. Lemeshow S, Teres D, Klar J, Avrunin JS, Gehlbach SH, Rapoport J (1993) Mortality probability models (MPM II) based on an international cohort of intensive care unit patients. JAMA 270:2478–2486
34. Suter P, Armaganidis A, Beaufils F, et al (1994) Predicting outcome in ICU patients. Consensus conference orgnaized by the ESICM and the SRLF. Intensive Care Med 20:390–397
35. Thibault GE, Mulley AG, Barnett GO, et al (1980) Medical intensive care: indications, interventions and outcomes. New Engl J Med 302:938–942
36. Zimmerman JE, Wagner DP, Draper EA, Knaus WA (1994) Improving intensive care unit discharge decisions: supplementing physician judgment with predictions of next day risk for life support. Crit Care Med 22:1373–1384
37. Morrow BC, Lavery GG, Blackwood BM, Ball IM, McLeod HN, Fee JP (1996) The provision of adult intensive care in Northern Ireland with reference to the role of high dependency care. Ulster Med J 65:39–46
38. Ryan DW, Bayly PJ, Weldon OG, Jingree M (1997) A prospective two-month audit of the lack of provision of a high-dependency unit and its impact on intensive care. Anaesthesia 52:265–270
39. Zimmerman JE, Junker CD, Becker RB, Draper EA, Wagner DP, Knaus WA (1998) Neurological intensive care unit admissions: identifying candidates for intermediate care and the services they receive. Neurosurgery 42:91–101
40. Goldhill DR, Summer A (1998) Outcome of intensive care patients in a group of British intensive care units. Crit Care Med 26:1337–1345
41. Jacobs S, Chan RWS, Lee B, Lee B (1989) An analysis of the utilisation of an intensive care unit. Intensive Care Med 15:511–518
42. Keenan SP, Massel D, Inman KJ, Sibbald WJ (1998) A systematic review of the cost-effectiveness of noncardiac transitional care units. Chest 113:172–177
43. Bone RC, McElwee NE, Eubanks DH, Gluck EH (1993) Analysis of indications for intensive care unit admission. Chest 104:1806–1811
44. Kollef MH, Canfield DA, Zuckerman GR (1995) Triage considerations for patients with acute gastrointestinal hemorrhage admitted to a medical intensive care unit. Crit Care Med 23:1048–1054
45. Marinac JS, Mesa L (2000) Using a severity of illness scoring system to assess intensive care unit admissions for diabetic ketoacidosis. Crit Care Med 28:2238–2241

46. Engelhardt, H Jr, Rie MA (1986) Intensive Care Units, scarce resources, and conflicting principles of justice. JAMA 255:1159–1164

Preventing Nosocomial Infections
to Improve Outcomes of Intensive Care

C. Brun-Buisson

Introduction

There are few topics that have been subjected to such controversy as the question of the influence of nosocomial infections on outcomes, especially mortality, of critically ill patients. The topic is indeed of importance, since nosocomial infection (similarly to other 'iatrogenic' events) is a frequent event [1-3] and probably the most frequent drawback of intensive care, and determining outcomes attributable to nosocomial intensive care unit (ICU)-acquired infections is going to bear heavily on the design and interpretation of studies aimed at prevention or treatment of such infections. Therefore, the question whether prevention of nosocomial infection will result, or not, in improved outcome from intensive care is undermined by the uncertainty surrounding the consequences of infection on outcome. For example, it is apparent that if nosocomial infections do not influence mortality, there is no point in attempting to show a difference in mortality through implementation of a preventive or therapeutic intervention. In this circumstance, the impact of the intervention on other end-points such as length of stay or antibiotic use will be examined, and this has important implications in terms of study design and sample size needed. In this chapter, we shall examine the available data for the most common nosocomial infections occurring in ICU patients, in terms of their impact on mortality, length of stay and resource use, including antibiotics when available. Most such studies have focused on specific sites of infection, and these will be examined separately, after a brief overview of the problem. We shall then examine the evidence, if any, regarding to what extent preventing nosocomial infection may impact on outcome of critically ill patients, and the indicators that may be used for the purpose of quality improvement processes and follow-up.

An Overview of the Impact of ICU-acquired Infections
in Critically Ill Patients

Nosocomial infection affects approximately one-fifth of all patients admitted to critical care units. Respiratory or urinary tract, and bloodstream infections altogether account for more than three-quarters of all infections; the vast majority of these infections are device-associated. For example, the recent report from ICUs participating in the National Nosocomial Infection Surveillance (NNIS) program, showed that 83 % of ICU-acquired respiratory tract infections were associated with mechanical ventilation, 97 % of urinary tract infections (UTIs) occurred in catheterized patients, and 87 % of primary bloodstream infection (BSI) in patients with a central line. A few studies have examined the global impact of nosocomial infections on the outcomes of ICU patients. In the European Prevalence of Infection in Intensive Care (EPIC) study dating back 10 years [4], the occurrence of bacteremia or sepsis and of pneumonia was associated with an increased risk of mortality. Likewise, in the recent European sepsis survey conducted in 1999 by Alberti and Le Gall [5], nearly 20 % of patients acquired infection during the ICU stay; infection occurred more frequently when patients were infected on admission, and even more so when infection at ICU admission was hospital acquired. In that study, it appeared that ICU-acquired infection and sepsis had a more severe impact on outcome of patients than their community-acquired counterparts.

Another important feature of current nosocomial infection in the ICU is the increasing prevalence of antimicrobial resistance among species causing infection. Surveillance data from various sources show that overall resistance rates among prevalent pathogens is increasing, both in Gram-positive and Gram-negative organisms [6]. This evolution has a major impact on outcome of infection, since prevalence of resistance increases the risk of inappropriate antibiotic therapy and poor outcome from infection, as shown recently by Kollef et al. [7]. These authors found that about 25 % of empiric therapy was inappropriate; this rate increased from about 15 % in community-acquired infection to about 40 % in nosocomial infection. Most (80 %) of such inadequate empiric therapy was due to resistant species or acquired resistance that was not anticipated.

Obviously, many factors contribute to determining outcomes of ICU patients, some of which have a major impact such as the severity of underlying disease and acute illness, organ failures recorded on admission, etc. [8–10]. Therefore, it is apparent that events occurring subsequently during the ICU stay, such as nosocomial infection, can only marginally affect the overall outcome (mortality) of patients. Such effects may thus be difficult to delineate and require large cohort studies to sort out. While a global impact of nosocomial infection on mortality likely exist, there are variations in the magnitude of this impact depending on selected characteristics of patients. The severity of acute illness is one of these characteristics modulating the impact of ICU-acquired infections. Early studies by Britt et al. [11] and Gross et al. [12–14] made two points: 1) that nosocomial infection primarily affects the more ill or those having more comorbidities; and 2) that nosocomial infections are more likely to impact on outcome of the less severely ill patients. These concepts were later confirmed by subsequent studies performed in critically ill patients [15–18]. Bueno-Cavanillas et al. [15] explored the relationship between severity indexes (acute physiology score and therapeutic activity score) and the occurrence of nosocomial infection; they demonstrated that the largest impact on mortality of infection was recorded in patients presenting with mid-range APACHE II severity scores. In a matched-paired study of 41 ICU patients, Girou et al. [17] also found that nosocomial infection was associated with increased or persistently high therapeutic activity index, as measured by the therapeutic intervention scoring system (TISS).

Two preliminary conclusions can be drawn from these studies:
1) nosocomial infections occur at a high rate in ICU patients, mostly in association with the presence of multiple invasive devices and a high level of therapeutic activity; and
2) they may impact on the outcomes of patients, depending on their underlying condition and associated co-morbidities, and on the severity of their acute illness.

The relationship between intense therapeutic activity or high severity of illness scores and nosocomial infections is not however, a simple one. This question has been addressed recently by several authors, and specifically applied to catheter-related infections. Di Giovine et al. [19] matched 68 patients having catheter-related bacteremia to 68 controls on several variables including comorbidities and diagnosis, and severity of illness on the day before the occurrence of bacteremia. These authors reported that catheter-related bacteremia was not associated with a significant attributable mortality (35.3 % in cases vs. 30.9 % in controls). Confirmation of this unexpected finding was brought by Soufir et al. [20] in another case-control (1:2) study of 43 cases and 86 controls, where the crude mortality of cases and controls were 50 % and 21 %; the relative risk (RR) for death of cases was 2.1 [1.08–3.73, p=0.03] after adjustment on baseline variables of severity, but decreased to only 1.14 [0.76–2.61, p=0.21] after adjustment on severity of illness indexes recorded within 3 days prior to the onset of bacteremia. While these results are consistent with a mortality attributable to catheter-related bacteremia of 5 to 10 % [21, 22], they also suggest that the increased therapeutic activity and severity of illness recorded in patients prior to nosocomial infection may reflect both a risk for and a consequence of infection.

Perhaps the most controversial site of infection in terms of impact on mortality has been infection of the lower respiratory tract (i.e., pneumonia). This question has been addressed using two approaches: the cohort and case-control study. Both are subjected to biases, especially depending on the choice of other variables of prognostic importance explored in the cohort studies, and on the variables used for matching in the case-control studies. Since it is almost impossible to control for all variables of prognostic importance in cohort studies examining heterogeneous groups of ICU patients, case-control studies are more likely to give more precise estimates of attributable mortality when appropriate variables are controlled for. However, the latter usually examine selected groups of patients, and the generalizability of their findings is questionable. Another problem relates to the methods used to diagnose pneumonia: stringent criteria (e.g., respiratory tract samplings via bronchalveolar lavage [BAL], protected specimen brush [PSB]) may select a group with high disease severity, while more lenient criteria (e.g., Centers for Disease Control and Prevention [CDC] criteria) may include patients who do not have pulmonary infection. In addition, the therapeutic approach used and appropriateness of antimicrobial therapy may largely influence the results [23]. Perhaps the largest well-controlled study in non-ICU patients was performed by Leu et al. [24], who analyzed a cohort of 890 patients with hospital-acquired pneumonia (diagnosed by CDC criteria) and matched 74 randomly selected cases with 74 controls. These authors found a crude mortality in cases of 33 % and a 6.8 %

mortality attributable to pneumonia (p=0.09); the mean excess length of stay in cases was 7 days. Pneumonia thus accounted for one third of the mortality in cases. By multiple regression analysis, mortality of patients with pneumonia was associated with age, time from admission to pneumonia, neoplastic disease, and prior use of mechanical ventilation. Subsequent studies performed in critically ill, mechanically ventilated patients have provided results consistent with these estimates. Fagon et al. [25] described another case-control study of 48 pairs in which crude mortality was 57 % and attributable mortality was 27 % [25]. Similar to Leu et al. [24], Heyland et al. [26] found a 5.8 % crude increase in mortality attributable to pneumonia, corresponding to a 33 % increased relative risk of mortality in their mixed ICU population. The impact on mortality of pneumonia was more apparent in medical than in surgical patients, and in patients receiving inappropriate antibiotic therapy. Interestingly, in that study, outcomes were similar whether pneumonia was diagnosed using the more specific 'invasive' techniques (e.g., PSB or BAL) or using clinical criteria and tracheal aspirates. Similarly, Bregeon et al. reported that outcomes did not differ whether patients had pneumonia diagnosed using PSB or bronchial aspirates [27], although they did find that in patients having a medical diagnosis, mortality was higher when pneumonia was diagnosed using PSB. In a subsequent case-control study of 85 pairs, the same group reported that they were unable to detect an excess mortality attributable to pneumonia [28]. Likewise, Timsit et al. [29] found no difference in mortality among patients with clinically suspected pneumonia whether infection was subsequently confirmed or not [29], indicating that in such patients, factors other than pneumonia may be associated with mortality.

Although these data are somewhat conflicting, it would appear that deep tissue infection occurring at any site (e.g., pulmonary infection) in a fragile patient can cause death, especially when treated with delay or inadequately. However, therapy has not been accounted for adequately in most of the above studies. Thus, and despite these conflicting results, a reasonable estimate of the overall impact of pneumonia on mortality of ICU patients receiving mechanical ventilation is one third crude mortality, ranging from 5 to 30 % crude excess mortality.

On the other hand, it is apparent that in specific subgroups of patients, such as trauma patients, pneumonia only marginally increase the risk of death. This is especially the case when the underlying disease has such a large impact on outcomes that any superimposed event is unlikely to act as a prognostic modifier, e.g., after head trauma [30, 31] or during acute respiratory distress syndrome (ARDS) [32–34]. As mentioned above, other important modifiers of prognosis include the timeliness and appropriateness of antimicrobial therapy and severity of underlying chronic disease if any.

Despite these disputes on mortality, a consistent finding across studies is that nosocomial pneumonia incurs a prolongation of length of ICU stay (and/or mechanical ventilation) by about 7 to 10 days.

Evidence that prevention of infection can improve the outcome of critically ill patients

Although numerous studies have shown some effects of an intervention on infection rates, the direct evidence that prevention of infection bears substantially on patient-centered outcomes such as mortality, length of stay, or other sequelae of ICU care is sparse. However, many such studies have been conducted in critically ill patients, and both direct and indirect evidence suggest that prevention of infection can indeed improve outcomes of patients. Many such studies have, however, been conducted in specific subgroups of patients, and/or have focused on specific infections, and it is difficult to generalize from these to all critically ill patients or all nosocomial infections.

Perhaps the most compelling evidence of the positive impact of nosocomial infection prevention on outcomes of patients comes from the numerous trials on selective digestive tract decontamination (SDD) and lower respiratory tract prevention in critically ill patients. These studies have been aggregated in several meta-analyses, the most recent and comprehensive of which [35, 36] conclude that administration of a combination of early systemic and topical antimicrobials is associated with reduced pneumonia rates and mortality, especially in surgical/trauma patients; topical antimicrobials only did not provide such an effect on mortality, although they were able to prevent pneumonia. It should be noted that the reduction in mortality recorded in these studies is in the expected range of 3 to 5 % absolute reduction, which implies very large randomized trials (or meta-analyses) would be required to confirm effects of this small magnitude. None of the SDD studies has adequately shown a reduction in duration of mechanical ventilation or length of ICU stay, however. The results from the SDD studies are also consistent with those from a recent randomized controlled trial conducted in patients with acute exacerbation of chronic obstructive pulmonary disease (COPD), in whom administration of 'prophylaxis' or 'preemptive therapy' with ofloxacin was associated with a reduction of secondary (mainly pulmonary) infection, antibiotic use and mortality [37]. Therefore, the available evidence to date suggest that systemic antimicrobial prophylaxis may improve mortality and overall outcomes of patients, at least in specific groups of critically ill patients. This measure is, however, not recommended because of the concerns regarding increased risk of resistance if all mechanically ventilated patients routinely receive antibiotics, and because antibiotic costs have not been shown to be reduced.

The first simple approach to avoid infection occurring in the ICU patient often means avoiding or limiting the use of invasive devices, and substituting 'non-invasive ones' [38]. Much of the controversy surrounding the use of the pulmonary artery catheter (PAC) is based on weighing the risk (of infection and other risks) associated with insertion of a PAC against the potential benefits of better hemodynamic management to the patients. At present the data are inconclusive regarding this issue, and results of large randomized trials are awaited, ideally comparing hemodynamic monitoring using PAC versus echocardiography [39]. Along the same line, substituting 'non-invasive' ventilation (NIV) for invasive mechanical ventilation delivered via an endotracheal tube whenever possible can lead to substantial benefits in terms of duration of mechanical ventilation, length of ICU stay, and nosocomial infections [40]. In a case-control study [40], the use of NIV rather than of conventional mechanical ventilation in patients with COPD or cardiogenic pulmonary edema was associated with a lower overall incidence rate of nosocomial infections (18 vs 60 %, p<0.001) and of pneumonia (8 vs 22 %, p=0.04), and a lower daily risk of nosocomial infection (19 vs 39 episodes /1000 patient-days, p=0.05); mortality was lower (4 vs 26 %, p=0.02) as well as length of ICU stay (9 vs 15 days, p=0.02). Although it is difficult to ascribe all the benefits in terms of outcomes to the prevention of infection, this study does show an association between the use of non-invasive devices, lower nosocomial infection rates, and improved outcomes.

Another indirect line of evidence stems from a study of prevention of catheter-related infection. Using a multi-faceted interventional approach emphasizing barrier precaution during catheter insertion and care as well as hand hygiene with alcohol-based handrub solutions, Eggimann et al. [41] were able to obtain a marked reduction in catheter-related sepsis and bacteremia (from 22.9 to 6.2 episodes/1000 catheter-days). Although this before-after intervention study did not document improvement of outcomes of patients, since sepsis and bacteremia are associated with poor outcome [4], such preventive strategies are likely to improve outcomes of patients.

As mentioned earlier, prevention of antimicrobial resistance is currently a major objective, since increasing antimicrobial resistance mostly affects nosocomial infection, and likely impacts on both our ability to treat such infection and the risk of mortality in patients affected. The approach to control of antimicrobial resistance in the ICU involves both stewardship of antibiotic use and control of cross-transmission. Low compliance to handwashing in ICUs has been a vexing problem for a long time. Recent studies emphasize the difficulties experienced by health care workers to comply with handwashing recommendations, a large part of which is simply due to lack of time and the high number of opportunities for hand hygiene during routine patient care [42]. New strategies, however, exist to overcome these practical problems associated with poor compliance, especially via implementation of waterless alcohol-based solutions, which are much more simpler to use, available at the bedside, and require less time for efficacy. Pittet et al. [43] have shown that making these solutions available in their hospital resulted in gradual improvement of compliance to hand hygiene; more importantly, this improvement was associated with a reduction of nosocomial infection rates, as well as of the attack rate of methicillin-resistant *Staphylococcus aureus* (MRSA) [43]. Given the impact of both of these factors on patient outcome, such a strategy is likely to have a substantial impact on outcome and costs of care.

In summary, nosocomial infections, particularly pneumonia, bacteremia, and sepsis are associated with poor outcomes, although this may not be apparent in all subgroups of patients. Preventing these infections will improve the outcomes of patients, especially in those with intermediate severity. Antimicrobial prophylaxis in selected subgroups is one of these approaches. Attention to hygiene practices and prevention of cross-transmission is another strategy, which has proved effective for catheter-related infections and sepsis. Other approaches aimed at improving host defenses are awaited, but the evidence for effective preventive strategies is still lacking at this time.

References

1. Richards MJ, Edwards JR, Culver DH, Gaynes RP (2000) Nosocomial infections in combined medical-surgical intensive care units in the United States. Infect Control Hosp Epidemiol 21:510–515
2. Richards MJ, Edwards JR, Culver DH, Gaynes RP (1999) Nosocomial infections in medical intensive care units in the United States. National Nosocomial Infections Surveillance System. Crit Care Med 27:887–892
3. CDC. Nosocomial Infections Surveillance Activity, Hospital Infection Program, National Center for Infectious Diseases (2000) Monitoring hospital-acquired infections to promote patient safety – United States, 1990–1999. Morbidity and Mortality Weekly Report MMWR 49:149–153
4. Vincent JL, Bihari D, Suter PM, et al (1995) The prevalence of nosocomial infection in intensive care in Europe. Results of the European prevalence of infection in intensive care (EPIC) study. JAMA 274:639–644
5. Kauffman CA, Vazquez JA, Sobel JD, et al (2000) Prospective multicenter study of funguria in hospitalized patients. Clin Infect Dis 30:14–18
6. Hanberger H, Garcia-Rodriguez J-A, Gobernado M, et al (1999) Antibiotic susceptibility among aerobic Gram-negative bacilli in intensive care units in 5 European countries. JAMA 281:67–71
7. Kollef MH, Sherman G, Ward S, Fraser VJ (1999) Inadequate antimicrobial treatment of infections: a risk factor for hospital mortality among critically ill patients. Chest 115:462–474
8. Le Gall JR, Klar J, Lemeshow S, et al (1996) The logistic organ dysfunction system: A new way to assess organ dysfunction in the intensive care unit. JAMA 276:802–810
9. Le Gall JR, Lemeshow S, Saulnier F (1993) A new simplified acute physiology score based on a European-North American multicenter study. JAMA 270:2957–2963
10. Brun-Buisson C, Doyon F, Carlet J, et al (1995) Incidence, risk factors, and outcome of severe sepsis and septic shock in adults. A multicenter prospective study in intensive care units. JAMA 274:968–974
11. Britt MR, Schleupner CJ, Matsumiya S (1978) Severity of underlying disease as a predictor of nosocomial infection. Utility in the control of nosocomial infection. JAMA 239:1047–1051
12. Gross PA, DeMauro PJ, van Antwerpen C, Wallenstein S, Chiang S (1988). Number of comorbidities as a predictor of nosocomial infection acquisition. Infect Control Hosp Epidemiol 9:497–500
13. Gross PA, van Antwerpen C (1983) Nosocomial infections and hospital deaths. A case-control study. Am J Med 75:658–662
14. Gross PA, Neu HC, Aswapokee P, van Antwerpen C, Aswapokee N (1980) Deaths from nosocomial infections: experience in a university hospital and a community hospital. Am J Med 68:219–223
15. Bueno-Cavanillas A, Delgado-Rodriguez M, Lopez-Luque A, Schaffino-Cano S, Calvez-Vargas R (1994) Influence of nosocomial infection on mortality rate in an intensive care unit. Crit Care Med 22:55–60
16. Bueno-Cavanillas A, Contreras RR, Lopez-Luque A, Delgado-Rodriguez M, Galves-Vargas R (1991) Usefulness of severity indices in intensive care medicine as a predictor of nosocomial infection risk. Intensive Care Med 17:336–339
17. Girou E, Stephan F, Novara A, Safar M, Fagon JY (1998) Risk factors and outcome of nosocomial infections: results of a matched case-control study of ICU patients. Am J Respir Crit Care Med 157:1151–1158

18. Girou E, Pinsard M, Auriant I, Canonne M (1996) Influence of the severity of illness measured by the simplified acute physiology score (SAPS) on occurrence of nosocomial infections in ICU patients. J Hosp Infect 34:131–138
19. Digiovine B, Chenoweth C, Watts C, Higgins M (1999) The attributable mortality and costs of primary nosocomial bloodstream infections in the intensive care unit. Am J Respir Crit Care Med 160:976–981
20. Soufir L, Timsit JF, Mahe C, Carlet J, Regnier B, Chevret S (1999). Attributable morbidity and mortality of catheter-related septicemia in critically ill patients: a matched, risk-adjusted, cohort study. Infect Control Hosp Epidemiol 20:396–401
21. Renaud B, Brun-Buisson C (2001) Outcomes of primary and catheter-related bacteremia. A cohort and case-control study in critically ill patients. Am J Respir Crit Care Med 163:1584–1590
22. Mermel LA (2000) Prevention of intravascular catheter-related infections. Ann Intern Med 132:391–402
23. Wenzel RP (1998) Perspective: attributable mortality – the promise of better antimicrobial therapy. Clin Infect Dis 178:917–919
24. Leu HS, Kaiser DL, Mori M, Woolson RF, Wenzel RP (1989) Hospital-acquired pneumonia: attributable mortality and morbidity. Am J Epidemiol 129:1258–1267
25. Fagon JY, Chastre J, Domart Y, Trouillet J-L, Gibert C (1996) Mortality due to ventilator-associated pneumonia or colonization with Pseudomonas or Acinetobacter species: assessment by quantitative culture of samples obtained by a protected specimen brush. Clin Infect Dis 23:538–542
26. Heyland DK, Cook DJ, Griffith L, Keenan SP, Brun-Buisson C, The Canadian Critical Care Trials Group (1999) The attributable morbidity and mortality of ventilator-associated pneumonia in the critically ill patient. Am J Respir Crit Care Med 159:1249–1256
27. Bregeon F, Papazian L, Visconti A, Gregoire R, Thirion X, Gouin F (1997) Relationship of microbiologic diagnostic criteria to morbidity and mortality in patients with ventilator-associated pneumonia. JAMA 277:655–662
28. Papazian L, Bregeon F, Thirion X, et al (1996) Effect of ventilator-associated pneumonia of mortality and morbidity. Am J Respir Crit Care Med 154:91–97
29. Timsit JF, Chevret S, Valcke J, et al (1996) Mortality of nosocomial pneumonia in ventilated patients: influence of diagnostic tools. Am J Respir Crit Care Med 154:116–123
30. Baker AM, Meredith JW, Haponik EF (1996) Pneumonia in intubated trauma patients. Microbiology and outcome. Am J Respir Crit Care Med 153:343–349
31. Hsieh AHH, Bishop MJ, Kubilis PS, Newell DW, Pierson DJ (1992) Pneumonia following closed-head injury. Am J Respir Crit Care Med 146:290–294
32. Chastre J, Trouillet J-L, Vuagnat A, et al (1998) Nosocomial pneumonia in patients with acute respiratory distress syndrome. Am J Respir Crit Care Med 157:1165–1172
33. Delclaux C, Roupie E, Blot F, Brochard L, Lemaire F, Brun-Buisson C (1997) Lower respiratory tract colonization and infection during severe acute respiratory distress syndrome. Incidence and diagnosis. Am J Respir Crit Care Med 156:1092–1098
34. Markowicz P, Wolff M, Djedaini K, et al (2000) Multicenter prospective study of ventilator-associated pneumonia during acute respiratory distress syndrome. Incidence, prognosis, and risk factors. ARDS Study Group. Am J Respir Crit Care Med 161:1942–1948
35. D'Amico R, Pifferi S, Leonetti C, Torri V, Tinazzi A, Liberati A (1998) Effectiveness of antibiotic prophylaxis in critically ill adult patients: systematic review of randomised controlled trials. Br Med J 316:1275–1285
36. Nathens AB, Marshall JC (1999) Selective decontamination of the digestive tract in surgical patients. A systematic review of the evidence. Arch Surg 134:170–176
37. Nouira S, Marghli S, Belghith M, Besbes L, Elatrous S, Abroug F (2001) Once daily oral ofloxacin in chronic obstructive pulmonary disease exacerbation requiring mechanical ventilation: a randomised placebo-controlled trial. Lancet 358:2020–2025

38. Maki DG (1989) Risk factors for nosocomial infection in intensive care. 'Devices vs. nature' and goals for the next decade. Arch Intern Med 149:30–35
39. Vieillard-Baron A, Girou E, Valente E, et al (2000) Predictors of mortality in acute respiratory distress syndrome. Focus On the role of right heart catheterization. Am J Respir Crit Care Med 161:1597–1601
40. Girou E, Schortgen F, Delclaux C, et al (2000) Association of non-invasive ventilation with nosocomial infections and survival in critically ill patients. JAMA 284:2361–2367
41. Eggimann P, Harbarth S, Constantin MN, Touveneau S, Chevrolet JC, Pittet D (2000) Impact of a prevention strategy targeted at vascular-access care on incidence of infections acquired in intensive care. Lancet 355:1864–1868
42. Pittet D, Mourouga P, Perneger TV (1999) Compliance with handwashing in a teaching hospital. Ann Intern Med 130:126–130
43. Pittet D, Hugonnet S, Harbarth S, et al (2000) Effectiveness of a hospital-wide programme to improve compliance with hand hygiene. Lancet 356:1307–1312

Preventing Iatrogenic Complications

J. Bion, G.K.Hart, and Z. Khan

'Human error should be seen as a consequence, not a cause, of failure'.
An organisation with a memory. Department of Health, London 2001

Introduction

When Ignac Semmelweis tried to convince the medical community that the contagion of puerperal sepsis was transmitted on the hands of attending medical staff, one of the arguments adduced against his evidence was that doctors, being well-intentioned almost by definition, could not therefore be maleficent agents. Such paternalistic attitudes have changed since the mid-nineteenth century, but only in recent years has there been a willingness to accept that iatrogenic disease is frequent, serious, and most importantly, often preventable. There is also a growing understanding that medical error as a subset of iatrogenic disease, represents a failure of the system, not just the individual, and the prevention of error therefore requires a systems approach.

Medical error is a subject with blurred borders. The focal point is the day-to-day quality of care delivered at the bedside to individual patients, and it spreads from here to include the education and professional accreditation of health care workers, the development of standards for benchmarking, and local and national systems of quality assurance. Making mistakes is an everyday occurrence and is an important part of human learning, so that in complex systems like medical care which have imprecise methods of measurement it can be easy to accept error as a normal (and thus 'acceptable') part of clinical practice. Data collection on the frequency of medical errors may be laborious, costly and inaccurate, while a culture of blame, guilt and litigation inhibits remedial action. Medical error also lacks a robust and universal taxonomy, making prior definition essential.

In this chapter we include as our subject matter all adverse events that arise from medical treatment in critically ill patients, but focus mainly on errors and adverse events that can arise from health care processes. We will start with a brief taxonomy, then examine current estimates of the scale of the problem in acute hospital care, review some of the speciality- and disease-specific surveys, and consider common patterns and causes of error. We will discuss the role of critical care medicine in contributing, and preventing, medical error and examine the relationship between changing medical knowledge with respect to what is natural history of disease

Table 1. Taxonomy of error

Term	Definition	Comment or example
Accident	An event that involves damage to a defined system that disrupts the ongoing or future output of that system [1]	Commonly used examples include Bhopal, Challenger, Chernobyl, Herald of Free Enterprise, Three Mile Island, warfare, and many others. Usually a consequence of a chain of causation.
System	A set of interdependent elements, human or non-human, which interact to achieve a common aim [2]	
Error	The failure of a planned action to be completed as intended (execution error), or the use of a wrong plan to achieve an aim (planning error) [2–4].	Errors can include problems in practice, products, procedures and systems. Medical error requires intent (not the result of random events) and implies preventability.
Mistake	Wrong action plan properly conducted, resulting in an unintended outcome	Wrong diagnosis results in wrong treatment plan.
Slip or lapse	Execution errors in which the action conducted differs from that intended. Slips are observable, lapses are not [2]	Incorrect drug drawn up (slip). Forgetting to review patient (lapse)
Active error	A fault in performance at the level of the operator [2]	Giving the wrong drug.
Latent error	A fault in design, installation, management or maintenance which may subsequently result in harm [2]	Two different drugs with very similar packaging which are easily confused.
Criticalt inciden	A pivotal event with the potential to cause an adverse event. [5]	Failure to tighten connectors on a central venous catheter.
Adverse event	An injury caused by medical management that resulted in measurable disability [6]	Cellulitis or bacteremia from central venous catheter. Peptic ulceration from non-steroidal anti-inflammatory analgesics.
Negligent adverse event	A preventable adverse event caused by medical management which did not meet the standard of care expected of that practitioner [6]	Air embolism from failure to observe and correct a disconnection in a central venous catheter.
Iatrogenic disease	Injury produced or caused by doctors .	Also used to include harm resulting from any group of health care workers, or from the health care system as a whole.
Patient safety	Freedom from accidental injury [2]	Maximizing benefit, reducing risk, eliminating harm to patients.

Table 2. The spectrum of harm

Criminal injury	Negligent error	Potentially avoidable adverse event	Unavoidable side effect of treatment or disease
Deliberate harm	Incompetent care	Nosocomial infection	Muscle wasting
Intent to shorten life rather than alleviate distress when withdrawing treatment	Wrong drug	Thromboembolism	Tracheostomy scar
	Failure to attend patient, or seek help	Persisting with futile care	Post-traumatic stress disorder

rather than a consequence of therapy. Finally, we will explore methods of prevention, including local practice standards, education and dissemination of best practice, and the development of national monitoring and reporting mechanisms.

A Taxonomy of Error

Table 1 lists the terms used to describe different types of error and consequences of errors, with the source of their definitions where available, and comments or examples. Although there is no universally agreed system of definitions, there is a reasonable degree of consistency of approach in the publications on this subject. The major potential differences of approach reflect the quest in some quarters to confine the scope of the error discussion to that where causality between medical error and adverse outcome can be established.

It should be noted however, that attributability (causation) and avoidability (potential for prevention) are neither synonymous nor static properties of iatrogenic disease. Table 2 provides examples of the spectrum of harm associated with treatment processes. With advances in medical care, some adverse events, which would have been regarded as unavoidable, are now perceived not only as preventable but also as demonstrating negligent care, nosocomial infection being one example of many.

Medical Error: Common, Serious, and often Preventable

Superficially, medical care has never been better. And yet during the last decade of the past century, an increasing number of reports have emerged suggesting that medical error and avoidable harm to patients have reached epidemic proportions when considered across the entire patient population. These reports include:

- The Harvard Medical Practice Study [6, 7] identified an adverse event rate amongst New York hospital admissions of 3.7 %, of which 27.6 % were negligent, 2.6 % caused permanent disability and 13.6 % were fatal. The elderly were more susceptible to adverse events overall, and to negligent adverse events. The authors estimated that among the 2,671,863 patients discharged from New York hospitals in 1984 there were 98,609 adverse events, of which 27,179 would have been negligent

- A survey from Utah and Colorado in 1992 [8, 9] randomly sampled 15,000 hospital discharges, and found an adverse event rate of 2.9 %, of which 30 % were negligent and 6.6 % resulted in death. Surgeons contributed 46.1 % of adverse events of which 22.3 % were considered negligent, and physicians contributed 23.2 %, of which 44.9 % were negligent. Adverse drug events accounted for 19.3 % of all adverse events. If these results were generalizable to the whole of the USA, approximately 44,000 patients would die each year from medical errors; the Harvard Medical Practice study would suggest that the figure is in the region of 98,000 deaths annually.

- The Quality in Australian Health Care Study [10] reviewed the medical records of over 14,000 admissions to 28 hospitals in New South Wales and South Australia. The authors found that 16.6 % of admissions were associated with an adverse event, of which 51 % were considered preventable. In 13.7 % the disability was permanent and in 4.9 % the patient died. They estimated that adverse events cost the Australian healthcare system $4.7bn a year.

- In the UK, a pilot study [11, 12] reviewing 1014 medical and nursing records in two London hospitals found that 110 (10.8 %) patients experienced an adverse event, of which 48 % were considered preventable and 8 % contributed to death. If extrapolated to the whole of the UK, this would suggest that around 425,000 patients each year would suffer an avoidable adverse event at an additional cost of over £1 billion.

These reports from three different health care systems provide a consistent message, that errors in medical care are not rare, not innocuous, and – most importantly – not inevitable. The message is reinforced by many other studies, confidential inquiries, infection surveillance systems, and small scale surveys from other countries.

A selection of these sources is presented in Table 3. Several features stand out when reviewing this literature. First, although mortality is an unambiguous and clinically relevant outcome that is usually accurately recorded, it will detect only a small proportion of complications arising from medical care. Adverse event reports will offer a more accurate estimate of the scale of the problem, but require careful definition, and data collection is more laborious. Heinrich studied industrial accidents in the 1940s, and identified a ratio of non-injury accidents (near misses) to minor adverse events to major adverse events of 300:29:1 [13]. Second, there are substantial variations in error rates and adverse events between these studies, reflecting differences in methodology, definitions, and patient populations as well as in standards of practice. Third, it is evident that even where adverse events may appear to be low in percentage terms, because of the volume of activity the number of patients who may suffer harm is large. Third, the financial (and emotional) costs of error are high, and this represents a substantial loss of resource for the health care system that would be better invested in prevention.

It is important to note that there has been a vigorous dialog between the authors of the above studies and others who dispute the methodology and the scale of the

Table 3. Selected studies and reports of error in health care

Reference	Type of study	N	Adverse event or error rate	% adverse events or errors preventable	Comments	AE mortality
Beecher HK, Todd DP (1954) Ann Surg 140:2–34	Prospective 5 yr study deaths after anesthesia	600,000 anesthetics	Anesthesia contributed to death 1:1,560			Anesthesia caused death in 1:2,680
Trunet P et al (1980) JAMA 244:2617–2620	Prospective study 1 yr, France	325 ICU admissions	12.6 %	46.3 %	All required ICU admission	19.5 %
Steel K (1981) N Engl J Med 304:638–642	General medical wards USA	815	293 (36 %)		25% morbidity	5.4 %
Lakshmanan MC (1986) Arch Intern Med 146:1931–1934	Medical admissions to hospital USA	834 admissions	5.4 % iatrogenic admissions	50 %		
Lesar TS (1990) JAMA 263:2329–2334	Prospective 1 yr study hospital prescribing errors, USA	289 411 medication orders	905 errors (3.1/1000). 522 (57.7 % = 1.8/1000) serious		Juniors more likely to make errors	
Classen DC (1991) JAMA 266:2847–2851	Modeling of drug errors		1.7 % of admissions			
Brennan TA et al (1991) N Engl J Med 324: 370–376 and LL Leape TA (1991) N Engl J Med 324:377–384	Case record review, New York 1984	30121 in-patients, 51 hospitals	3.7 %		69 % of injuries caused by errors	6.6 %

Table 3. (*Continued*)

Reference	Type of study	N	Adverse event or error rate	% adverse events or errors preventable	Comments	AE mortality
O'Neil AC (1993) Ann Intern Med 119:370–376	USA Physician reporting + concurrent record review	3146 hospital admissions	89 (2.8 %) physician-reported, 85 (2.7 %) case note review; only 41 same patients	62.5 % physician-reported, 32 % case review	Physician-reporting cheaper, found more preventable AEs	
Muckart DJ et al (1994) S Afr J Surg 32:69–73	Surgical ICU, 1 yr	657 patients	229 (34.8 %) suffered 369 adverse events		AEs per patient = 1–4	Mortality in AE+ve = 29.3, 20.3 % in AE -ve $p < 0.02$
Vincent JL, et al (1995) JAMA 274:639–644	One-day European point prevalence survey	1417 ICUs, 10038 patients	20.6 % ICU-acquired infection			ICU-acquired pneumonia OR death = 1.91
Donchin Y (1995) Crit Care Med 23:294–300	Prospective study of ICU clinicians	554 errors in 4 months	1.7 errors per patient per day	s	2 serious errors per day overall	
Wilson RM (1995) Med J Aust 163:458–471	Case record review Australia	14179 patients, 28 hospital	16.6 %	51 %	Permanent disability in 13.7 % of patients	4.9 %
Stambouly JJ (1996) Intensive Care Med 22:1098–1104	Prospective, pediatric ICU	1035 s admission 18-months	115 complications in 83 (8.0 %) admissions		2.7 AEs per 100 PICU days	

Table 3. (*Continued*)

Reference	Type of study	N	Adverse event or error rate	% adverse events or errors preventable	Comments	AE mortality
Andrews LB (1997) Lancet 349:309 –313	Prospective study, surgical wards USA	1047 patients	185 (17.7 %)	63.2 %	17.7 % Risk of AE ↑ 6 % per day	
Bates DW (1997) JAMA 277:307–311	Prospective drug error study, USA	4108 med/surg admissions	50 % of admissions	60/190 errors (31.5 %)	Increased costs, LOS	
McQuillan P, et al (1998) Br Med J 316:1853–1858	Case note review of pre-ICU care	100 admissions to 2 UK ICUs	54 % received suboptimal care before admission			SMR 1.4 for suboptimal group
Bhasale AL (1998) Med J Aust 169:73–76	20 month study, anonymous reporting	324 Australian general practitioners	805 errors or incidents	76 %	27 % potential for severe harm	
Gawande AA, et al (1999) Surgery 126 :66–75 and Thomas EJ, et al (2000) Med Care 38:261–271	2-state case record review 1992 USA	15,000 cases	3 % (66 % surgical)	27.4 %–32.6 % AEs negligent	44.9 % AEs perioperative; 16.6 % → permanent disability	6.6 %
Darchy B (1999) Arch Intern Med 159:71 –78	Prospective study, 1 yr, France	623 ICU admissions	10.9 %	51 %	All required ICU admission	13 %
Richards MJ, et al (1999) Crit Care Med 27:887–892	USA National Nosocomial Infections Surveillance System	Medical ICUs, 181, 993 patients	UTI 31 %, Pneumonia 27 %, Bacteraemia 19 %		86-90 % infections device-related	

Table 3. (*Continued*)

Reference	Type of study	N	Adverse event or error rate	% adverse events or errors preventable	Comments	AE mortality
NHS Ombudsman	UK NHS complaints by patients	86,013 hospital complaints			285 referred independent review	
Medical Devices Agency (UK), 1999	Adverse events relating to equipment	National voluntary reporting	6610 AEs in 1999 caused by equipment failures		64 % device related, 12 % user error	
Plowman, et al 1999, and National Audit Office report, 2000.	Prospective survey UK hospital-acquired infection	3980 patients in community hospital	7.8 % HAI in hospital. 19.1 % after discharge	30 %	↑ LOHS × 2.5 ↑ costs × 3.2 Excess cost nationally ~ £1000M	↑ risk of death × 7.1
National Audit Office Report 2000	Clinical negligence claims in UK	10,000 new claims in 1999–2000	23,000 claims outstanding		£3,900M required to cover all claims	
Vincent C, et al (2001) Br Med J 322:517–519 and Neale G, et al (2001) J R Soc Med 94:322–330	Case record review, UK	2 hospitals, 1014 patients	110 (10.8 %)	48 %	53 % of preventable AEs involved ward care	8 %

AE: adverse event; UTI: urinary tract infection; LOS: length of stay reported adverse outcomes. Issues such as inter-rater concordance, outcome bias, failure to define or rate likelihood of causality are raised by those who believe the 'error industry' over states the case [14]. Countering, are claims that the published figures actually understate the problem because the selection criteria of the studies excluded many patients and care environments which are likely to have errors, and that the medical record is notoriously poor at providing all relevant information [15].

The Development of Standards for Medical Care

Internal (Personal) Standards

Hippocrates laid the foundations for 'good' and ethical medical practice, including the first stated maxim of harm avoidance. Within this and other cultural, social and political environments, medical practitioners have generally worked in a beneficent manner. The transition of the doctor from someone who observed and documented diseases while providing reassurance and placebo effect, to practitioners within health care systems offering treatments and interventions of considerable potency, has been accompanied by an increase in expectations amongst patients, practitioners and society. This has inevitably brought with it an increase in accidents, errors and adverse outcomes, and the need for improved monitoring of the processes of care, which in turn exposes more error. Clinicians, being human, have a variety of intrinsic, ethno-cultural and medico-cultural mechanisms for coping with the realization of imperfection. The training medical students receive has not, to date, provided mechanisms for students to appropriately rationalize adverse outcomes [16]. This training has been provided by peers and mentors and is therefore open to 'institutionalized' reactions that may not be beneficial to individual practitioners, patients or the care system itself. Medico-legal considerations at personal and institutional levels also impact on the responses to adverse outcomes.

In the last decade, a growing awareness of the imperfections of the institutional structures under which health care is provided, together with increased attention to the lessons learned after both medical and industrial disaster, has focused attention on the psychological basis of human performance in both individual and group environments.

A variety of institutional structures have evolved to address concerns about the quality of medical practice. Structures for monitoring standards of medical training and practice are a legal requirement and a pre-requisite for professional self-regulation in virtually all countries.

Standards of Medical Care in Hospital

The hospital quality assurance movement developed in the 19th century through the efforts of people like Florence Nightingale in the UK, Theodore Fliedner in Germany, and Jean Henri Dunant in Switzerland. In the USA, the rapid increase in

Table 4. Useful web-based sources of information including national reports with information relating to adverse events in medical care

Kohn LT, Corrigan JM, Donaldson MS (Eds). To Err is Human. Building a safer health system. Institute of Medicine. National Academy Press, Washington 2000	http://www.iom.edu/iom/iomhome.nsf/WFiles/ToErr-8pager/$file/ToErr-8pager.pdf
The Australian Council on Healthcare Standards	http://www.achs.org.au/
Dr Foster (UK)	http://home.drfoster.co.uk/
Solucient (USA)	http://www.100tophospitals.com/
Commission for Health Improvement (UK)	http://www.chi.nhs.uk/
Medical Devices Agency (UK)	http://www.medical-devices.gov.uk/
Department of Health performance indicators (UK)	http://www.doh.gov.uk/nhsperformanceindicators/2002/
National Audit Office (UK)	http://www.nao.gov.uk/
Audit Commission (UK)	http://www.audit-commission.gov.uk/home/
Critical to Success: The Place of Efficient and Effective Critical Care Services within the Acute Hospital. Audit Commission. London 1999	http://www.audit-commission.gov.uk/publications/brccare.shtml
Comprehensive Critical Care. Department of Health 2000. (UK)	http://www.doh.gov.uk/compcritcare/index.htm
The Report of the Public Enquiry into children's heart surgery at the Bristol Royal Infirmary 1984–1995	http://www.bristol-inquiry.org.uk
National Institute for Clinical Excellence (UK)	http://www.nice.org.uk
National Confidential Enquiry into Maternal Deaths (UK)	http://www.doh.gov.uk/cmo/mdeaths.htm
National Confidential Enquiry into Perioperative Deaths. NCEPOD 2000 (UK)	http://www.ncepod.org.uk/
Task Force. Doing what counts for patient safety: federal actions to reduce medical errors and their impact. Report of the quality interagency coordination taskforce (QuIC). February 2000. (USA)	http://www.quic.gov/

Table 4. *(Continued)*

Australian Incident Monitoring Program	http://www.archi.net.au/toolkit/canberra–toolkit-Apr2001/pdf/01-Barraclough.pdf
National Health Priorities and Quality Branch (Australia)	http://www.health.gov.au/hsdd/nhpq/pubs/pquality.htm
Department of Health. An organisation with a memory. London 2000. (UK)	http://www.doh.gov.uk/pdfs/org.pdf
Handling Clinical Negligence Claims in England.	http://www.nao.gov.uk/guidance/chiefexec2d.htm
American Hospitals Directory	http://www.ahd.com/
National Audit Office. The Management and Control of Hospital-Acquired Infection in Acute NHS Trusts in England. London 2000	http://www.nao.gov.uk/publications/nao_reports/9900230.pdf
National Health Service Complaints: Health Services Commissioner (UK)	http://www.ombudsman.org.uk/publications.html
National Nosocomial Infection Surveillance (USA)	http://www.cdc.gov/ncidod/hip/Surveill/nnis.htm
Canadian nosocomial infection surveillance	http://www.hc-sc.gc.ca/hpb/lcdc/publicat/ccdr/97vol23/dr2306ea.html#
Hospitals in Europe Links for Infection Control through Surveillance, HELICS)	http://helics.univ-lyon1.fr/surv_net/surv_net.htm
Evidence-based guidelines for preventing Healthcare associated infections) Journal of Hospital Infection (2001) 47 (Supplement)	http://www.doh.gov.uk/hai/epic.htm
National Nosocomial Infection Surveillance scheme (UK)	http://www.phls.co.uk/ and http://www.phls.co.uk/publications/NINSS-Bacteraemia.pdf
Leapfrog Group (USA)	http://www.leapfroggroup.org/
The General Medical Council (UK)	http://www.gmc-uk.org/
The Society of Cardiothoracic Surgeons of Great Britain and Ireland	http://www.scts.org/doc/3811
The Society of Thoracic Surgeons (USA)	http://www.sts.org/
Institute for Healthcare Improvement	http://www.ihi.org

the number of hospitals at the beginning of the 20th century and the variations in standards between them resulted in the development of five minimum standards for hospital practice by the American College of Surgeons in 1924 [17]. These standards were based on the College's survey in 1919 and on surgical audit by Dr Ernest Codman of the Massachusetts General Hospital [18]. The standards encompassed professional organization, medical qualifications and competence, monthly meetings to review clinical work, documentation of clinical care, and appropriate supervision of laboratory services. By 1952, this method had evolved into a formal system of hospital accreditation involving colleges and associations in North America, now referred to as the Joint Commission on Accreditation of Healthcare Organizations. The Commission publishes comprehensive accreditation standards for the organization and processes of medical care [19], determined by on-site inspection.

In the United Kingdom, nationwide hospital standards were slow to develop, perhaps because nationalization of the health service encouraged the assumption that quality of care was uniformly high. The tradition of charitable health care which preceded the National Health Service, and the removal thereafter of a direct link between payment and service, has until recently tended to minimize consumer criticism, which is more usually directed towards the government and away from health service professionals. The responsibility for maintenance of standards has traditionally been devolved to Royal Colleges and other professional organizations. With the exception of laboratory services, these standards have tended to focus on process aspects of speciality training programs, rather than on clinical outcomes.

Recent Developments

A Proliferation of Control Agencies

This situation has changed following certain high-profile reports of medical error. In the UK, the most notable was that involving pediatric cardiac surgery at the Bristol Royal Infirmary [20]. The UK is of course not the only country so affected: in the USA the Institute of Medicine [2] has recommended the establishment of a Center for Patient Safety within the Agency for Healthcare Research and Quality. Corporate purchasers of health care have also had an important impact on health care in the USA: Solucient, an organization that provides health care information to other organizations, now publishes reports on the best 100 hospitals using benchmarks which include intensive care [21]. The Leapfrog Group, a consortium of the 500 largest US corporations, has begun an attempt to improve the quality of care for those workers insured by them. It has increased reimbursement for healthcare providers that use technologies proven to reduce error or improve outcome. The first three criteria are: use of electronic prescribing system with decision support, use of an intensivist to co-ordinate ICU care, and evidence based referral patterns.

In Australia, the Australian Council on Healthcare Standards [22] has responsibility for accreditation and benchmarking of health care services together with professional organizations. It has moved from triennial audit to a process of continuous monitoring of KPIs and indicators with hospitals having to provide evidence of structures and process for continuous improvement.. The Australian Incident Monitoring Program [23, 24] targets adverse events in anesthesia and intensive care medicine; and the National Health Priorities and Quality Branch of the health service produces reports [25] on many aspects of the health service including safety and hospital organization. In 2000, The Australian Council for Safety and Quality in Health was formed to promote better use of data to identify, learn from and prevent error or system failure, promote effective clinical govern-ance and accountability of individuals and organizations, re-design systems, create a culture of safety within health care organizations and to put consumers first. The Victorian Department of Human Services has now mandated hospitals to imple-ment a formal risk management program based on Australian/New Zealand Stand-ard 4360:1995. This incorporates sentinel event reporting, root cause analysis of reportable incidents and formal examination by each hospital of coronial inquest findings to ensure that lessons are learned and assimilated into practice.

In the UK, the role of the Royal Colleges has been augmented (or diminished from some points of view) by the creation of the National Institute for Clinical Excellence (NICE) [26], and the Commission for Health Improvement (CHImp) [27]. The role of NICE is "to provide patients, health professionals and the public with authoritative, robust and reliable guidance on current 'best practice'" which includes guidance on health technologies and the treatment of specific conditions. The role of CHImp is to "assure, monitor and improve the quality of patient care" through clinical governance reviews, and on-site visits to every NHS trust and health authority in England and Wales. It also has responsibility for investigating serious service failures in the NHS at the request of the Secretary of State for Health, an activity that was traditionally the role of the Royal Colleges. There are many other bodies with varying responsibilities for differing aspects of medical practice. The General Medical Council and General Nursing Council are responsible for standards of professional practice, the Royal Colleges for standards of education and training, the Medical Devices Agency [28] coordinates reports of adverse events relating to healthcare equipment, the Audit Commission [29] is an inde-pendent body responsible for ensuring the proper use of public monies by all public services, and the National Audit Office [30] has a similar role but reports through the Auditor General directly to Parliament. More recently an independent com-pany called 'Dr Foster' has been set up by a group of non-medical individuals supported by senior clinicians, to provide information about all hospitals in the UK and Ireland [31]; this is similar in scope to the American Hospital Directory [32], except that the latter provides detailed information only to subscribers. Dr Foster is free, and offers benchmarking on all hospitals using mortality, waiting times, and complaints response times.

It is evident that one of the challenges for those working in health care services, whether as front line staff or as managers, is knowing how to respond to the various agencies, auditors, reports, and standards, all of which have interlinking interests or responsibilities for the various processes which focus finally on the delivery of medical and nursing care to specific individuals. In the USA the Quality Interagency Coordination Task Force (QuIC) [4] was established in 1998 to undertake this task, to "ensure that all Federal agencies involved in purchasing, providing, studying, or regulating health care services are working in a coordinated manner toward the common goal of improving quality care". In the UK the seminal report, "An organization with a memory" [33], produced by the chief medical officer recommends the development of coordinated reporting mechanisms for learning from medical error and adverse events.

Speciality-Specific Surveys and Confidential Enquiries

Perinatal Mortality

One of the earliest standing surveys of mortality was the report by the Committee on Maternal Morbidity and Mortality in the UK, published in 1930 by the Ministry of Health with the collaboration of the (Royal) College of Obstetricians and Gynaecologists [34]. Since 1952 the report, The Confidential Enquiry into Maternal Deaths, has been published triennially [35]. These reports incorporate the two key elements of confidentiality and peer review. Over the years they have shown a continued trend towards lower mortality and morbidity rates.

Perioperative Mortality

Another seminal survey, of deaths relating to anesthesia in the USA, was that of Beecher and Todd in 1964 [36], who examined prospectively nearly 600,000 anesthetics over a five-year period, separating anesthetic causes of mortality from those attributable to surgery. Anesthesia could be identified as a factor contributing to death in 1:1,560 procedures, and causative in 1:2,680. This survey had been preceded in the UK by that commissioned by the Association of Anaesthetists in 1949 [37] which collected 1,000 voluntary reports of deaths occurring over five and a half years; the authors stated that "in the great majority of reports there were departures from ideal practice" although they could not determine the size of the problem as the study did not provide denominator data. This was followed by Dinnick in 1964 [38], who reviewed a further six hundred deaths. Again no denominator information was available, but the results of this second report confirmed the finding of the first, and went on to highlight the presence of important surgical factors in high-risk patients whose deaths had been attributed to anesthesia. Poor physical health had also been identified as an independent risk factor by Dripps et al [39]. In 1977, the Association of Anaesthetists, funded by the Nuffield Provincial Hospitals Trust, initiated a study of anesthetic deaths in Britain. The objectives were to establish a system of confidential and anonymous reporting, to determine current standards for future comparative analyses, to identify factors related to anesthetic deaths, and to improve standards. Surgical collaboration was initially not obtained, and this made it difficult to interpret the results, which were published in 1982 by Lunn and Mushin [40, 41]. Subsequent studies gained the participation of the Association of Surgeons, and the survey has evolved into the National Confidential Enquiry into Perioperative Deaths (NCEPOD), which publishes annual reports examining factors contributing to deaths within the first thirty days following surgery [42–44].

Table 5. Type and incidence of serious adverse events (SAEs) (from [45] with permission)

Serious adverse event	Number (%)
Emergency admission to ICU	95 (22.9 %)
Death	80 (19.3 %)
Respiratory failure	52 (12.6 %)
Readmission to ICU	37 (8.9 %)
Sepsis	27 (6.5 %)
Cardiac arrest	27 (6.5 %)
Unscheduled tracheostomy	26 (6.3 %)
Acute pulmonary edema	19 (4.6 %)
Continuous hemofiltration	16 (3.8 %)
Stroke	16 (3.8 %)
Acute myocardial infarction	15 (3.6 %)
Pulmonary embolism	4 (1.2 %)
Total	414

These surveys use deaths as the denominator, not all operations or anesthetics, so the incidence of attributable mortality is an estimate. Data collection is retrospective, and the burden of data is not inconsiderable. There has been a commendable reduction in deaths attributable to anesthesia and surgery over the years, and improvements in sub-optimal practices, but the pace of change is slow, and the methods for diffusing information not well defined.

Large numbers of adverse events occur in surgical patients, but many of the studies documenting this are retrospective. A recent, prospective study in a large Australian medical center documented the incidence of pre-defined serious adverse events (Table 5) in surgical patients expected to remain in hospital longer than 48 hrs [45]. There were 414 serious adverse events in 190 of 1125 surgical inpatients between 1998 and 1999. Serious adverse events were more common after unscheduled surgery and in patients over 75. A mortality rate of 20 % pertained if both factors were present compared to an overall mortality of 7.1 %. These data are supported by studies from Colorado and Utah [8, 9] and in the UK [11] where similar incidences of adverse events were documented.

The overall mean hospital stay was 21.8 days: for those with no serious adverse event it was 18.4 days and for those with one or more serious adverse event mean hospital stay was 38.5 days (p<0.001).

These adverse events occur in what are accepted as 'good' hospitals but reflect care processes which have not adapted to the current realities of economic contraction, shorter medical working hours and the concentration of sicker more at risk patients by the devolution of simpler cases to outpatient care. There is often a lack of skills to cope with the sick ward patient that can be a consequence of non-availability of sufficiently senior staff (otherwise occupied in outpatients or operating room) or to the use of inexperienced junior staff covering at night and at weekends. This produces boundary zone transition problems that result in a mismatch between patient acuity and medical/nursing resources and skill sets. This can occur either during pre-ICU [46] or post-ICU care. Unfamiliar medical hardware (e.g., tracheostomy, central venous catheters) combined with reduced patient tolerance of 'stress', and unfamiliarity with the potential complications of such devices – obstruction from poor humidification and line sepsis – are major impact areas where follow up and education may be very successful.

The question remains, how many of these adverse events on the wards are preventable? The Bellomo group instituted a prospective intervention study (Bellomo et al personal communication) using the Medical Emergency Team (MET) concept [47, 48]. An intensive care based team responds to calls to patients initiated by ward staff according to a set of pre-determined simple physiological criteria. These criteria are well-documented precursors of cardiac arrest if uncorrected [49]. There were 8,974 medical admissions during the control period and 8,377 during the MET intervention period. In the control period there were 33 cardiac arrests among these patients, which decreased to 11 during the intervention period (relative reduction: 66.6 %; p=0.0022). There were 12,116 surgical admissions during the control period and 12,544 during the intervention period. Cardiac arrests in these patients decreased from 30 to 11 (relative reduction: 63.3 %; p=0.0026). Overall, there were 37 deaths due to cardiac arrests in the control period and 16 during the intervention period (relative reduction: 56.7 %; p=0.0084). After their cardiac arrest, survivors in the control period required a total of 163 ICU bed days versus 33 in the intervention period (relative reduction: 79.7 %; p<0.0001) and a further 1353 hospital bed days versus 159 in the intervention period (relative reduction: 88.2 %; p<0.0001). There were 302 in-patient deaths during the control period and 222 during the intervention period (relative reduction: 26.5 %; p<0.0042). It therefore appears that a 'hospital wide system re-engineering process' to enable a systematic response to signs of physiological instability in surgical and medical in-patients is capable of significantly reducing the morbidity, mortality and (probably) cost of care.

Several other studies demonstrate the potential for a system-based factor to promote poor outcomes for hospital patients: for example, night-time discharge from ICU increases mortality [50], more than 50 % of ICU emergency admissions receive inadequate pre-ICU care [46], and a decreased nurse-patient ratio increases complications after esophagectomy [51].

Cardiac surgery is a special case in terms of audit. Surgeon-specific outcomes are published in the USA, and will shortly be published in the UK, a move long-resisted but no longer defensible following the Bristol inquiry. It is difficult to measure the effect that this approach might have on surgical practice even within large databases such as those of the Society of Cardiothoracic Surgeons of Great Britain and Ireland [52], or the Society of Cardiothoracic Surgeons in the USA [53]. Personal experience indicates that such data will increase the frequency of prolonged and futile intensive care treatment, and a disinclination to operate on high-risk cases.

In Australia, several regional and national peer group audit processes are being conducted which have a formal feedback capability. Examples are the Melbourne

Vascular Surgical Association which receives data on all surgical procedures conducted by its members, collates and compares outcomes and is able to counsel surgeons whose results are two standard deviations below the group mean results for particular procedures. There is a national joint replacement outcomes register and the Australian and New Zealand Intensive Care Society Patient Database supervises collection, collation and reporting of aggregated ICU patient outcomes. These data are returned to State intensive care committees that represent State or Area health authorities and the intensive care constituencies and advise on the validity of outlier results with a view to specific inquiry and improvement.

Nosocomial infection is also subject to standardized – but voluntary – reporting in the USA [54] and the UK [55–58], both systems of surveillance demonstrating substantial risks to patients from hospital-acquired infection, much of which is device-related. Canada [59] and Australia [60] also have surveillance systems. In the UK, around 100,000 hospitalized patients (one in eleven hospital admissions) acquire a nosocomial infection each year, most frequently the elderly and children. Patients so affected spend 2.5 times longer in hospital at an increased cost of almost £1 billion each year. It is estimated that 30 % of these nosocomial infections are avoidable; if only half were prevented, this would save the health service around £150M.

Intensive care infections are identifiable separately in the USA database. Surveys of infection in intensive care have been reported in France [61, 62], and the European Prevalence of Infection in Intensive Care (EPIC) survey across 17 European countries [63]. The HELICS group [64] provides a degree of European coordination of nosocomial infection surveys and reports. However, those relating to intensive care – the area of the hospital with the highest levels of nosocomial infection – are generally dependent for their continuance on the commitment of individuals and the vagaries of research funding.

Medical Error in Critically Ill Patients

Intensive care medicine has to some extent been protected from the public exposure of medical error accorded to other disciplines. There are several likely reasons for this. The heterogeneity of case mix makes it more difficult to determine causation. Adverse outcomes are often expected, and are frequently the reason for admission to intensive care in the first place. Sub-speciality status in many countries means that analysis of intensive care activity may be subsumed in that of the base speciality. Finally, the intensity of supportive care may deflect attention from other aspects of quality such as appropriateness or diagnostic accuracy.

There have been several surveys of medical error in ICUs and in the care of critically ill patients. The results of such surveys are inevitably weighted towards the greater likelihood of detection of error, given the greater severity of illness of the patients, higher levels of therapeutic dependence and interventions, and (once inside the ICU) more opportunities for detection from more intensive monitoring. These factors should be taken into account when interpreting differences between ICU and non-ICU rates, when examining the effect of complication rates on mortality, and when planning comparative studies.

Outside the ICU

Studies of patients outside the geographical confines of the ICU have focused on inter- or intra-hospital transport, and on patients receiving care in ordinary wards before or after ICU admission. Fifty critically ill patients transferred by a dedicated transport team suffered no adverse events during the journey [65], compared with eight life-threatening complications in seven of 50 patients being transported by non-specialist staff [66]. Similar findings apply to pediatric transfers [67, 68] A survey of 100 consecutive admissions to two ICUs in the UK [46] identified suboptimal care in 54 patients before admission, and an increase in the stand-ardized mortality ratio in this group. An earlier study from France found a pre-ICU adverse event rate of 12.6 %, half of which were preventable [69]. Death following discharge from intensive care may also be a measure of suboptimal discharge decisions or poor ward care. Discharge from the ICU at night, as a surrogate from premature discharge driven by rationing, is associated with a 73 % increase in mortality risk [48]. The impact of post-ICU care on ICU-attributed outcomes is important, since post-ICU mortality varies substantially between ICUs and coun-tries; a unit with a high standardized mortality ratio may be providing adequate care in the unit, but acquire surplus mortality because of premature discharge decisions or poor post-ICU care.

Inside the ICU

There are several studies of adverse event rates in adult ICUs, from the UK [70], France [71], Israel [72], and South Africa [73]. These suggest that patients suffer an adverse event rate in the region of 30 %, most of which are attributable to human error involving drug prescribing and communication failures, followed by techni-cal and equipment-related errors. Patients suffering an adverse event have an increased mortality risk of between 30–90 %. A survey of complications in pediatric intensive care in the USA [74] demonstrated an adverse event rate of 8 %; risk was higher early in the patients' stay, and in the more severely ill children, and increased the risk of death. Excessive workload [75], and inadequate specialist nursing and medical involvement in patient care [51, 76–78], have been identified as important factors contributing to adverse outcomes. Prospective observational studies and data reported from the AIMS-ICU (voluntary anonymous incident reporting in Australian ICUs) have demonstrated that communication failures, medication errors, staff shortages and to a lesser extent equipment failure or misuse, contribute to actual safety reductions or near misses. In most cases it is possible to institute system wide processes to reduce the incidence of, or mitigate the results of such events.

An important complication of medical care in the ICU is nosocomial infection, as mentioned above. At least 20 % of critically ill patients acquire an infection in the ICU [63] and this is usually device-related [79]. Encouraging staff to adopt proper hand disinfection techniques remains a challenge [80]. Education is likely to be the most effective component in modifying this risk [81]. The high incidence of methicillin-resistant *Staphylococcus aureus* (MRSA) in ICUs and hospitals around the world has almost become accepted by practitioners (though not by patients and their families) as an inevitable part of clinical practice. It is not true, however, that such infections are inevitable or resistant to remediation. Bacteriological surveillance studies using phage and DNA typing have demonstrated the contamination of pre-operative wards from fomites such as blood pressure cuffs and bedside curtains. Increased attention to ward cleanliness, allocation of specific equipment to individual patients, cohort nursing of identified cases, streaming of pre- and post-operative patients into different ward areas and use of chlorhexidine in alcohol hand rinses have all reduced the incidence of colonization and subsequent infection rates.

At what point does the natural history of a disease become indiscernible from the complications of treatment? An example of this is acute respiratory distress syndrome (ARDS). Undeniably, a complex set of inflammatory responses is set in train by many types of primary lung injury. When the physiological dysfunction is sufficient, medical intervention such as endotracheal intubation and mechanical ventilation are required. Undoubtedly these interventions have saved many lives, but there is increasing evidence to suggest that well intentioned, but ill informed, treatment modalities may have exacerbated the disease process. Even if mortality rates were not increased, potentially salvageable patients (given better subsequent knowledge regarding ventilation technique) will have died. The debate over the use and abuse of the pulmonary artery catheter is another case in point.

Causes and Prevention of Error

Table 6 lists some of the main causes of error. As patient care is usually mediated through human contact, the traditional approach to error management has been to identify and blame the member of staff who was involved in the final common pathway. However, adverse events in medicine are rarely, if ever, caused by a single factor, whether related to staff, equipment, or the organization. Reason's 'Swiss cheese' model of accident causation [3] demonstrates graphically how hazards of various types may be realized as adverse events through a chain of causation

Table 6. Factors contributing to medical error

System factors	Human factors
Suboptimal organizational culture	Failure to apply knowledge
Inadequate resources	Communication errors
Inadequate investment in audit	Inexperience
No investment in staff training or support	Technical inadequacy
Failure to learn from experience	Overwork and fatigue
	Denial, fear and guilt
	Inability to collaborate
	Lack of supervision, support

involving latent errors in the system, organizational deficits, faults in error recognition and detection, and human slips and lapses. The human element is usually the final common pathway, and much of the time institutional or system errors are prevented from becoming realized as adverse events by corrective action taken at this stage.

System Factors

The system in which people work has a profound effect on outcomes. Examples from industry demonstrate that an organizational culture which is supportive, open, collaborative, eager to learn, and committed to quality will do much to reduce the incidence of avoidable error. Most health care organizations are themselves part of larger systems, and will have difficulty in creating a successful culture unless they are themselves supported from the top. The key to success is leadership by example, combined with adequate investment in structures and people. A knowledge base is essential, but will be insufficient if it is not accompanied by dissemination of information and support for the introduction of best practice.

Human Factors

Expressions such as "to err is human", and "A comedy of errors" indicate that humans have come to accept the inherent fallibility of their activities. Such fallibility is manifest in errors of judgement or interventions. In turn these errors are promoted by the intrinsic neuronal and functional characteristics of our brains, lack of knowledge, and by environmental factors which modify attention span, concentration, or physical performance. When people work together towards a common goal, communication of intent, required activities and outcomes is an intrinsic part of achieving the desired group goal. Communication errors are frequent co-factors in adverse events where human beings interact. The book edited by Marilyn Sue Bogner, "Human Error in Medicine" covers a wide range of scenarios where human behavioral frailties impact on clinical care [82].

The Interaction Between Individuals and the System

Since the pioneering works of Reason [3] and Rasmussen [83] in studies on industrial accidents, a large body of work has been generated about the role of 'human factors' and error. As a general construct, it is widely agreed that clinicians generally do their best to achieve a desirable outcome for their patients. Individuals work within an environment which will impact on their performance. The environment consists of a knowledge space, a physical space, cultural space, rules space and an inter-personal interaction space.

Absence of knowledge (e.g., 'the Earth is flat') leads to logical but inappropriate behavior ('don't fall off the edge'). Similarly, prior to knowledge of germ activity in causation of disease and sepsis, 'laudable pus' was seen as the normal curative process following wounding or surgery, and therefore a desirable outcome. Translating advances in knowledge into sustained changes in behavior remains a major challenge, and infection control and cross infection prevention are good examples of the problem. Hospitals do not need to be dirty and dangerous places; the fact that many are is an indication of both personal and institutional failures that require a systems approach for correction. One of the problems of the current adversarial approach to analyzing mistakes and adverse events is that blame is attributed to individuals rather than the system. Sleep deprivation and impaired individual performance is an example [84, 85]. The complexity of adopting a systems approach to this problem is easily demonstrated by the consequences which flow from the desirable aim of limiting long working hours, but at the price of reduced training time and clinical experience, impaired team working, reduced continuity and responsibility for patient care, and a diminished sense of personal responsibility and professionalization.

Reporting Systems

The Australian Incident Monitoring Study in intensive Care-AIMS-ICU is a voluntary anonymous reporting system to identify incidents which result in harm, or have the potential to reduce patient safety. Over a 4-year period 4000 incidents were submitted to a central repository that collated and published the data. The following is a small selection of information that has already been or is being prepared for publication [86, 87]. Further details should be sought from sources sited in the reference section. The AIMS-ICU program has received reports in the major categories shown in Fig. 1 and Table 7.

Information from AIMS type programs has revealed that failure to follow agreed protocols and forgetfulness are important factors in equipment and drug related errors. Many of the simplest and most mundane sounding bedside processes can have a major effect in reducing the chance of error; for example, aircraft pilot type checklists and algorithms have been a major factor in reducing anesthesia morbidity and mortality. These processes can be adopted for ICU patient bay equipment, 'doctors orders', medication and infusion checks prior to patient admission and again at change of nursing shift. Check lists for other complex devices/processes such as hemofiltration machines, balloon pumps, temporary pacemakers are examples. Double checking of drugs prior to administration is also effective in reducing medication events. Communication failures have repeatedly been identified as central to adverse events in complex care environments. One of the benefits of the intensivist is as a co-ordinating individual who can prevent discrepant therapies being instituted by various members of the team, and ensuring that therapeutic goals are enunciated frequently and targets achieved. Explicitly stated and written objectives increase the likelihood that all members of the bedside team – senior and junior medical staff, nurses, physiotherapists, dietitians, and relatives where appropriate – are aware of the daily plan of management and this is a major benefit in ensuring that conflicting therapies are avoided.

The AIMS process has been adopted and modified in the US. By implementing a web based ICU Safety Reporting System (ICUSRS), the participants aim to

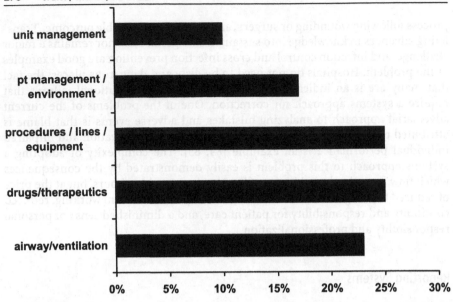

Fig. 1. AIMS-ICU Summary of the First 4000 reports. Proportion of reports in each of the major categories. From [25] with permission.

Table 7. AIMS-ICU. Details of the first 4000 reports. Each of the major categories has been broken down into more descriptive sub-categories. By collating events in this way, low frequency high impact events may be found as having a systematic cause rather than being a random event. From [25] with permission.

Airways/Ventilation - Total 1594					
Airway related incidents	378	Airway equipment systems	834	Airway complications	382
Accidental extubation	115	Incorrect setup	179	Hypoxia/desaturation	140
Inadequate airway securing	79	Faulty equipment	56		
Unplanned reintubation	77				
Nasal/facial trauma	63				

Drugs/Therapeutics – Total 1762			
Treatment planning	203	Administration problems	1559
Portal of entry error	41	Delayed administration	213
Inappropriate preparation	21	Wrong infusion rate	162
Failure to cease	21	Incorrect dose/frequency	159
		Labeling error	111
		Wrong concentration	110

Table 7. *(Continued)*

Procedures/Lines/Equipment – Total 1772			
Vascular access line related	693	Other procedures/equipment systems	1079
Incorrect set up	164	Incorrect set up	150
Dislodgement	154	Faulty equipment	112
Inadequate securing	190	Power/battery problem	35

Patient Management/Environment Total 1214		Unit Management Total 695	
Moving/positioning patient	85	Insufficient nursing staff	100
Pressure care	72	Staff inexperience	88
Inadequate patient supervision	60	Communication/handover	71
Infection control	57	Liaison with team outside ICU	65
Missed diagnosis/incorrect treatment	47	Incorrect allocation of staff/patient	48
Care of confused patient	47		
Fall/physical injury	47		

Most frequently chosen contributing factors: *(multiple selections possible)*			
Error of problem recognition	1,124	Distraction	624
Failure to follow protocol	874	Inadequate patient assessment	617
Failure to check equipment	712	Error of judgement	613
Communication problem	657	High unit activity	599

identify high-risk situations and working conditions, to help change systems and reduce the risk of error. The analysis and feedback of reports will inform the design of interventions to improve patient safety. The effort is aided substantially by collaboration with the 30 participating ICUs. Important stakeholders include the Society of Critical Care Medicine, the American Society for Healthcare Risk Management (ASHRM), the FDA Center for Devices and Radiologic Health; the Foundation for Accountability (FACCT), and the Leapfrog Group. A demonstration and evaluation of the system is under way, funded by the Agency for Healthcare Quality and Research.

One of the problems cited by critics of voluntary anonymous schemes is that the denominator rate of events is unknown and that 'good' units which use AIMS effectively would have many more events reportable than units in which the system was not working well. Both comments are true but miss the fundamental point that the process engenders a safety oriented focus in the unit which is cognizant of risk related situations and operates to minimize or mitigate such events. AIMS was never designed to provide a league table for inter-unit comparisons. Nevertheless it is true that the effectiveness of error reduction strategies is hard to gauge using an AIMS process alone. The Institute of Healthcare Improvement (Boston Mass, USA) has designed a number of collaborative exercises involving emergency departments and ICUs amongst others. Using a random sampling of ICU patients' charts and tabulating the occurrence of pre-defined trigger events, a time series sample can be obtained to give some idea of the efficacy of quality/safety improvement exercises. This process could potentially be used as a comparative index between units. However, in the same way that severity scoring systems like APACHE II and SAPS II may fail to explain differences in care processes and outcomes between institutions, this trigger index is also likely to be affected by factors which may not be under the direct influence of the unit under examination.

Human error usually comes at the end of the chain of causation. A common factor is failure to take appropriate action even though with hindsight the individual knows what he or she should have done. Underlying reasons for this are inexperience, failure to take proper care, errors in communication, and lack of senior support and supervision. Many of these problems can be addressed through training, and it is essential that appropriate attitudes to safe practice are taught as early as possible in the undergraduate curriculum, and reinforced subsequently.

Forces for Change

Consumer-lead Pressure

A combination of cost-containment, consumer pressure groups, and litigation has made patient safety a political priority. In the USA the Leapfrog Initiative [88] initiated by the chief executives of the country's 500 most influential and largest companies, directs patients for whose medical insurance they are responsible to those hospitals which make the fewest mistakes and provide the best standards of care. They have identified three key indicators: computerized prescribing, evidence-based referral patters, and the presence of properly trained intensive care doctors. They state that 'intensivists', physicians specially trained to care for critically ill patients in intensive care units (ICUs), should staff ICUs. More than four million patients are admitted to ICUs each year in the US and more than 500,000 of these patients die. Studies reveal that at least one in ten patients who die every year in ICUs would have an increased chance to live if intensivists were present in the ICU and managing their care for at least eight hours per day. While not every hospital's ICU can assure 8 hours per day of intensivist care because there is a shortage of intensivists in the United States, this staffing level is an important factor to consider when choosing a hospital if your doctor expects that you are likely to stay in an ICU during your hospitalization". At the same time, Solucient, an organization that provides health care information to other organizations [21], now incorporates information about intensive care in its benchmarking process to identify the best 100 hospitals in the USA. This type of pressure is a potent force for change, and it also brings with it some challenging responsibilities for health care planning.

Education

Medical education is changing rapidly. The two most important components are the drive towards outcome-based methods [89], and the development of competency-based learning. In the UK it is now a requirement for clinical negligence insurance cover for hospitals that doctors in training have their competence assessed in those areas in which they practice. This has had the beneficial effect of directing the emphasis on training away from exam-based methods and towards workplace-based methods of training and assessment. The UK's competency-based training program in intensive care medicine is the first fully comprehensive such scheme for any speciality [90]. Competency-based methods allow trainers and trainees to focus on those aspects of knowledge, skills and attitudes that directly affect the delivery of patient care, including aspects of patient safety.

Information and the Role of Databases

It is evident from the multiplicity of organizations and agencies with responsibility for different but inter-related aspects of healthcare that there is a real need for adequate support for the collection and dissemination of accurate information collected once, and as close to the point of care as possible. Duplication of data collection for different agencies, inadequate support for the process of data collection, and the absence of methods for dissemination and implementation, are real problems.

In this respect, intensive care has demonstrated significant commitment to data collection and analysis of outcomes in a manner that has found favor with politicians at least. Several countries now have important observational databases containing case mix-adjusted outcomes, and are using these to inform and improve practice through education and research. Examples include the Intensive Care National Audit and Research Center in the UK, Project Impact in the USA, the ANZICS Patient Database for Australia and New Zealand, and the Canadian Collaborative Critical Care Trials Group. These activities were established by the efforts and commitment of intensive care practitioners, with somewhat variable support from the health services that they are designed to benefit.

Health Informatics

The massive change in the system of health care delivery and the knowledge explosion have led to increasing fragmentation of the partners in care. Multiple care providers mean multiple opportunities for miscommunication, failure to follow up, potential for contradictory care plans and drug interactions. The advent of stronger privacy legislation in many parts of the world may have the unintended result of increasing this fragmentation of patient information by restricting information flow about patients. In many countries, political sensitivity to unique patient identifiers has prevented development of information systems to facilitate patient care across multiple locations and providers. One of the major problems associated with the rapid increase in knowledge is the failure of the medical community to use new information – failure to adopt new 'proven' therapies and failure to discard familiar 'disproved' therapies. This can be seen, e.g., in the widespread failure to use beta-blockers in at risk peri-operative patients with ischemic heart disease, or the often patchy use of heart failure therapy or asthma prophylaxis.

Identification of these patients and recommendations for therapy based on hospital policy and the increasing evidence base can be facilitated by models of care. Over the last 20 years, pioneers in health informatics [91, 92] have developed unique institution based computer systems which have far reaching implications. There are many reasons why the lessons learned have been slow to gain foothold in routine clinical practice. Modern web browser technology, the internet and open systems databases, together with reducing cost/computing power ratio, reduced cost of data storage, and data showing efficacy together with an increasingly safety conscious public and governments, have opened the way for computer based electronic health records. These records will not only record information but assist the disparate care providers to communicate with each other more freely, assimilate evidence based guidelines into the care process and reduce drug error. In so doing they will also be able to facilitate real time education of staff and patients and provide aggregate data about individual clinician performance and patient outcome as a natural corollary of the care process. Hospital wide clinical information systems can improve the feed back of information about patient outcome to medical care 'silos' such as emergency departments [93] and ICUs, where follow up is difficult. Significant funding, political, privacy, standards, coding and technological hurdles exist, but already the lessons learnt by the informatics pioneers can be readily assimilated in the new technology.

Confidentiality and Ownership of Data

Patients have a right to information about the quality of care they will receive, to justify the trust they must have in the clinical staff to whom they entrust themselves. Clinical staff must also have the freedom to review and improve their practice without fear of litigation in the absence of negligence. The collection of case mix-adjusted data on medical performance requires commitment and integrity; the ability to recognize and correct deficiencies requires courage. The move towards publication of doctor-specific outcomes is probably detrimental to these parallel processes, and negates the recognition that error is usually a systems problem, not a person-specific problem. Individual performance should be a matter for local clinical governance; performance of groups and of services should be in the public domain. Intensive care can contribute to this process by making outcomes data more freely available, and stimulating public discussion about the aims and processes of care. This would do much to enhance the trend towards a culture of greater openness and partnership with our patients.

Conclusion

Medical error is common, and represents a significant source of avoidable injury to patients. A systems approach is required to reduce the current level of adverse events, through investment in coordinated systems of data gathering and reporting, education, and encouraging a focus on quality and leadership at a local level. At this point, the interaction between our knowledge of human factors, the widespread application of clinical risk management programs, development of clinical information systems, evidence based medicine and the electronic health record hold the promise of improved systems safeguards to reduce the burden of medical error. The key to success lies in transdisciplinary collaboration and an institutional focus on quality.

References

1. Perrow C (1984) Normal Accidents. Basic Books, New York
2. Kohn LT, Corrigan JM, Donaldson MS (2000) To Err is Human. Building a Safer Health System. Institute of Medicine Report. National Academy Press, Washington
3. Reason J (1990) Latent Errors and System Disasters. In: Human Error. Cambridge University Press, Cambridge, pp 173–216
4. Quality Interagency Coordination Task Force (QuIC) (2000) Doing What Counts for Patient Safety: Federal Actions to Reduce Medical Errors and their Impact. At http://www.quic.gov/report/errors6.pdf. Accessed 7/5/02
5. Cooper JB, Newbower RS, Long CD, McPeek B (1978) Preventable anesthesia mishaps: A study of human factors. Anesthesiology 49:399–406
6. Leape LL, Brennan TA, Laird N, et al (1991) The nature of adverse events in hospitalized patients. Results of the Harvard Medical Practice Study II. N Engl J Med 324:377–384
7. Brennan TA, Leape LL, Laird NM, et al (1991) Incidence of adverse events and negligence in hospitalized patients. Results of the Harvard Medical Practice Study I. N Engl J Med 324:370–376
8. Gawande AA, Thomas EJ, Zinner MJ, Brennan TA (1999) The incidence and nature of surgical adverse events in Colorado and Utah in 1992. Surgery 126:66–75
9. Thomas EJ (2000) Incidence and types of adverse events and negligent care in Utah and Colorado. Med Care 38:261–271
10. Wilson RM, Runciman WB, Gibberd RW, Harrison BT, Newby l, Hamilton JD (1995) The Quality in Australian Health Care Study. Med J Aust 163:458–471
11. Vincent C, Neale G, Woloshynowych M (2001) Adverse events in British hospitals: preliminary retrospective record review. Br Med J 322:517–519
12. Neale G, Woloshynowych M, Vincent C (2001) Exploring the causes of adverse events in NHS hospital practice J R Soc Med 94:322–330
13. Heinrich HW (1941). Industrial Accident Prevention: A Scientific Approach. McGraw-Hill, New York
14. Hofer TP, Kerr EA (2000) What is an error? Institute of Healthcare Improvement, Boston
15. Leape LL (2000) Institute of Medicine medical error figures not exaggerated. JAMA 284:95–97
16. Lester H, Tritter JQ (2001) Medical error: a discussion of the medical construction of error and suggestions for reforms of medical education to decrease error. Med Education 35:855–861
17. American College of Surgeons (1924) The Minimum Standard. Bulletin of the American College of Surgeons 8:1–4
18. Codman EA (1916) Report of a Committee on Hospital Standardisation. Surg Gynecol Obstet 22:119–120

19. http://www.jcaho.org
20. http://www.bristol-inquiry.org.uk
21. http://www.100tophospitals.com
22. http://www.achs.org.au
23. http://www.archi.net.au/toolkit/canberra-toolkit-Apr2001/pdf/01-Barraclough.pdf
24. http://www.health.gov.au/hsdd/nhpq/pubs/pquality.htm
25. Hart GK (1999) Error in medicine: adverse events in intensive care. Schweiz Med Wochenschr 129:1583-1591
26. http://www.nice.org.uk
27. http://www.chi.nhs.uk
28. http://www.medical-devices.gov.uk
29. http://www.audit-commission.gov.uk/home
30. http://www.nao.gov.uk
31. http://home.drfoster.co.uk
32. http://www.ahd.com
33. http://www.doh.gov.uk/pdfs/org.pdf
34. Report on Confidential Enquiries into Maternal Deaths in England and Wales 1952-1954 (1957). HMSO, London
35. http://www.doh.gov.uk/cmo/mdeaths.htm
36. Beecher HK, Todd DP (1954) A study of the deaths associated with anaesthesia and surgery. Ann Surg 140:2-34
37. Edwards G, Morton HJV, Pask EA, Wylie WD (1956) Deaths associated with anaesthesia. Anaesthesia 11:194-220
38. Dinnick OP (1964) Anaesthetic deaths. Anaesthesia 19:536-556
39. Dripps RD, Lamont A, Eckenhoff JE (1961) The role of anaesthesia in surgical mortality. JAMA 178:261
40. Lunn JN, Mushin WW (1982) Mortality Associated with Anaesthesia. Nuffield Provincial Hospital Trust, London
41. Mushin WW (1983) Mortality associated with anaesthesia: The background to the British study. In: Vickers MD, Lunn JN (eds) European Academy of Anaesthesiology Proceedings. Springer-Verlag, Heidelberg
42. Buck N, Devlin HB, Lunn JN (1987) The Report of a Confidential Enquiry into Perioperative Deaths. Nuffield Provincial Hospitals Trust and the King's Fund, London
43. NCEPOD (1990) National Confidential Enquiry into Perioperative Deaths Report 1989. NCEPOD, London
44. http://www.ncepod.org.uk
45. Bellomo R, Goldsmith D (2002) Postoperative serious adverse events in a teaching hospital: a prospective study. Med JAust 176:216-218
46. McQuillan P, Pilkington S, Allan A, et al (1998) Confidential inquiry into quality of care before admission to intensive care. Br Med J 316:1853-1858
47. Buist MD, Moore GE, Bernard SA, Waxman BP, Anderson JN, Nguyen TU (2002) Effects of medical emergency team on reduction of incidence of and mortality from unexpected cardiac arrests in hospital: preliminary study. Br Med J 324:387-390
48. Hurihan F, Bishop G (1995) The medical emergency team: a new strategy to identify and intervene in high risk patients. Clin Intensive Care 6:269-272
49. Schein RM, Hazday N, Pena M, Ruben BH, Sprung CL (1990) Clinical antecedents to in hospital cardiopulmonary arrest. Chest 98:1388-1392
50. Goldfrad C, Rowan K (2000) Consequences of discharges from intensive care at night. Lancet 355:1138-1142
51. Amaravadi RK, Dimick JB, Pronovost PJ, Lipsett PA (2000) ICU nurse-to-patient ratio is associated with complications and resource use after esophagectomy. Intensive Care Med 26:1857-1862
52. http://www.ctsnet.org/section/outcome Accessed 7/5/02

53. http://www.sts.org
54. http://www.cdc.gov/ncidod/hip/Surveill/nnis.htm
55. National Audit Office 2000: http://www.nao.gov.uk/publications/nao_reports/9900230.pdf
56. Plowman R, Craves N, Griffin M, et al (2000). The socio economic burden of hospital acquired infection. Public Health Laboratory Service, London
57. http://www.doh.gov.uk/hai/epic.htm
58. http://www.phls.co.uk/publications/NINSS-Bacteraemia.pdf
59. http://www.hc-sc.gc.ca/hpb/lcdc/publicat/ccdr/97vol23/dr2306ea.html
60. http://www.med.unsw.edu.au/hiss/Default.htm Accessed 7/5/02
61. REANIS (1999) Guide pour la Prevention des Infections Nosocomiales en Reanimation. 2eme edn. EDK, Paris
62. Lelale A, Savey A, Pinzaru G, Fabry J (1995, 1996, 1997) Rea Sud-Est. Reseau de Surveillance des infections nosocomiales en reanimation. Rapports annuels
63. Vincent JL. Bihari DJ. Suter PM, et al (1995) The prevalence of nosocomial infection in intensive care units in Europe. Results of the European Prevalence of Infection in Intensive Care (EPIC) Study. EPIC International Advisory Committee. JAMA 274:639–644
64. http://helics.univ-lyon1.fr/surv_net/surv_net.htm
65. Bion JF, Aitchison TC, Edlin SA, Ledingham IM (1988) Sickness Scoring and response to treatment as predictors of outcome from critical illness. Intensive Care Med 14:167–172
66. Bion JF, Wilson IH, Taylor PA (1988) Transporting critically ill patients by ambulance: audit by sickness scoring. Br Med J 296:170
67. Barry PW, Ralston C (1994) Adverse events occurring during interhospital transfer of the critically ill. Arch Dis Child 71:8–11
68. Edge WE, Kanter RK, Weigle CG, Walsh RF (1994) Reduction of morbidity in interhospital transport by specialized pediatric staff. Crit Care Med 22:1186–1191
69. Trunet P, Le Gall JR, Lhoste F, et al (1980) The role of iatrogenic disease in admission to intensive care. JAMA 244:2617–2620
70. Wright D, Mackenzie SJ, Buchan I, Cairns CS, Price LE (1991) Critical incidents in the intensive therapy unit. Lancet 338:676–678
71. Giraud T, Dhainaut JF, Vaxelaire JF, et al (1993) Iatrogenic complications in adult intensive care units: a prospective two-center study. Crit Care Med. 21:40–51
72. Donchin Y, Gopher D, Olin M, et al (1995) A look into the nature and causes of human errors in the intensive care unit. Crit Care Med 23:294–300
73. Muckart DJ, Bhagwanjee S, Aitchison JM (1994) Adverse events in a surgical intensive care unit-a cause of increased mortality. S Afr J Surg 32:69–73.
74. Stambouly JJ, McLaughlin LL, Mandel FS, Boxer RA (1996) Complications of care in a pediatric intensive care unit: a prospective study. Intensive Care Med 22:1098–1104
75. Tarnow-Mordi WO, Hau C, Warden A, Shearer AJ (2000) Hospital mortality in relation to staff workload: a 4-year study in an adult intensive-care unit. Lancet 356:185–189
76. Blunt MC, Burchett KR (2000) Out-of-hours consultant cover and case-mix-adjusted mortality in intensive care. Lancet 356:735–736
77. Dimick JB, Pronovost PJ, Heitmiller RF, Lipsett PA (2001) Intensive care unit physician staffing is associated with decreased length of stay, hospital cost, and complications after esophageal resection. Crit Care Med 29:753–758
78. Pronovost PJ, Jenckes MW, Dorman T, et al (1999) Organizational characteristics of intensive care units related to outcomes of abdominal aortic surgery. JAMA 281:1310–1317
79. Richards MJ, Edwards JR, Culver DH, Gaynes RP (1999) Nosocomial infections in medical intensive care units in the United States. National Nosocomial Infections Surveillance System. Crit Care Med 27:887–892
80. Nishimura S, Kagehira M, Kono F, Nishimura M, Taenaka N (1999) Handwashing before entering the intensive care unit: what we learned from continuous video-camera surveillance. Am J Infect Control 27:367–369

81. Maas A, Flament P, Pardou A, Deplano A, Dramaix M, Struelens MJ (1998) Central venous catheter-related bacteraemia in critically ill neonates: risk factors and impact of a prevention programme. J Hosp Infect 40: 211–224
82. Bogner MS (1994) Human Error in Medicine, Lawrence Erlbaum Associates, Hillsdale
83. Rasmussen J (1990) Information Processing and Human-machine Interaction. Cambridge University Press, Cambridge
84. Olson LG, Ambrogetti A (1998) Working harder-working dangerously? Fatigue and performance in hospitals. Med J Aust 168:614–616
85. Nocera A, Khursandi DS (1998) Doctors working hours: can the profession afford to let the courts decide what is reasonable? Med J Aust 168:616–618
86. Beckmann U, Baldwin I, Hart GK, Runciman WB (1996) The Australian Incident reporting in Intensive care: Aims-ICU. An analysis of the first year reporting. Anaesth Intensive Care 26:320–329
87. Beckmann U, Carless R (1998) Incidents relating to central venous line usage in intensive care: Analysis of the first 4000 reports submitted to the Australian Incident Monitoring Study in intensive care (AIMS-ICU). Anaesth Intensive Care 26:396–400
88. http://www.leapfroggroup.org
89. http://www.acgme.org/index.htm
90. Intercollegiate Board for Training in Intensive Care Medicine: Competency-based training programme. At http://www.ics.ac.uk
91. Bates DW, Leape LL, Cullen DJ, et al (1998) Effect of computerized physician order entry and a team intervention on prevention of serious medication errors. JAMA 280:1311–1316
92. Shortliffe EH, Perrault LE (2000) Medical Informatics: Computer Applications in Healthcare and Biomedicine. Springer, New York
93. Croskerry P (2000) The Feedback Sanction. Acad Emerg Med 7:1232–1238

Changing ICU Behavior To Focus On Long Term Outcomes

J. McMullin and D.J. Cook

Introduction

Implicit in the title of this chapter is the belief that currently in the intensive care unit (ICU), our focus is restricted to short term outcomes. We hypothesize that there are several reasons for this. The appellation of critical care medicine underscores the serious illnesses from which most of our patients suffer. We provide advanced life support of a technological and pharmacological nature in the ICU, resuscitating and stabilizing patients. We invasively and non-invasively monitor physiology, usually intervening in an effort to normalize pathophysiology. Traditionally, critical care interventions have been highly intensive, expensive and brief, ending when patients are discharged from the ICU.

Figure 1 shows four typical time courses of illness leading to admission to the ICU. Dispositions of death or discharge can occur at any time. Critical illness is often presented as occurring only within the confines of an ICU, as shown in these schematics.

We believe that to change ICU behavior to focus on long term outcomes, we need to:
A) increase global awareness of disability post-ICU discharge, and
B) expand the involvement of the ICU team in key management decisions outside the ICU.

This alternative model of health care reflects the reality that critical illness is but an episode in the continuum of a patient's illness. In addition, it reflects the fact that critical illness has its own continuum, and it is not constrained by the ICU. Critically ill patients are cared for in many venues, including the emergency room, on the wards, in coronary care units and intermediate care units [1]. The notion of a health care continuum is one of the foundations of disease management [2]. The continuum concept lends itself well to considering critical illness more broadly than from the perspective of an ICU patient, and helps to concentrate our efforts on long term outcomes.

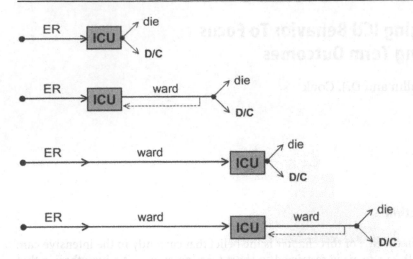

Fig. 1. This shows four different typical time courses of critical illness involving an ICU admission. The critical care delivered has primarily short term goals of resuscitation, stabilization and monitoring. ER: emergency room; D/C: discharge

Increased Awareness of Post-ICU Disability

Increased awareness of a problem is the first step towards change (although not always sufficient to result in change, or sustain change). Although a recent phenomenon, awareness of post-ICU disability has been relatively recent. Examples of diverse types of research attending to post-ICU disability has focused on analyzing the rates and reasons for ICU readmissions as a marker of ongoing or re-emergence of critical illness [3], a systematic review of studies measuring quality of life post-ICU discharge [4], and a description and costing of long term ventilation [5]. International consensus conferences and workshops about ICU outcomes [6] and end of life care [7] have also helped to shape our thoughts about the importance of health status following critical illness and ultimate outcomes. These meetings shape opinion and future research, culminating in academic milestones such as this Roundtable Meeting on Surviving Critical Illness (Brussels, 2002).

However, to increase awareness of post-ICU disability, we must:
1) acknowledge its relation to the original critical illness, and
2) acknowledge its relation to the interventions that we use in the ICU.

Acknowledging the Relation Between Post ICU Disability and Critical Illness

Many complications of critical illness have long term sequelae for ICU survivors. A simple and common example of this phenomenon is myocardial infarction sustained in the ICU which causes left ventricular dysfunction and subsequent functional limitation. The quintessential ICU complication of serious illness is acute respiratory distress sydnrome (ARDS), the study of which has demonstrated a commitment of intensivists to document the consequences of critical illness [8]. In an ongoing longitudinal multicenter cohort study, Herridge and colleagues are following ARDS survivors well beyond the conventional duration of follow-up, carefully documenting the patterns of receding organ dysfunction [9].

While it is obvious that recovery from critical illness is not immediate, factors less obvious are the extent of disability following critical illness experienced by some patients, and the scope and cost of rehabilitation that they require. The link between post-ICU disability, and the severity and duration of the original critical illness is challenging to quantitate, acknowledged somewhat in clinical practice, and worthy of further investigation. ICU clinicians may refer to this relationship when prognosticating for the families of ICU patients. Rigorous matched cohort studies estimating the hospital length of stay and functional outcomes attributable to critical illness would be welcome, since research examining attributable morbidity and mortality has tended to focus on ICU length of stay and mortality.

Acknowledging the Relation Between Post-ICU Disability and Critical Care Interventions

Care delivered in the ICU (comprised of monitoring devices, diagnostic tests, preventive and therapeutic interventions) can also have a direct effect on post-ICU disability. Necessary devices for diagnosis, monitoring and treatment such as internal jugular central venous catheters have associated complications such as catheter-related bacteremia, thrombosis, and pneumothorax. These apparently short-lived problems may nonetheless result in further complications in the ICU such as antibiotic associated diarrhea, a painful swollen limb, and chest tube insertion. These events may also have longer term sequelae such as the emergence of resistant organisms and pulmonary embolism. Fortunately, the ubiquitous central venous catheter rarely results in serious post-ICU disability.

Treatments administered in the ICU can have serious downstream effects. For example, neuromuscular blockers and corticosteroids may contribute to critical illness neuromuscular abnormalities. Inattention to the prevention of future clinical events during the ICU stay can have life threatening consequences on the ward (e.g., neglecting unfractionated heparin for venous thromboembolism prophylaxis resulting in pulmonary embolism). Adverse events in the ICU may also have long term sequelae, such as esophageal intubation during urgent reintubation resulting in anoxic encephalopathy. These latter three phenomena could all constitute 'medical errors' in the popular new lexicon. The first could be viewed as occurring because of too protracted a period of neuromuscular blockade (i.e., act of comission), the second occurring because of failure to attend to prevention (i.e., act of omission), and the third due to an iatrogenic complication (i.e., act of comission).

Acknowledging the links between these post-ICU disabilities (profound weakness, pulmonary embolism, and anoxic encephalopathy) and the interventions received by patients (or not) while they are in the ICU is fundamental to having a long term perspective of critical illness. General inattention to prophylaxis may

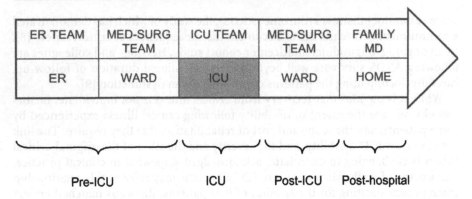

Fig. 2. This shows the traditional model of critical illness in which critical care is delivered only by ICU clinicians in the ICU. Patient management is delivered according to distinct clinical roles during distinct, usually short term, episodes of illness. ER: emergency room

partly reflect the fact that preventing future theoretical events is less compelling than managing real and present problems. The contemporary emphasis on classifying and remediating medical errors in the ICU may distinguish the short from the long term ICU outcomes associated with care delivered in the ICU.

Involvement of the ICU Team Outside the ICU

Conventionally, patients (whether or not they develop critical illness) are managed by different health care teams in different venues. A traditional course for a patient who develops critical illness during hospitalization is represented in Figure 2. A patient presents to the emergency room with a diagnosis of community acquired pneumonia, and is admitted to the ward. Her initial care is from the emergency room health care team, then the ward team. When her condition worsens and she develops respiratory failure, she is admitted to the ICU, intubated, ventilated and cared for by the ICU team. When she no longer requires life support and is stable for transfer, she is transferred back to the ward where the ward team takes over her care. Upon hospital discharge, the family physician takes over her care.

We propose an alternative model for caring for the critically ill patient, as represented in Figure 3. This involves an expanded role for clinicians with expertise in critical illness at several points along the continuum of care, identified by hatch marks.

Pre-ICU Critical Care Consultations

In this alternative model proposed in Figure 3, ICU clinicians may be called upon for critical care consultations, to help in the management of seriously ill, but not necessarily critically ill patients before they require ICU. The objectives of these

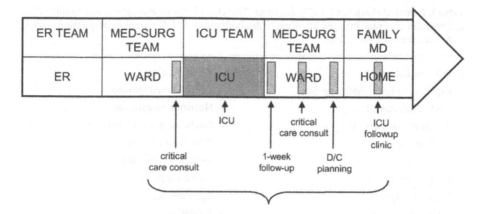

Expanded role of critical care

Fig. 3. This shows an alternative model of caring for the critically ill patient. Critical illness is viewed on a continuum. Patient management related to critical illness is offered at several points in the illness continuum. The focus is on optimizing long term outcomes.ER: emergency room; D/C: discharge

consultations may include clarifying diagnoses, and directing early treatment strategies, and preventing the development of critical illness. These consultations may recommend specific tests or changes in drug and other therapy. They may help to establish the short and long term goals of care, encouraging documentation of patients' resuscitation preferences.

Such a critical care consultation service has been described by Hillman and others in Australia (K Hillman, personal communication). Depending upon the foci of these critical care consultations, they may change the number of patients admitted to ICU and the level of care administered therein.

Critically Ill Patients in the ICU

In this alternative model, ICU clinicians would coordinate the care of critically ill patients while they are in the ICU, as usual.

The trigger for ICU discharge for many critically ill patients is ability to breathe spontaneously, ability to protect the airway, and hemodynamic stability without vasoactive drug infusion. Other considerations before discharge may include the match between the nursing workload associated with a transferable patient, and the workload capacity of the ward to which the patient is being transferred. Reconceptualizing ICU discharge is another way to change behavior to focus on long term outcomes.

For example, use of administrative interventions such as discharge checklists can symbolize the need for better transitioning between venues of care, and can foster recognition of long term consequences of critical illness. Such checklists can

Table 1. Potential check-list for ICU discharge. This checklist is an example of an administrative intervention that may increase attention to disability post-ICU discharge by requesting explicit orders for post-ICU discharge.

– Problem list	– Rehabilitation
– Expected hospital discharge date	– Occupational therapy
– Goals of treatment	– Nutrition assessment
– Resuscitation directives	– Swallowing assessment
– Medications	– Depression screen
– Device care	– Psychiatric evaluation
– Respiratory therapy	– Social supports
– Physiotherapy	– Spiritual needs
– Occupational therapy	– Palliative care

focus recommendations of the ICU team on clinical assessments, formal tests and services that are needed at the early stage of recovery from critical illness (Table 1).

ICU Follow-up Rounds

In this alternative model, ICU clinicians would round on selected patients discharged from ICU within the last week. These patients may be targeted using criteria such as: i) chronic comorbidities before ICU admission; ii) ICU admission for at least 72 hours; or iii) severe multiple organ dysfunction while in ICU. Patients may be excluded from a one week follow-up visit if their post-ICU care is highly routine, and they have a low probability of long term complications (e.g., the majority of elective cardiac surgery patients). In other words, the patients suitable for one week follow-up rounds would be those patients whose critical illness, or critical care interventions, make them susceptible to protracted disability following ICU admission.

One focus of ICU follow-up rounds could be critical illness neuromuscular abnormalities, which are well established complications of the ICU stay. This is a heterogeneous condition affecting nerve, muscle, or both, and may be a major contributor to protracted convalescence following critical illness [10]. More common and less serious is the disuse atrophy experienced by many bedridden patients, which usually recovers with time, optimal nutrition and graduated activities. These problems may have very serious long term consequences for patients who are elderly or deconditioned before hospitalization. We propose that each ICU patient is formally evaluated for acquired neuromuscular abnormalities while they are in the ICU. However, because such assessment ideally involves voluntary movement, this assessment may not be optimal until patients have spent a few days on the ward. We believe that physiotherapists may be more suitable assessors than physicians for this task, and obviously they are more skilled at targeted rehabilitation for affected patients.

These one week post-ICU follow-up rounds could be educational and interactive, occurring weekly as part of the portfolio of teaching sessions in a residency rotation. During these rounds, socratic methods could be used to elicit specific recommendations for helping the transition from critical illness to recovery.

Post-ICU Critical Care Consultations

In this alternative model, in addition to the one week post-ICU follow-up rounds, ICU clinicians may be called upon for critical care consultation at any point during the patients' hospitalization. These patients may be selected by the ward team because they are at risk of needing readmission to the ICU. The consultations may recommend intensified treatment for the same problem that necessitated their index ICU admission, thereby preventing recidivism to the ICU. Alternatively, these consultations may recommend new treatment strategies for new hospital-acquired problems (non-invasive mechanical ventilation for COPD patients just developing an exacerbation).

With the passage of time and as mentation improves, patients on the ward may begin to reflect on their ICU experiences. Another way to change ICU behavior to focus on long term outcomes is to increase awareness of ICU workers about the experiences that patients remember from their ICU stay. Limited recall of ICU events is not universal, and several investigators have described patients' disturbing memories of weaning from mechanical ventilation using qualitative methods. Qualitative research aims to interpret data to develop theoretical insights that describe and explain phenomena such as interactions, experiences, roles, perspectives and organizations. These qualitative studies used primarily in-depth personal interviews as a data collection method, grounded theory as an analysis method. Important experiences of weaning from mechanical ventilation included frustration, uncertainty, hopelessness, fear and lack of mastery [11]. The extent to which, in at least some patients, these experiences are determinants or consequences of weaning failure, or both, is difficult to establish. An assumption of this genre of research is that if clinicians understand the lived experiences of patients, they can better appreciate patient needs during the weaning process, and by inference, their role as clinicians during weaning from mechanical ventilation. We suggest that this research is also important for its role in highlighting the psychological aftermath of the ICU stay.

A reminder-based system for drug therapy could be an integral part of post-ICU critical care consultations. Computer decision supports or simple paper reminders could be used to prompt weekly review of each patient's medication profile to promote individualized pharmcotherapy appropriate for each patient's stage of critical illness. When we implemented this in our own institution for 20 patients discharged from ICU, we found three patients who needed drug discontinuation. Ranitidine had been continued post-ICU discharge when it had been originally prescribed for stress ulcer prophylaxis based on the presence of the risk factor of mechanical ventilation for more than 48 hours. In one patient, aspirin was discontinued, which had been started in ICU for electrocardiographic signs of coronary ischemia. Instead, the patient was ambulated and a stress test conducted; no sign of coronary artery disease was identified. For three other patients with diabetes, a prokinetic was restarted, which had been discontinued upon ICU discharge when nasoduodenal enteral nutrition was changed to oral feeds; two of these three patients had nausea and vomiting on the ward likely related to diabetic gastroparesis exacerbated by their critical illness.

Hospital Discharge Rounds

In this alternative model, ICU clinicians would attend hospital discharge rounds for selected patients who were in the ICU. These patients may be targeted using criteria as outlined earlier. At this time, prognosis may be discussed regarding their specific critical illness disabilities such as cardiorespiratory dysfunction and neuromuscular abnormalities of critical illness. Recommendations would be formulated about outpatient physiotherapy and other rehabilitation requirements. Patients and their families would be approached to ask whether they would like to attend the ICU follow-up clinic.

Like all of the foregoing suggestions for increasing attention to long term outcomes following critical illness, attendance of ICU clinicians at hospital discharge rounds could be formally evaluated in terms of decisions made, new services offered, patient and family satisfaction, and return to hospital rates. Attendance of ICU clinicians at these discharge rounds may have a substantial impact on discharge arrangements in the first 6 months, and it may become redundant over time. Research itself can be a powerful change strategy, and identifying situations in which interventions can be short lived, without reinforcing strategies, and yet still effective would be worthwhile.

ICU Follow-up Clinic

In this alternative model, selected ICU patients as outlined above would be invited to return as an outpatient for an ICU follow-up clinic. During this clinic visit, patients would be reassessed regarding the original condition that necessitated the ICU admission, and the specific problems they acquired during their critical illness. Emphasis would be placed on secondary prevention of critical illness. At this outpatient visit, the patient could also debrief about their experience in the ICU.

It is well accepted now that people who have suffered catastrophic illnesses are prone to develop anxiety disorders, post-traumatic stress, mood disorders, and major depression. These problems may surface during the ICU stay, during the post-ICU hospitalization, or occur many months remote from the hospitalization. We propose that screening for these psychological problems be undertaken through an in-depth interview and use of validated instruments at least once during the post-ICU hospitalization. However, the potential advantage of doing this during the ICU follow-up visit is a greater perspective due to the opportunity to reflect on recovery and residual disability. The ICU follow-up visit also provides a more relaxed opportunity to alert patients and family members of the possibility of delayed development of these disorders so that early recognition and necessary treatment can be offered, perhaps later by the family physician.

This meeting also provides an opportunity to explore any role redefinition or other readjustment (personal or familial) as the patient returns to the family unit or community. Many patients, particularly those who are elderly or debilitated before their ICU admission may be unable to cope with their previous living arrangements. Some patients discharged from hospital following an ICU admission may initially be considered suitable for their prior living arrangement, but after hospital discharge, delayed recognition of functional decline and cognitive impairment may make may prior arrangements unsuitable. An ICU follow-up clinic could provide an opportunity to identify this inability to cope with the prior living arrangement, and may avert the need for readmission to hospital.

Conclusion

Temporal trends suggest that the demand for critical care will increase in future years. Limited ICU bed availability will necessitate earlier ICU discharge, resulting in sicker patients being cared for on the wards. A growing number of elderly ICU patients will have premorbid disability, meaning that more ICU survivors will have post-ICU disability.

Insufficient attention to the long term outcomes of critical illness is contributed to by many modifiable factors. Successful change strategies require an analysis of the real and perceived deterrents to change.

Change usually requires introducing enabling and reinforcing strategies. Several different initiatives may refocus the attention of ICU clinicians, educators, and researchers on long term outcomes following critical illness. Specific effective behavior change strategies include interactive education, reminders and feedback, audits, evidence based practice guidelines, benchmarking and multifaceted approaches [12–18].

When change is proposed, it is important to define who has decisional responsibility for the change, who is responsible for maintaining the change strategy, and who is responsible for evaluating it. This is imperative when implementing interventions by several different ICU clinicians from different disciplines.

With respect to other educational initiatives, profiling post-ICU disability more prominently in daily ICU rounds, local teaching sessions, post-graduate courses, symposia and conferences would further increase global awareness of post-ICU disability, particularly if the education is interactive. This awareness could strengthen the foundation for future change. Qualitative research on how clinicians perceive the link between critical illness and ICU interventions – and the long term outcomes we seek to optimize – would be useful. This work could increase attention to short term and long term outcomes of critical illness inside and outside the complex, dynamic multidisciplinary ICU environment. A research program to implement cognitive, behavioral and administrative strategies for changing behavior is necessary.

To change ICU behavior to focus on long term outcomes, we need to increase global awareness of disability post-ICU discharge, and expand the involvement of the ICU team in key management decisions outside the ICU. This model of health care reflects the reality that critical illness is but an episode in the continuum of a patient's illness, and that critical illness is itself a continuum.

References

1. Cook DJ (1998) Caring for critically ill patients: Past, present and future. JAMA 280:181–182
2. Ellrodt AG, Cook DJ, Lee J, Cho M, Hunt D, Weingarten S (1997) Evidence-based disease management. JAMA 278:1687–1692
3. Chen LM, Martin CM, Keenan SP, Sibbald WJ (1998) Patients readmitted to the intensivd care unit during the same hospitalization: Clinical features and outcomes. Crit Care Med 26:1834–1841
4. Heyland DK, Guyatt GH, Cook DJ, et al (1998) Frequency and methodologic rigor of quality-of-life assessments in the critical care literature. Crit Care Med 26:591–598
5. Gracey DR, Gillespie D, Nobrega F, et al (1987) Financial implications of prolonged ventilator care of Medicare patients under the prospective payment system: A multicenter study. Chest 91:424–427
6. Suter P, Armagandis A, Beautils F, et al (1994) Predicting outcome in ICU patients. European Consensus Conference Report. Intensive Care Med 20:390–397
7. Rubenfeld DG, Curtis JR for the End-of-Life Care in the ICU Working Group (2001) End of life care in the intensive care unit: A research agenda. Crit Care Med 29:2001–2006
8. Davidson TA, Caldwell ED, Curtis JR, et al (1999) Reduced quality of life in survivors of acute respiratory distress syndrome compared with critically ill control patients. JAMA 281:354–360
9. Herridge MS, Cheung AM, Tansey C, et al (2001) Long term clinical outcomes in survivors of ARDS. Am J Resp Crit Care Med 163:A253 (abst)
10. DeJonghe BD, Cook DJ, Sharshar T, LeFaucheur JP, Carlet J, Outin H (1998) Neuromuscular disorders in critically ill patients: A systematic review. Intensive Care Med 24:1242–1250
11. Cook DJ, Meade MO, Perry AG (2001) Qualitative studies on the patient's experience of weaning from mechanical ventilation. Chest 120 (Suppl 6):469S–473S
12. Bero LA, Grilli R, Grimshaw JM, et al (1998) Closing the gap between research and practice: An overview of systematic reviews of interventions to promote the implementation of research findings. Br Med J 317:465–468
13. Grimshaw J, Freemantle N, Wallace S, et al (1995) Developing and implementing clinical practice guidelines. Qual Health Care 4:55–64
14. Oxman AD, Thomson MA, Davis DA, et al (1995) No magic bullets: A systematic review of 102 trials of interventions to improve professional practice. Can Med Assoc J 153:1423–1431
15. Davis D, Thompson-O'Brien MA, Freemantle N, et al (1999) Impact of formal continuing medical education: Do conferences, workshops, rounds and other traditional continuing education activities change physician behavior or health care outcomes? JAMA 82:867–874
16. Soumerai SB, Avorn J (1990) Principles of educational outreach ('academic detailing') to improve clinical decision making. JAMA 263:549–556
17. Hunt DL, Haynes RB, Hanna SE, et al (1998) Effects of computer-based clinical support systems on physician performance and patient outcomes: A systematic review. JAMA 280:1339–1346
18. Kiefe CI, Allison JJ, Williams OD, et al (2001) Improving quality improvement using achievable benchmarks for physician feedback: A randomized controlled trial. JAMA 285:2871–2879

L.O.V.E. and Quality of Life within the ICU: How can it improve Patient Outcome?

J. Carlet, M. Garrouste-Orgeas, and B. Guidet

Introduction

Many factors potentially able to influence outcomes in critically ill patients have been described and widely explored. These include, besides therapeutic issues and quality of care [1], the underlying condition of the patient, the acute severity of illness, as well as organizational and managerial issues in the intensive care unit (ICU) [2–4]. Each of these areas is discussed in this book. However, quality of life of the ICU team, or of the patient or relatives during or after their ICU stay, which are heavily influenced by the quality of the relationship between the team and the patients/relatives, and could theoretically influence patient outcomes or be responsible for severe psychological sequelae, have been poorly studied. For simplification, we will regroup all those managerial, sociologic, and behavioral issues in the ICU under the term L.O.V.E. (Leadership, Ownership, Values and Expectations). L.O.V.E. will of course be influenced by many factors related to human polymorphism, occurrence of acute and painful events, before or during the ICU stay, but mostly by the managerial and governance profile within the unit, which determine the respect that people (both patient, relatives and health care workers) 'feel' during the part of their life that they spend in the ICU. Although very scarce in the hospital setting in general, a few data are available in the ICU [4–10]. More extensive data are available from the industrial world.

L.O.V.E. and Quality of life within the ICU: Theoretical Concept

As everywhere else, people in the ICU need, in order to be happy and thus efficient, to work in agreement with their personal values and to be both understood and respected [11–13]. Job satisfaction is an important parameter of team cohesion, nurses intent to stay in the team and quality of care [14–17]. However, it is likely that living in the ICU environment makes job satisfaction more difficult to achieve. Patients and their relatives are very anxious [18, 20]. Some of them show their anxiety clearly and it is rather easy to take care of them. Others are unable to communicate and often react in an 'aggressive' manner [18]. This feeling of anxiety, sometimes leading to aggressiveness is often amplified by a strong feeling of guilt in the relatives of certain patients (Fig. 1).

The most frequent example of this aggressiveness is when relatives have taken an important part in a surgical decision, and the surgical procedure is unfortunately followed by serious complications. In fact, it is likely, although not carefully studied, that aggressiveness in the relatives of ICU patients is a mixture of anxiety, lack of understanding of the medical situation, lack of communication with the team [21–24] and, eventually, guilt. Very few people are aggressive just for fun.

Similar reactions can occur in health care professionals. Many young nurses or residents coming into the ICU for the first time are very anxious and highly stressed [25]. Some of them understand quickly how to deal with these feelings and are able to ask for advice when needed. Others find this less easy and either react with excessive anxiety or give the wrong impression that they are not focused or even not motivated for the job. This leads usually to the departure of the nurses from the unit, which further increases nurse turnover [14, 15, 26] and can leave serious physiological sequelae and frustration, both in deciders and people involved (Fig. 2).

Fig. 1. Stress consequences in relatives of critically ill patients

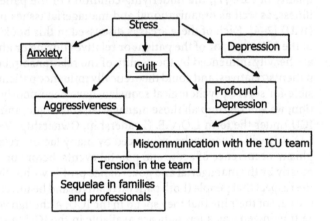

Fig. 2. The nurse turnover vicious circle

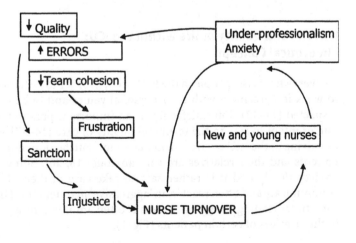

Fig.3. The team and patient
or relatives anxiety interaction

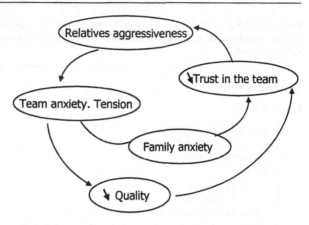

There are strong interactions between the levels of anxiety of the nurses and those of the patients and relatives (Fig. 3). Some of the families can, usually after an initial period of extreme anxiety and/or guilt, or in response to sometimes trivial events happening during the patient stay, lose confidence in the team.

Such relatives then usually check every therapy delivered, look at the charts, try to find abnormalities or hidden undesirable events, which will confirm in some kind of evidence based manner' their negative judgement of the team. Most of these behaviors are likely to be due to 'uncontrolled' anxiety and lack of communication. This can further increase anxiety or at least extreme discomfort in the team and lead to vicious circles (Figs. 1–3).

Most of these tensions and problems are probably preventable. The list of organizational or behavioral solutions, which of course is far from exhaustive, is shown in Table 1. The actions that can be implemented to improve quality of life of patients and relatives during the stay in the ICU are plotted on Table 2. Some actions are of paramount importance (not all of them have been carefully studied). This program includes:

1) The implementation of an appropriate program including dedicated nurses to teach the new professionals arriving in the ICU, in order to help them feel comfortable in the unit and decrease their stress. In some countries, including France, very inexperienced nurses are sent to the ICU just after obtaining their diploma. These additional programs are of paramount importance. Similar strategies must be implemented with residents.

2) The involvement of the complete team, including of course the nurses, for important decisions, in particular end of life decisions in patients. Regular discussions for the most difficult cases.

3) Strong collaboration between nurses and physicians. The unit must be like a family.

4) Freedom for any member of the team to mention their disagreement with decisions, contest the behavior of anyone, or mention any serious concern without being considered as a spy ('non punishment reporting'). Conflict management and trouble shooting systems.

Table 1. L.O.V.E. in the ICU: Managerial and behavioral aspects as important components of patient, relative and ICU team quality of life, potentially influencing patient outcomes (non exhaustive list)

Governance Style:

Leadership (L)

1. Example of team managers.
2. Management style (27–29)
3. Interpersonal warmth
4. Justice
5. Encouragement
6. Autonomy. Liberty
7. Conflict management. Trouble shooting [30]
8. Support of new nurses (teaching, psychological support…). Specific nurse for teaching
9. Team decision for end of life and ethical or difficult issues [31,32]
10. Rotation day/night for nurses and physicians, to avoid conflicts between the teams
11. Non punishing reporting

Recognition and valorization of each profession within the team (ownership) (0)

Respect and development of personal values and expectations (V, E)

Table 2. How to improve quality of life of patients and of relatives during their stay in the ICU)

Who is the patient?
 – Photos, hobbies, religious issues

Visiting hours for relatives [34, 35]:
 – Day and night visiting
 – The ICU room as an 'extension of their home'
 – Special organization for end of life

Compassion throughout the ICU stay [33]

Cooperation and transparency with the relatives :
 – Information
 – Charts available for close relatives
 – Family as 'part of the team'
 – Total transparency and honesty with patients and relatives [38, 40].
   Incident and error reporting

Quality of the end of life and death

Psychologist in the ICU team.

Free visiting hours (anytime, day or night) for the relatives. Efforts to help them 'make themselves at home'. Compassion.

6) Consistency in the information given to relatives between all professionals working in the unit (quality and stability of the transmission of the information).

7) Easy access to medical charts for the (close) relatives if they ask for it.
8) Total transparency concerning medical decisions with both the team and relatives.
9) Signaling of errors and undesirable events to relatives.
10) Continuous improvement of the communication program in the unit.

Such a program needs formalized and shared policies and a common philosophy, with a very strong involvement of the managers of the team (head nurse, senior medical staff, head of the unit, and department) and even more important a strong willingness of the hospital managers (human resources department) to implement and support this kind of program and behavior all over the hospital. Exemplary is determinant in this respect.

In fact, interconnected with the above 10 'commandments', love (not the acronym this time) is indubitably the most important issue, in order to improve quality of life for staff, patients, and relatives.

Influence of the ICU Governance Style on Patient Outcomes. Examples from the Industrial World and Application to the ICU

Different managerial styles has been described [5, 7, 27, 28, 41, 42]. The assessment of governance styles could be made through specific questionnaires such as the Organizational Culture Inventory (OCI) which has been used by several authors [5, 7, 28]. These authors define:
1) a 'constructive style', composed of self-actualizing, achievement, 'humanistic encouragement' and affiliation cultures
2) a passive/defensive style composed of approval, conventional, dependent, and avoidance cultures
3) an aggressive/defensive style composed of oppositional, power, competitive, and perfectionist cultures.

Each of those 'forces' can be graded and plotted on a scheme, summarizing the 'profile' of the given unit or structure.

A very complex and extensive questionnaire with 120 items is needed to determine these governance styles. This OCI has been used in several studies performed in the ICU. Shortell et al. [43] showed, in a multicenter study involving 1700 respondents in 42 ICUs, that the questionnaire was appropriate to the ICU environment. In another study, the same author [28] looked at the relationship between a series of parameters, including managerial ones, and mortality predicted by the APACHE III score. They found that after a careful risk-adjustment, the following items were related to a low mortality: technology availability, low diagnostic diversity, caregiver interaction comprising culture, leadership, co-ordination, communication and conflict management abilities, lower nurse turnover, high evaluated technical quality of care, and greater evaluated ability to meet family member needs. They proposed that some of these issues could be important 'leverage points' for caregivers, managers and external policy givers.

There are very few other studies showing a relationship between governance style or managerial issues and outcome. Miranda et al. [3] showed that organizational designs influence burn out and ICU team quality of life in a multicenter study involving 12 European countries.

Several studies have showed a positive influence of an appropriate and constructive nurse/physician co-operation and outcome [44-46]. Some other studies showed, on the contrary, that distance from the ideal-type discretionary pattern predicted organizational, but not clinical, outcomes [28]. In this study, units closer to the ideal-type had higher nurse retention, and were viewed as better places to work, higher perceived quality of care by both nurses and physicians. However, objectively measured quality of care, patient satisfaction, severity-adjusted mortality and length of stay were not consistently related to better structured units.

We have implemented most of the actions listed in Table 1 in our unit. A special emphasis has been put on free visitation for relatives, ability for families to participate in patient care, efforts to better know who is the patient (recent patient photograph required), teaching program for new nurses provided by a well trained, long time nurse member of the unit, regular ethical discussions, team work and common decisions for end of life, efforts to improve quality of death of the patients, triage policies, assessment of post-ICU quality of life of patients and families. Whether these actions have improved outcomes in our unit is not known yet, and a study has been designed to look at this issue. Moreover, we intend to look prospectively at the sequelae in relatives of the most severely ill ICU patients, which has been poorly studied, in order to use it as one of the outcomes to be followed. A multicenter study is ongoing in France, co-ordinated by one of us (BG PHRC n° 98-124), and aimed at correlating outcomes, in particular mortality predicted by case mix and severity adjusted severity scores (SAPS II), with organizational, managerial and governance styles (assessed by OCI) in the participating units. The data will be available shortly.

In conclusion, we think the way people behave within an ICU team is an important determinant of patient outcome, health care workers and patient/relative's quality of life. Although, some data are already available, additional studies are mandatory in order to move this concept from logic- and heart-based to evidence based medicine.

References

1. Clemmer TP, Spuhler VJ, Oniki TA, et al (1999) Results of a collaborative quality improvement program on outcomes and costs in a tertiary critical care unit. Crit Care Med 27:1768-1774
2. Pronovost PJ, Jenckess MW, Dorman T, et al (1999) Organizational characteristics of intensive care units related outcomes of abdominal aortic surgery. JAMA 14:1310-1317
3. Reis Miranda D, Ryan DW, Schanfeli WB, Fidler V (1997) Organizational and Management of Intensive Care: a Prospective Study in 12 European Countries. Springer, Heidelberg
4. Zimmerman JE, Shortell SM, Rousseau DM, et al (1994) Improving intensive care units : Observations based on organizational case studies in nine intensive care units. Crit Care Med 10:1443-1451

5. Cooke RA, Szumal JL (1993) Measuring normative beliefs and shared behavioral expectations in organizations: The reliability and validity of the Organizational Culture Inventory. Psychol Rep 72:1299–1330
6. Xenikou A, Furnham A (1996) A correlational and factor analytic study of four questionnaire measures of organizational culture. Hum Rel 49:349–371
7. Cooke RA, Rousseau DM (1988) Behavioral norms and expectations: A quantitative approach to the assessment of organizational culture. Group and Organization Studies 13: 245–273
8. Rousseau DM (1990) Normative beliefs in fund-raisins organizations: Linking culture to organizational performance and individual responses. Group and Organization Studies 15:448–460
9. Klein AS, Masi RJ, Wiedner CK (1995) Organizational culture, distribution and amount of control and perceptions of quality. Group and Organization Studies 20:122–148
10. Bennett D, Bion J (1999) ABC of intensive organization of intensive care. Br Med J 318:1468–1470
11. Devidhizar R (1989) Retention technique # 1. Developing managerial warmth. Dimens Crit Care Nurs 8:28–37
12. Rushton CH (2001) Caregiver suffering is a dimension of end-of-life care. Am Nurse 33:9–23
13. Rushton CH, Scanlon C (1995) When values conflict with obligations: safeguards for nurses. Pediatr Nurs 21:260–261
14. Al-Ma'aitah R, Cameron S, Horsburgh ME, Armstrong-Stassen M (1999) Predictors of job satisfaction, turnover, and burnout in female Jordanian nurses. Can J Nurs Res 31:15-30
15. Boyle DK, Bott MJ, Hansen HE, et al (1999) Managers' leadership and critical care nurses' intent to stay. Am J Crit Care 8:361–371
16. Sohl-Kreiger R, Lagaard MW, Scherrer J (1996) Nursing case management: relationships as a strategy to improve care. Clin Nurse Spec 10:107–113
17. Demerouti E, Bakker AB, Nachreiner F, et al (2000) A model of burnout and life satisfaction. J Adv Nurs 32:454–464
18. Caine RM (1989) Families in crisis: making the critical difference. Focus Crit Care 16:184–189
19. Azoulay E, Pochard F, Chevret S, et al (2001) Meeting the needs of intensive care unit patient families. Am J Respir Crit Care Med 163:135–139
20. Pochard F, Azoulay E, Chevret S, et al (2001) Symptoms of anxiety and depression in family members of intensive care unit patients: ethical hypothesis regarding decision-making capacity. Crit Care Med 29:1893–1897
21. Fins JJ, Solomon MZ (2001) Communication in intensive care settings: the challenge of fuel disputes. Crit Care Med 29:N10–N15
22. Lilly CM, De Meo DL, Sonna LA, et al (2000) An intensive communication intervention for the critically ill. Am J Med 109:469–475
23. Fetters MD, Churchill L, Danis M (2001) Conflict resolution at the end of life. Crit Care Med 29:921–925
24. Wright S, Bowkett J, Bray K (1996) The communication gap in the ICU – a possible solution. Nurs Crit Care 1:241–244
25. Severinsson EI, Kamaker D (1999) Clinical nursing supervision in the workplace – effects on moral stress and job satisfaction. J Nurs Manag 7:81–90
26. Cavanagh SJ (1988) The conflict management style of intensive care nurses. Intensive Care Nurs 4:118–123
27. Shortell SM, Zimmerman JE, Rousseau DM, et al (1994) The performance of intensive care units : Does good management make a difference? Med Care 32:508–525
28. Mitchell PH, Shannon SE, Cain KC Hegyvary ST (1996) Critical care outcomes : linking structures, processes and organizational and clinical outcomes. Am J Crit Care 5:353–363
29. Volk MC, Lucas MD (1991) Relationship of management style and anticipated turnover. Dimens Crit Care Nurs 10:35–40
30. Thijs LG (1997) Continuous quality improvement in the ICU: general guidelines. Task force of the European Society of Intensive Care Medicine. Intensive Care Med 23:929–930

31. Mularski RA, Bascom P, Osborne M (2001) Educational agendas for interdisciplinary end of life curricula. Crit Care Med 29 (Suppl):N16–N23
32. Puntillo KA, Benner P, Drought T, et al (2001) End-of-life issues in intensive care units : a national random survey of nurses' knowledge and beliefs. Am J Crit Care 10:216–229
33. Levy MM, Carlet J (2001) Compassionate end-of-life care in the intensive care unit. Crit Care Med 29 (Suppl): N1
34. Whitis G (1994) Visiting hospitalized patients. J Adv Nurs 19:85–88
35. Roland P, Russell J, Richards KC, Sullivan SC (2001) Visitation in critical care : processes and outcomes of a performance improvement initiative. J Nurs Care Qual 15:18–26
36. Bijttebier P, Vanoust S, Delva D, Ferdinande P, Erans E (2001) Needs of relatives of critical care patients : perceptions of relatives, physicians and nurses. Intensive Care Med 27:160–165
37. Prost SG, Puchalski CM, Larson DB (2000) Physicians and patient spirituality : professional boundaries, competency, and ethics. Ann Intern Med 132:578–583
38. Patrick DL, Danis M (1989) Patients' and families' preferences for medical intensive care. JAMA 13:242–243
39. Danis M, Patrick DL, Southerland LI, Green ML (1988) Patients' and families' preferences for medical intensive care. JAMA 260:797–802
40. Danis M, Jarr SL, Southerland LI, Nocella RS, Patrick DL (1987) A comparison of patient, family, and nurse evaluations of the usefulness of intensive care. Crit Care Med 15:138–143
41. Brilli RJ, Spevetz A, Branson RD, et al (2001) Critical care delivery in the intensive care unit : defining clinical roles and the best practice model. Crit Care Med 29:2007–2019
42. Adams A, Bond S (2000) Hospital nurses' job satisfaction, individual and organizational characteristics. J Adv Nurs 32:536–543
43. Shortell SM, Rousseau DM, Gillies RR, et al (1991) Organizational assessment in intensive care units (ICUs) : construct, development, reliability, and validity of the ICU Nurse-Physician Questionnaire. Med Care 29:709–723
44. Sirio CA, Rotondi AJ (1999) The value of collaboration: quality improvement in critical care units. Crit Care Med 27:2034–2035
45. Baggs GJ, Schmitt MH, Faan RN, et al (1999) Association between nurse-physician collaboration and patient outcomes in three intensive care units. Crit Care Med 27:1991–1998
46. Bushnell MS, Dean JM (1993) Managing the intensive care unit: physician-nurse collaboration. Crit Care Med 21:S389–S390

Re-organizing Health Care Systems to Optimize Critical Care Outcomes

M. Hartleib and W. J. Sibbald

Introduction

Short-term health outcomes may be an attractive measure of success for individual hospital departments. For example a coronary care unit (CCU) may feel that improvements in morbidity and mortality following cardiac catheterization are valuable, while an intensive care unit (ICU) physician may feel that a decrease in the rate of ventilator-acquired pneumonia (VAP) represents a significant improvement in care. While both of these outcomes do represent short-term quality, they may be meaningless to downstream health care workers if these same patients are suffering adverse long-term outcomes because of or related to their initial treatment. For example, a patient who is significantly malnourished and suffering from 'critical care polyneuropathy' may represent a significant burden to downstream medical staff, and to the hospital as a whole. This is especially worrisome if these problems were preventable during the treatment for a patient's initial illness. Moreover, the initial treating physicians may be unaware of these long-term complications, because their effects and treatment do not affect short-term quality outcomes.

The business community has demonstrated success through the integration of services, the elimination of duplicated effort, and the concentration by all departments on the company mission or long-term outcomes. We believe that health care systems can improve the quality of patient care by re-organizing their services to optimize long-term outcomes. It is our goal in this chapter to examine the theoretical framework for change, and to use the ICU as a model to demonstrate how the shift in focus from short-term to long-term outcomes can improve the quality of care delivered by a health care system as a whole. We will examine the meaning of a health care system, examine lessons from the business world, discuss the integration of services, briefly examine a conceptual framework for change, and then provide examples of how an ICU physician can utilize these lessons both before and during admission to an ICU, as well as following discharge, to integrate care and improve both short and long-term outcomes.

Health Care Systems

Health care has become increasingly complex, in pace with rapid advancements in science and technology. However, because or in spite of this increased complexity, health care systems have generally failed to translate advances into meaningful improvements in clinical practice. In fact, health care not infrequently harms patients, persists in using ineffective treatment, is slow to adopt effective therapies, and continues to be overly tolerant of delays and unacceptably high levels of error [1–3]. Improving quality in health care is a goal shared by managers attempting to guide institutions, as well as clinicians seeking to provide the best care for their patients. Quality is defined by The Institute of Medicine as the "degree to which health services for individuals and populations increase the likelihood of desired health outcomes and are consistent with current professional knowledge" [4].

Healthcare often refers to its care delivery models as 'systems'. A system can be defined as the integration of parts that become interconnected to achieve a common purpose. While each part may be able to function independently, and may be analyzed separately from the whole, it is the interconnection of the various parts which creates the real power by which systems achieve their goal. Health care systems are a classic example of 'interconnectedness' and can be analyzed according to component micro-systems (e.g., a doctors office), or larger macro-systems (e.g., a hospital or a community based health maintenance organization [HMO]). Intuitively, levels of interconnectedness increase dramatically in macro- versus micro-systems. In successful macro-systems, such as when care is delivered by an HMO, each of the parts (e.g., hospitals, outpatient clinics, community care, and the laboratory) ideally integrate both vertically and horizontally to smoothly achieve a common goal. In the same way, smaller macro-systems, such as hospitals, require integration of the various services involved in care delivery (e.g., emergency departments, critical care units, medical wards, labs, etc.,) to achieve an acceptable end product.

Lessons from the Business World

There are many examples of success in the private, non-health related sector where safety and productivity of complex macro-systems have been improved through quality improvement initiatives [5]. There are also examples of the private sector translating their penchant for quality initiatives into the health system. For example, the Leapfrog consortium is an alliance of large US based companies that have collaborated on an effort to promote quality improvement in the US healthcare system (www.leapfroggroup.org). This initiative is based on the presumption that efficiencies and improved quality can be created in the delivery of health services. The important message in this initiative is that change in the way that we manage the healthcare delivery business is being driven by outside forces because we have ignored the need for fundamental change. Healthcare managers increasingly appreciate the urgency of narrowing performance gaps between health care and non-health related industries.

Another trend in health care has been the examination of non-health industry to translate examples of best practices with regards to improving efficiency and quality in health care. One approach that has proved successful in the private sector (and even in a few health related areas) is General Electric's "Six Sigma Quality Improvement Strategy" [5]. Briefly, the Six Sigma program requires that: a) workers are empowered to define and optimize processes, which are both meaningful and measurable, and b) that reorganization of systems is driven by data and facts. In this approach, the most successful examples of change occur when service boundaries are broken down and micro-systems become more fully integrated. Optimizing each building block before another is tackled ensures structural integrity. This program ultimately requires proof that quality has been improved (i.e., change must be measurable).

Integrating Services and Using Data to Promote Quality Improvement

While there are many barriers to implementing quality improvement, the majority of quality improvement programs fail because they are not aligned under a shared framework for performance improvement, not supported by existing infrastructure, and do not cross anachronistic organizational boundaries [6]. Systematically coordinated improvement initiatives that impose order, strategy and priority on change and break down inter-departmental barriers by harmonizing the needs of artificial 'silos' are the most successful.

Regardless of the processes adopted, health care systems need to promote quality improvement and performance initiatives by integrating services and abandoning the concept that physician groups can function as separate 'silos'. In a silo approach, physicians act without either complete information regarding a patient's condition or current best management practices. Health care managers need to radically redesign care delivery by incorporating current evidence through the promise of information technology in an environment where quality improvement and reduction of error are systemic priorities [7]. In such an environment, these data can be reevaluated consistently to ensure that care delivery continues to improve.

One example where data can drive quality improvement in health care is 'benchmarking', a process in which comparisons of selected outcomes are made with peer hospitals [8, 9]. The ideal outcome for all health care systems is to return patients to their pre-existing state of health, or to a state expected for a person of the same age and medical condition. However, measuring this outcome is somewhat more complex in that the outcome measures chosen (e.g., indices for the measurement of physical functional status) must be demonstrated to be both relevant to patients and dependent on the quality of health care delivery, in much the same way as a surrogate outcome (e.g., ventilation/perfusion [V/Q] scan) should accurately reflect a gold standard test (e.g., pulmonary angiogram). Only by providing such validation can outcomes data be used to promote quality improvement [10].

A traditional outcome assessment of providing critical care is mortality rate [11]. While living versus dying is clearly unambiguous, the use of such data to compare across different units is complicated by the requirement to appropriately adjust such data for factors which vary between ICUs (for example, patient population and case mix). Regardless of the process used to validate appropriateness, mortality rate has been widely promoted as a short-term outcome that reflects the quality of care patients receive in an ICU. Mortality rate may also reflect the quality of care delivered by the macro-system as a whole (e.g., the hospital or the HMO).

However, short-term outcomes may not tell the whole story. While it has been assumed that long-term mortality is unrelated to care received during an ICU stay [12], evidence is now accumulating to suggest that the quality of ICU care influences both short-term (e.g., during or immediately post admission) and longer-term mortality rates [13]. For a group of patients with similar baseline characteristics who are treated for a similar condition, quality of life following an ICU admission (another 'outcome') may also be dissimilar [14]. A poor quality of life resulting from an ICU admission will not usually affect the ICU as a micro-system, but can have significant implications for the macro-system in which the ICU participates. Patients who survive with a poor quality of life may increase demand on components of the health care system downstream from the ICU (e.g., physiotherapy, long term care units, family doctors), thus increasing demand on the system as a whole. Managers concerned about efficiency and effectiveness of health care delivery are therefore beginning to learn that each component of the system can impact on both short- and long-term outcomes. As a corollary, ICU management may therefore be asked to implement strategies which have little or no impact on either the ICU's budget or on quality of ICU care, but will be expected to generate significant improvements in mortality, morbidity, as well as cost savings for the perfectly integrated system in the long term [15].

Lessons Learned by Studying Complex Adaptive Systems

Some of the recent theory behind the redesign of health care systems originates in the study of complex adaptive systems [3]. In contrast to largely mechanical systems (e.g., the space shuttle) whose various components are integrated in a highly predictable manner to complete a given objective, complex systems have components (e.g., people) possessing many degrees of freedom in response to various inputs. Complex systems are therefore highly unpredictable in behavior. Not only do complex systems have adaptable elements, but they also demonstrate emergent behavior, are not predictable in detail, and are non-linear in response to input. These same systems, however, have inherent order despite central control (e.g., the Internet) and can demonstrate complex outcomes through the local application of simple rules. Simple rules allow integral freedom of response that can manifest as either innovation or error. Mechanical-systems thinking posit that complex rules are required to govern complex systems such as health care. In contrast, the science of complex adaptive systems allows that simple rules have a higher likelihood of success. Thus, successful high technology firms were more likely to have fewer rules, structures and policies than their competitors [3].

Applying the study of complex adaptive systems to the redesign of health systems suggests simple plans that allow complex systems to adapt and evolve are often the most elegant and successful. However, health care managers must apply these plans in a system where patient safety is a fundamental and necessary restriction to freedoms of response. Some observers feel that the elimination of error is impossible given that people, who are inherently fallible, are responsible for the ultimate delivery of health care [16]. A highly safe system may be envisioned as one that is driven by protocol and delivered by infallible elements such as computers. Such a system would be inherently rigid and non-adaptive. And, physicians would be unlikely to accept a system that was inherently restrictive of professional freedoms. The reorganization of health systems will, therefore, necessitate less detailed restriction of response. We ultimately must evaluate health delivery in this context and strive to create an environment that balances the necessary tension between the elimination of error through restrictions at a systemic level, and the individual freedom of response that is fundamental, both to the practice of medicine and the proper evolution of health care systems.

Summary and Purpose

The ICU is frequently viewed as a stand-alone unit in which complex care is delivered to improve the health of acutely ill patients. Unquestionably, this micro-system approach can respond to short-term acute care issues. However, achieving good long-term outcomes requires a fully integrated macro-system approach. In this approach, acute issues are both managed *and* integrated into a plan of complete care in which short and long term outcomes are optimized. In the following sections, we will apply these concepts to the ICU as an instructive case study for the reorganization of health systems in general. We will also attempt to identify clear problems with meaningful and measurable outcomes and give special attention to those processes which cross intra- and inter-departmental priorities. We will, therefore, emphasize the opportunities to integrate and optimize the delivery of critical care both inside and outside of the ICU.

Care Systems Prior to ICU Admission – The Integration of Care

Case study

Mr. B was a 75 year-old male referred by his family doctor to an internist for a pre-operative assessment prior to planned surgery for liver resection. In the pre-operative clinic, Mr. B was seen by an internist and anesthesiologist who agreed he was in a high-risk category for peri-operative cardiovascular events and, therefore, prescribed a beta-blocker. Concerns were also noted regarding Mr. B's poor nutritional state. Unfortunately, Mr. B did not fill his prescription for the beta-blocker and neither his family doctor nor his surgeon received a consultation note regarding the pre-operative assessment until after the surgery was complete. Mr. B had his surgery, which was complicated and because of which Mr. B required post-operative ICU monitoring. Unfortunately the ICU was not aware that a bed might be required and was unable to accommodate Mr. B. A 'float' nurse was contracted from an agency to monitor Mr. B overnight in the post-anesthetic care unit. Because of complications related to post-op ventilation, an ICU physician and respiratory therapist spent considerable time outside the ICU assessing and treating Mr. B. Another patient was eventually discharged from the ICU late at night, and Mr. B. was admitted. Mr. B's post-op course was complicated by myocardial infarction and prolonged weaning from ventilation. An ICU resident wonders on rounds one day whether Mr. B's nutritional status may have had implications for his complications and recovery.

Error and Poorly Integrated Systems

Institute of Medicine

The (IOM) states that the elimination of error must be a priority in the re-shaping of the US health care systems [4]. The IOM also noted that safety practices within medicine are approximately a decade or more behind those of other high-risk industries. Although the elimination of error is a complex process, it is clear that systems can adapt and improve, as exemplified by the safety improvements in anesthesia (which now rival those of commercial aviation).

As the literature regarding error and patient safety is broad, an in-depth review of this area in the ICU is not possible. However, there are extensive data to suggest that many of the error issues in health care result from a decentralized and fragmented delivery system. This has resulted in many observers commenting on the 'non-system' approach to healthcare delivery supporting the notion that health care has many examples of a 'non-integrated, uncoordinated independent provider service'.

Medical errors are caused by faulty systems in which fallible people are allowed or, indeed, forced to make mistakes. Such faulty systems also have no mechanism for error detection or prevention [3, 4]. Errors are, therefore, most commonly caused by 'bad systems, not bad people'. The necessary conclusion is that attempts at error reduction should not focus on people, but rather on the systems in which they work. One such approach would focus on a more complete integration of service delivery so that communication breakdown between various providers is minimized or ideally prevented. Such an integrated system would also be expected to have multiply redundant error detection systems interwoven with the integration of services so that error is eliminated on a systemic basis.

Errors of Commission...Errors of Omission

For the ICU physician, the question remains how should the various components of the system be integrated to ensure that the delivery of my care is consistent with the goal of optimizing both short and long-term outcomes? The preceding case scenario provides examples of two types of error. There are errors of omission, or failing to do what would help, such as not prescribing a beta-blocker, or post-operative nutrition. There is also an example of an error of commission, or doing what has been shown to be unhelpful, such as discharging a patient from the ICU at night. Integration of service delivery and better communication can prevent both types of errors.

When ICU physicians are faced with an unexpected post-operative patient, they often feel pressure to discharge patients to accommodate such demands. Discharges may, therefore, be 'premature' and in response to attempts to balance the needs of acutely ill patients versus those patients recovering from acute illness. However, premature discharge might also put patients at risk. For example, patients discharged at night are less likely to be judged as fully ready for discharge and their discharge has been correlated with a significantly increased risk of death [17].

ICU readmission rates have also been proposed as an indicator of ICU care as they are felt to be related to a preceding inappropriate discharge [18]. Not surprisingly, patients readmitted to the ICU have a higher risk of death and a longer hospital stay than patients with similar physiologic indicators who are admitted for the first time [19]. The phenomenon of premature discharge from the ICU is also reflected in post-ICU discharge mortality rates, which currently remain high [20]. Failing to notify the ICU of a planned admission, as in the case example, puts the surgical patient at risk, and also increases the risk to patients who must be moved out of the ICU prematurely to accommodate a sicker patient.

Integration and communication should also protect against errors of omission. For example, prescribing beta-blockers to high-risk surgical patients will decrease peri-operative mortality. There is also consensus that patients in the ICU should receive nutritional support [21]. Malnourished patients have increased infectious morbidity, mortality and prolonged hospital stays. Postoperative and ICU patients who are not malnourished experience significant stress and are likely unable to meet all of their caloric needs [22, 23]. Providing nutritional support to critically ill patients positively influences outcomes [24]. Despite this preponderance of evidence for something as simple as feeding in the post-operative period, recent literature suggests that the provision of nutritional support to these patients is less than optimal [25]. The use of care maps has been reported to improve the provision of nutritional support and decrease both morbidity and mortality [26, 27].

In a truly integrated health system, an assessment suggesting that a patient would benefit from nutritional support would be provided to both the surgeon and the ICU physician. Here, the outcome of this communication might lead to the patient having a feeding tube (for enteral nutrition) or central line (for potential nutrition) placed at the time of surgery, after which the ICU physician and attending surgeon would agree on when to begin nutritional support.

Returning to the case example, integration of the services between physicians involved in the patient's care would have ensured: a) the patient's risk was minimized, b) services were not duplicated, and c) likelihood for error was minimized by creating redundancies at multiple levels (e.g., the patient may have received a beta-blocker had there been appropriate communication between all involved service providers). We even posit there is a role for an ICU physician in the pre-operative assessment period. While the prediction of who will require ICU care is an imperfect science, an ICU physician might be able to more accurately predict the necessity for resource provision. Although this may be debated, an intensivist could also provide more realistic information to patients and family members so that expectations might be optimized.

ICU Physicians Consulting Outside the ICU

Withdrawal or withholding of life-sustaining therapies to patients who either do not want this therapy or cannot be expected to benefit from it, would respect patient autonomy while simultaneously creating resource savings [28]. Advanced care planning may create realistic expectations for an ICU admission and define appropriate levels of care. This means that the patient, the patient's family and the ward staff will be appropriately prepared should clinical deterioration occur [29].

In contrast to what should be done, we now understand that frank discussions with patients regarding prognosis are poor and the prevalence of advance directives is low [30, 31]. Physicians may be unwilling to discuss prognosis and obtain advanced directives because of uncertainty about prognosis, limited time, the desire to maintain hope and/or the desire to avoid a difficult topic [32]. Subsequently, physicians seem likely to initiate such discussions with only the sickest patients. Further, these discussions often involve only family members, and paradoxically exclude patients who are now too ill to participate [32]. For the ICU physician, this often means spending long hours initiating discussions about care plans with families with whom they have no prior relationship under less than ideal clinical circumstances.

One approach to deal with this problem is to ensure that conversations regarding prognosis and advanced care planning occur early in the stage of a patient's illness. Of interest to critical care physicians is a study in which advanced care planning discussions were held with surgical patients during their preoperative evaluations [33]. This intervention was effective in increasing the rate of these discussions, as well as the rate of completion of advanced directives.

The question remains, should ICU physicians, as those most likely to have an appreciation for the outcome of conditions requiring a critical care admission, be involved in the early stages of these discussions with both surgical and medical patients? Would it be in a hospital's best interest to have an ICU consult team available to attend discussion with pre-operative patients as well as upon admission of terminally ill patients to the hospital? Such a plan would require a time commitment up front, but may result not only in time saved when patients suffer clinical deterioration, but also improve patient and family satisfaction. This approach means that 'upfront' integrating for the critical care physician would require a crossing of traditional boundaries of care to contribute to patient welfare and hospital resource management.

While there is support for involving ICU physicians in the planning of admissions to the ICU, other data suggests that service integration might also improve the care of patients admitted to the ICU on an emergent basis. Poor care prior to admission to the ICU can increase mortality after ICU admission [34]. For the ICU clinician, early identification of patients likely to require ICU intervention allows forward planning. For example, identifying patients receiving non-invasive ventilation in step down units [35] permits forward planning between the ICU and step down unit staff, as to what clinical parameters should be followed to determine when the non-invasive approach is failing and intubation (thereby requiring ICU admission) is needed. For the ICU physician-manager, an early warning of potential or impending ICU admissions allows better resource allocation.

Care pathways have successfully identified both medical and surgical patients likely to require admission to an ICU [36]. Information derived from applying such a pathway allows for early modification of clinical management in an attempt to prevent ICU admission. Should clinical deterioration occur, this approach allows that nurses and clinicians would be sufficiently warned so as to prevent cardio-respiratory arrest. Should ICU admission be required, it is expected that ICU physicians will be sufficiently warned to allow for appropriate resource allocation. Such a program need not be inherently restrictive of clinician response. The benefit would be to provide necessary information to point of care staff as well as non-involved specialists so that ultimately acute care is provided by a system rather than by individuals acting on an independent basis.

Summary

Although examples provided are by no means exhaustive, one can appreciate how the concept of integrating the ICU with care in advance of admission can change the philosophy of care provided by individuals usually working in silos. Care would no longer be fragmented and decentralized, but can be provided by a system in which service boundaries are broken down, communication is improved and services are appropriately integrated to optimize both the short and long term outcomes important to patients. Such a system would also have multiply redundant error detection strategies so that medical error is eliminated.

While integrating care processes may work well for a hospital, outcomes may continue to vary between hospitals because of factors such as inadequate staffing or lack of expertise. While a dedicated intensivist staff reduces mortality in patients admitted to the ICU [37], only a minority of critical care units now utilize an intensivist model for ICU patient care [38]. Until there is a distribution of ICU physicians to non-teaching hospitals, restructuring in large hospital systems may, therefore, require the centralization of ICU services into hospitals that can provide such expertise. Other solutions may also be considered, for example increasing the use of hospitalists, protocol driven care and tele-medicine conferencing. Whatever the approach, sub-optimal service delivery should be analyzed, optimized and integrated into highly functioning systems.

Incorporating Evidence into Practice during an ICU Admission

Case study

Ms. N is a 66-year-old female admitted to the ICU following a massive anterior myocardial infarction (MI) and subsequent congestive heart failure that required intubation for respiratory failure. While in the ICU, Ms. N's care was complicated by an episode of VAP. Unfortunately, she suffered a significant adverse drug reaction to antibiotics prescribed because of a penicillin allergy (which had been documented on the chart). She subsequently suffered an ischemic stroke presumably of cardio-embolic origin from a ventricular thrombus. She had not been started on anticoagulation following her anterior MI. Ms. N spent four weeks in the ICU that was complicated by significant skin breakdown and de-conditioning. She spent two more months in hospital and ultimately had to be discharged to a long-term care facility because of heavy care demands.

Medical Error and Evidenced Based Practice

Medical error remains an important source of mortality and morbidity in the ICU. Recent studies demonstrate that approximately 16% of patients admitted to the ICU experienced a human error, and that these errors prolonged ICU stay by 425 patient-days over the course of the year, and contributed to an increase of about 15% of ICU running costs [39]. Services that deal with complicated patients on an emergent basis such as ICUs or emergency departments may be particularly susceptible to human error [4]. The corollary is that one obstacle to perfection in the system is the fallibility of its human operators. Once again, the dichotomy between fallibility and perfection or between rigidity and freedom of action is the tightrope that needs to be negotiated to create a system that safeguards patients but is flexible enough to adapt and evolve.

The IOM suggests that one approach to optimizing health services is to match current best knowledge with patient need [3]. As previously mentioned, care may not match knowledge either as a result of omission (failing to do what would help) or due to waste (doing what cannot help) [3]. Unfortunately, it takes about 18 years for data from well conducted randomized trials to be incorporated into clinical practice [40]. Even then, treatments with proven efficacy are not universally implemented in practice [41]. In contrast to many other industries, the health care system has been slow to embrace information technology as a way to integrate the myriad sources of information (e.g., patient specific, current best practice) required to make appropriate and informed decisions about patient care [42].

Care Pathways and the ICU

Care pathways are guidelines that target specific processes in care delivery. They usually integrate multidisciplinary approaches to care, are often evidence based, and may be integrated with currently accepted practice guidelines. The implementation of care pathways would be expected to provide systematically acquired knowledge to point of care staff to help guide clinical decision making. In this way, errors of omission would be reduced by providing information on effective treatment, and errors of commission would be reduced by eliminating treatments which are known to be ineffective [43, 44].

An example can be found in antibiotic prescribing practices in the ICU. Incorrect antibiotic selection is an important predictor of mortality in the ICU [45]. Information technology might be utilized to provide data regarding local pathogens, local antibiotic resistance patterns, medication dosing, current best practice as well as patient specific information such as allergies and drug interactions to point of care staff to aid in decisions about antibiotic selection [46]. Not only might these systems be designed to be synchronous with point of care delivery (as aids in decision-making), but may also be designed to be asynchronous and more downstream from care delivery (to screen orders after they have been entered). What is clear is that the provision of such decision support improves dosing, decreases adverse drug combinations and improves antibiotic selection [46].

Adopting practice guidelines would be expected to improve short-term outcomes and impact significantly on ICU workload, mortality and budget, outcomes of immediate importance to ICU manager. Such practices might include those identified by the Agency for Healthcare Research and Quality as those with the evidence to support their widespread use such as prophylaxis for DVT; sterile barriers to prevent infection while inserting central lines; continuous aspiration of subglottic secretions to prevent ventilator acquired pneumonia; real time ultrasound to guide insertion of central lines; the prevention of skin injury with special beds; and use of nutritional support in critically ill patients.

What might not be so intuitively obvious is that such pathways would also support the implementation of practices that would be unlikely to affect directly the short-term outcomes important to ICU physicians, but that would be highly effective in improving the long-term outcomes important to patients and systems, for example, the use of anticoagulation, beta-blockers, angiotensin converting enzyme (ACE) inhibitors, and aspirin in patients following myocardial infarction.

Information Technology and the Electronic Patient Record

Along with an increased reliance on information technology to guide medication dosing or protocol driven care, there is also interest in using this technology in the development of electronic patient records. These electronic data systems would be utilized much like the daily clinical note [49]. The perceived advantage of electronic systems is that they will enhance legibility and data completeness, facilitate recall of patient information and reduce duplication of effort. In the ICU, where the integration of diverse sets of data is part of the daily routine, it is expected that electronic systems would facilitate not only the integration but also the dissemination of this data to multiple users. However, clinicians may not be willing to embrace this technology because they are unfamiliar or unconvinced about potential benefits. One of the most significant barriers to the incorporation of such information technology is the perception that, although high tech and flashy, this technology may in fact result in an increase in time and effort when compared to traditional paper based notes. Indeed, these systems are more likely to be accepted when benefits can be proven, especially when the benefit is time and effort saved [47]. One study that examined the effects of an electronic patient information system in an ICU environment found that it did not save any significant time for clinicians. However, it did not take any more time than traditional methods [48], while the use of structured data entry led to more detailed content and increased legibility of patient notes. Such findings are of value to those concerned with quality improvement because these records are more easily examined when providing administrative and patient-care reports, or linking process of care with patient outcomes.

Summary

Information technology provides the promise of the integration of care pathways with patient specific information to point of care staff [49]. A perceived benefit would be an increase in the dissemination of such data in a format that is expected to be user friendly and patient specific. Current technology may not support such an application, or applications using current technology may not be readily available. However, it is clear that any reorganization of health care systems will have to rely heavily on the elimination of error. Care pathways and decision support aids are system processes that would be expected to lower both errors of omission and commission, thereby resulting in improved short and long-term outcomes. Safety must be a system priority.

After the ICU – Re-involving the Patient in the Care Process

Case History

Mr. B is a 27 year-old man admitted to the ICU following a closed head injury from a motor vehicle accident. Because of the nature of his injuries Mr. B required prolonged ventilation and sedation. His family was concerned and had difficulty providing surrogate decision making because they received confusing and contradictory information from a number of different critical care staff. Mr. B eventually recovered but was unable to return to work and became socially isolated because he developed a significant post-traumatic stress disorder following his return home.

A Case for Better Communication

Physicians in the ICU setting appropriately concentrate on medical outcomes for their patients. Often patients are so acutely ill that the psychological needs of families and patients are overlooked. However, data are accumulating to suggest that these 'non-organic' needs are frequently not met, and may be important determinants of outcome.

Patients admitted to ICUs are often unable to participate in discussions about their diagnosis, proposed treatments and prognosis. In this case, family members are turned to as surrogate decision-makers with regard to consent for interventions and for end of life decision making. All of this occurs in a complex and poorly understood environment, at a time when family members are likely to be experiencing significant emotional strain. It is in this context that the critical care team needs to provide appropriate and unambiguous information so that family-members are in a position to make informed decisions. Unfortunately, poor communication between care providers and patient surrogates appears common in the ICU. For example, family members in one study frequently reported inadequate communication with their physicians [50]. While family members have reported conflict surrounding withdrawing or withholding care, this may in fact have more to do with doctor-family communication than with the decision about withdrawing or withholding care [51]. Inquiries established to understand and improve the limitations of current health care delivery have reinforced the concept that good communication is fundamental to delivering high quality care [2, 52].

Physicians must take seriously the concept that good communication with patients and families affects the perception of quality in health service delivery, and may reciprocally affect the delivery of care itself. For example, good communication between the physician and patient appears to reduce the risk of subsequent medical malpractice claims [53, 54]. Strategies such as multidisciplinary communication sessions with families that review and determine care plans for critically ill patients can reduce ICU resource utilization while not changing patient outcomes [55].

A recent intervention has been described which involves simply providing family member's of critical care patients with an information leaflet designed to provide general information about the ICU environment without providing patient specific information. The authors of this study were successful in demonstrating that this very simple intervention significantly improved both the comprehension and satisfaction of family members [56].

Non-organic Long Term Outcomes

Patients in the ICU frequently experience sedation, amnesia and partial or unpleasant recall. This fragmentation of memory may be a critical determinant in the development of long-term psychological problems such as post-traumatic stress disorder after a critical care stay [57]. Strategies have been employed to reach out to ICU survivors to support recovery and aid in reconstruction of memory surrounding the ICU stay. These have included community liaison programs and clinic follow-up with ICU staff [58]. Other novel programs have included the use of a personal diary written voluntarily each day by involved staff and relatives and which included elements from daily summaries of care to color photographs [59]. Such a program was found to be a successful adjunct to the debriefing process following intensive care admissions.

Summary

If we believe that psychological well being is an important contributor to long-term outcomes, then 'non-organic' interventions should play a role in the care plan of every patient who is treated in an ICU environment. Once again, the long term gain to patients may not be readily identifiable to ICU staff, or translate into improvements in the bottom line of ICU managers, but would be expected to provide significant improvements to resource utilization and efficacy of the system as a whole.

Conclusion

The preceding discussion has briefly analyzed some of the factors we believe should be considered when reorganizing health systems to improve long-term outcomes. While some examples, which draw most heavily on the ICU experience, were presented in support of the concepts discussed, they were not intended to be entirely inclusive or representative of all that is or could be done to improve health care systems. What is important is the incorporation of a few simple concepts into the reorganization of systems, including:

1. the elimination of anachronistic service boundaries;
2. the integration of currently fragmented and decentralized services;
3. the elimination of error through system wide initiatives;
4. the incorporation of evidence-based practice into everyday care; and
5. the re-involvement of the patient in their care process.

The ICU manager who sees their unit as only one of a number of non-integrated silos providing patient care may not be interested in initiatives that have little impact on his or her bottom line. However, the ICU manager who sees their unit as a fully integrated component of a health care system can realize significant improvements in both short and long-term outcomes. What is also apparent is that these concepts are becoming increasingly important to the managers of larger health care systems and in some cases, such as the Leapfrog group, these concepts are being used to drive change from outside the healthcare system itself. Although ICU physicians generally have been focused on short-term outcomes, significant restructuring is predicted both now and in the future - thus a change in focus offers the opportunity for critical care physicians to be involved in the change process in both the short and the long-term.

References

1. The Agency for Healthcare Research and Quality (1999) Making healthcare safer: A critical analysis of patient safety practices. AHRQ publication no. 01-E058
2. The Institute of Medicine (2001) Crossing the quality chasm. National Academy of Sciences, Washington
3. The Institute of Medicine (2000) To Err is Human: Building a safer health system. National Academy of Sciences, Washington
4. The Institute of Medicine (1990) Medicare: a strategy for quality assurance. National Academy of Sciences, Washington
5. Ettinger WE (2001) Six Sigma: Adapting GE's lessons to health care. Trustee 54:10–15
6. Clarke M, Hayduk M (1997) Putting it all together: Clinical performance improvement. Health Care Strateg Manage 15:1–20

7. Smith J (2001) Redesigning health care: radical redesign is a way to radically improve.Br Med J 322:1257–1258
8. Keenan SP, Doig GS, Martin CM, Inman KJ, Sibbald WJ (1997) Assessing the efficiency of the admission process to a critical care unit: does the literature allow the use of benchmarking? Intensive Care Med 23:574–580
9. Tweet AG, Gavin-Marciano K (1998) The Guide to Benchmarking in Healthcare. Practical Lessons from the Field. Quality Resources Press, New York
10. Weinberg M (2001) Using performance measures to identify plans of action to improve care. Jt Comm J Qual Improv 27:683–688
11. Hayes JA, Black NA, Jenkinson C, et al (2000) Outcome measures for adult critical care: a systemic review. Health Technol Assess 4:1–111
12. Dellinger RP (1997) From the bench to the bedside: The future of sepsis research. Chest 111:744–753
13. Davidson TA, Rubenfeld GD, Caldwell ES, Hudson LD, Steinberg KP (1999) The effect of the acute respiratory distress syndrome on long-term survival. Am J Respir Crit Care Med 160:1838–1842
14. Angus DC, Musthafa AA, Clermont G, et al (2001) Quality-adjusted survival in the first year after the acute respiratory distress syndrome. Am J Respir Crit Care Med 163:1389–1394
15. Shortell SM, Zimmerman JE, Rousseau DM, et al (1994) The performance of intensive care units: does good management make a difference? Med Care 32:508–525
16. McDonald CJ (1976) Protocol-based computer reminders, the quality of care and the non-perfectibility of man. N Engl J Med 295:1351–1355
17. Goldfrad C, Rowan K (2000) Consequences of discharges from intensive care at night. Lancet 355:1138–1142
18. Chen LM, Martin CM, Keenan SP, Sibbald WJ (1998) Patients readmitted to the intensive care unit during the same hospitalization: Clinical features and outcomes. Crit Care Med 26:1834–1841
19. Rosenberg AL, Hofer TP, Hayward RA, et al (2001) Who bounces back? Physiologic and other predictors of intensive care unit readmission. Crit Care Med 29:511–518
20. Rowan KM, Kerr JH, Major E, McPherson K, Short A, Vessey MP (1993) Intensive care society's APACHE II study in Britain and Ireland-I: Variations in case mix of adult admissions to general intensive care units and impact on outcome. Br Med J 307:977–981
21. Cerra FB, Benitez MR, Blackburn GL, et al (1997) Applied nutrition in ICU patients. A consensus statement of the American College of Chest Physicians. Chest 111:769–778
22. Beier-Holgersen R, Boesby S (1996) Influence of postoperative enteral nutrition on postsurgical infections. Gut 39:833–835
23. Daley J, Khuri SF, Henderson W, et al (1997) Risk adjustment of the postoperative morbidity rate for the comparative assessment of the quality of surgical care: results of the National Veterans Affairs Surgical Risk Study. J Am Coll Surg 185:328–340
24. Heyland DK (1998) Nutritional support in the critically ill patients. A critical review of the evidence. Crit Care Clin 14:423–440
25. Preiser JC, Berre J, Carpentier Y, et al (1999) Management of nutrition in European intensive care units: results of a questionnaire. Working Group on Metabolism and Nutrition of the European Society of Intensive Care Medicine. Intensive Care Med 25:95–101
26. Taylor SJ, Fettes SB, Jewkes C, Nelson RJ (1999) Prospective, randomized, controlled trial to determine the effect of early enhanced enteral nutrition on clinical outcome in mechanically ventilated patients suffering head injury. Crit Care Med 27:2525–2531
27. Martin CM, Doig GS, Heyland DK, Morrison T, Sibbald WJ for the Critical Care Research Network (2002) A multicenter, cluster randomized clinical trial of algorithms for critical care enteral and parenteral therapy (ACCEPT). JAMA (in press)
28. Sprung CL (1990) Changing attitudes and practices in foregoing life-sustaining treatments. JAMA 263: 2211–2215

29. Haidet P, Hamel MB, Davis RB, et al (1998) Outcomes, preferences for resuscitation, and physician-patient communication among patients with metastatic colon cancer. SUPPORT investigators. Study to understand prognoses and preferences for outcomes and risks of treatments. Am J Med 105:222–229

30. La Puma JL, Orentlicher D, Moss RJ (1991) Advance directives on admission: Clinical implications and analysis of the patient self-determination act of 1990. JAMA 266:402–405

31. Johnson RF, Baranowski-Birkmeier T, O'Donnell JB (1995) Advance directives in the medical intensive care unit of a community teaching hospital. Chest 107:752–756

32. Bradley EH, Hallemeier AG, Fried TR, et al (2001) Documentation of discussions about prognosis with terminally ill patients. Am J Med 111:218–223

33. Grimaldo DA, Wiener-Kronish JP, Jurson T, Shaughnessy TE, Randall-Curtis J, Liu LL (2001) A randomized, controlled trial of advance care planning discussions during pre-operative evaluations. Anesthesiology 95:43–50

34. McQuillan P, Pilkington S, Allan A, et al (1998) Confidential enquiry into quality of care before admission to intensive care. Br Med J 316:1853–1858

35. Moretti M, Cilione C, Tampieri A, Fraccia A, Marchioni A, Nava S (2000) Incidence and causes of non-invasive mechanical ventilation failure after initial success. Thorax 55:819–825

36. Stubbe CP, Kruger M, Rutherford P, Gemmel L (2001) Validation of a modified early warning score in medical admissions. Q J Med 94:521–526

37. Young M, Birkmeyer J (2000) Potential reduction in mortality rates using an intensivist model to manage intensive care units. Eff Clin Pract 3:284–289

38. Mallick R, Strosberg M, Lambrinos J, Groeger J (1995) The intensive care unit medical director as manager: impact on performance. Med Care 33:611–624

39. Bracco D, Favre JB, Bissonnette B, et al (2001) Human errors in a multidisciplinary intensive care unit: A 1 year prospective study. Intensive Care Med 27:137–145

40. Balas AE, Boren SA (2000) Managing clinical knowledge for health care improvement. In: Bemmel J, McCray AT (eds) Yearbook of Medical Informatics. Schattauer, Stuttgart, pp 65–70

41. Phillips KA, Shlipak MG, Coxson P, et al (2001) Underuse of beta-blockers following myocardial infarction. JAMA 285:1013

42. Becher EC, Chassin MR (2001) Improving quality, minimizing error: Making it happen. Health Affairs 20:68–81

43. Marrie TJ, Lau CY, Wheeler SL, Wong CJ, Vandervoort MK, Feagan BG (2000) A controlled trial of a critical pathway for treatment of community-acquired pneumonia. CAPITAL Study Investigators. Community-Acquired Pneumonia Intervention Trial Assessing Levofloxacin. JAMA 283:749–755

44. Hux JE, Melady MP, DeBoer D (1999) Confidential prescriber feedback and education to improve antibiotic use in primary care: a controlled trial. Can Med Assoc J 161:388–392

45. Kollef MH, Sherman G, Ward S, Fraser VJ (1999) Inadequate antimicrobial treatment of infections: A risk factor for hospital mortality among critically ill patients. Chest 115:462–474

46. Bailey TC, McMullin T (2001) Using information systems technology to improve antibiotic prescribing. Crit Care Med 29 (4 suppl):N87-N91

47. Lee F, Teich J, Spurr C, Bates D (1996) Implementation of physician order entry: User satisfaction and self-reported usage patterns. J Am Med Inform Assoc 3:42–55

48. Apkon M, Singhaviranon P (2001) Impact of an electronic information system on physician workflow and data collection in the intensive care unit. Intensive Care Med 27:122–130

49. Leonard K, Tan JK, Pink G (1998) Designing health care information systems for integrated delivery systems: where we are and where we need to be. Top Health Inf Manage 19:19–30

50. Azoulay E, Chevret S, Ghislaine L, et al (2000) Half the families of intensive care unit patients experience inadequate communication with physicians. Crit Care Med 28:3044–3049

51. Abbott KH, Sago JG, Breen CM, Abernathy AP, Tulsky JA (2001) Families looking back: One year after discussion of withdrawl or withholding of life-sustaining support. Crit Care Med 29:197–201

52. Bristol Royal Infirmary Inquiry (2001) Learning from Bristol: The report of the public inquiry into children's heart surgery at the Bristol Royal Infirmary 1984-1995. At http://www.bristol-inquiry.org.uk/final_report/the_report.pdf
53. Levinson W, Roter DL, Mulloly JP, Dull VT, Frankel RM (1997) Physician-patient communication: The relationship with malpractice claims among primary care physicians surgeons. JAMA 277:553-559
54. Moore P, Adler NE, Robertson PA (2000) Medical malpractice: The effect of doctor-patient relations on medical patient perceptions and malpractice intentions. West J Med 173:244-250
55. Lilly C, De Meo D, Sonna L, et al (2000) An intensive communication intervention for the critically ill. Am J Med 109:469-475
56. Azoulay E, Pochard F, Chevret S, et al (2002) Impact of a family information leaflet on effectiveness of information provided to family members of ICU patients: a multicenter, prospective, randomized, controlled trial. Am J Respir Crit Care Med 165:438-442
57. Griffiths RD, Jones C (1999) Recovery from intensive care. Br Med J 319:427-429
58. Hall-Smith J, Ball C, Coakley J (1997) Follow-up services and the development of a clinical nurse specialist in intensive care. Intensive Crit Care Nurs 13:243-248
59. Backman CG, Walther SM (2001) Use of a personal diary written on the ICU during critical illness. Intensive Care Med 27:426-429

Defining 'Success' in ICU Care

P. Pronovost, A. Wu, and C. G. Holzmueller

Introduction

The Institute of Medicine (IOM) Report, "Crossing the Quality Chasm", challenged physicians as part of the medical system to provide care that is safe, effective, efficient, timely, patient centered, and equitable [1]. Most intensive care physicians have little knowledge of whether they are achieving these aims. We generally do not systematically evaluate the quality of intensive care unit (ICU) care provided to patients and if we do, evaluation ceases when the patient leaves the ICU or hospital. With no capacity to evaluate the long-term impact of ICU care, it is difficult for intensivists to improve the care they provide, such that benefits are maximized and complications minimized. In this chapter, we will present a case of an 'ICU success story', review the gaps in knowledge and the available literature regarding the impact of ICU care, and propose an outline for research in this area.

Case

JS is a 65-year-old man admitted to the ICU for pneumonia with respiratory failure. He is intubated and then develops septic shock and the acute respiratory distress syndrome (ARDS), with an APACHE III predicted probability of hospital survival of 10 %. He is treated with activated protein C and a low tidal volume ventilator strategy. He receives a continuous insulin infusion to maintain serum glucose between 70–110 gm/dl, and two weeks of antibiotic therapy that includes an aminoglycoside.

JS survives and after one month in the ICU is discharged to the floor. A week later he is discharged to home. The team is commended for a job well done and believes that his survival is due to the application of evidence-based care. When the case is presented at a case conference, the team is congratulated for providing a salutary example of application of the six elements of high quality of care outlined above in the recent IOM report [1].

Six months later, the attending intensivist receives a call from the patient's primary care physician, an internist who is co-investigator with the intensivist on an ICU safety research grant. The internist describes the disheartening post-discharge course experienced by the patient. In the week following discharge to home, the patient continued to take the nortriptyline that had been prescribed as a sleep medication while in the ICU. As a result of daytime somnolence, he failed to complete the follow-up visit scheduled with the internist for one week after hospital discharge. When the appointment clerk called to reschedule the visit, he did not hear the phone because of aminoglycoside-induced hearing loss.

The patient also resumed taking the calcium channel blocker he had been prescribed prior to hospitalization in addition to the beta-blocker he was started on in the ICU. He had a syncopal episode and fell, sustaining a subdural hematoma. He was hospitalized for two weeks and now resides in a nursing home. The intensivist reconsiders the extent to which the patient's outcome can be considered 'a success'. He wonders if this scenario is common and realizes that he does not know. Indeed, he rarely receives the kind of follow-up that was available in this case and knows that this follow-up would be required to define 'success' or 'failure' of ICU care.

A committed adherent to evidence-based medicine, the intensivist searches the literature for guidance on how to improve the outcomes for his patients. He is dismayed to find that there is little published literature to inform him. Moreover, he realizes that he does not have a system to routinely evaluate the long-term impact of the ICU care he provides.

Existing Literature

An increasing number of studies have examined patient outcomes post-ICU discharge [2-23]. Early studies measuring quality of life after ICU care gave disparate findings [2–4]. More recent studies, however, suggest that despite high mortality rates, functional status and quality of life for survivors are often acceptable, and quality of life is often good [5–22].

A few studies have also attempted to identify risk factors for adverse outcomes post-ICU stays. Several studies have shown that poor baseline functioning is the strongest risk factor for subsequent disability [6, 7, 19, 23, 24]. Other studies report that although functional status and quality of life are generally correlated, there is discordance in these findings, presenting a need to further assess both of these concepts [5, 9, 10, 13, 14, 25, 26].

In one study, we evaluated the functional status and costs of patients who stayed in a surgical ICU for at least one week. We found that one-year survival was 45 % and the costs of care during that year were $282,618. Nonetheless, those who survived had a good quality of life [11]. As part of the SUPPORT study, Dr Wu and colleagues found that at 2 months, one third of patients who were seriously ill in an ICU had severe functional limitations. The patient's ability to perform activities of daily living prior to the ICU and degree of physiologic abnormalities during the ICU predicted functional outcome [7].

In addition to the personal burden, a serious illness also imparts a substantial burden on the patient's caregivers. As part of the SUPPORT study, Covinsky [27] found that 33 % of patients in this study required considerable caregiver assistance from a family member. In 20 % of patients, the caregiver had to quit work or make another major life change to provide care for the patient. As a result, 31 % of families reported a loss of most of their savings. Given the significant burden impact of serious illness on patients and their families, efforts to mitigate these effects are critical.

A few researchers have called for increased efforts to collect outcomes data on ICU patients [28–30], with a few encouraging efforts seen in this regard. The Australian Center for Documentation and Quality Assurance in Intensive Care Medicine assembled a cohort of ICUs to collect a set of 'interdisciplinary' data points and to evaluate performance in relation to severity of illness and care provided [31]. This data set, however, does not include functional or quality of life outcomes.

Fiser and colleagues reported on a 16-unit multicenter cohort study of pediatric ICUs (PICU) with a sample size of 11,106 patients [32]. The patients from this study represented all PICU admissions over 12 consecutive months. The investigators used clinician scored measures to assess functional outcomes, however, post-hospital follow-up data was not collected. The APACHE III severity assessment system is currently used in a large number of ICUs worldwide, but again does not include patient-reported or post-hospital data collection [33].

Our review suggests that there are virtually no concerted efforts to routinely follow ICU patients for short or long-term outcomes data. Though "Crossing the Quality Chasm" [1] challenges clinicians to deliver care that is safe, effective, efficient, patient-centered, timely and equitable, there are limited published resources or tools to help them evaluate their efforts in achieving these aims. Knowledge is almost exclusively limited to events that occur in the ICU, and even these data are not collected routinely. Intensivists lack data on the incidence of post-ICU outcomes and contributing factors, such as patient factors and ICU practices. In the absence of outcome data, it will be difficult for intensivists to improve the care they provide.

Expanding our Knowledge

What can be done to allow the intensivist to examine patient outcomes and how to improve them? The Framingham study provides one of the earliest examples of how this may be accomplished [34]. This study, which was the first to apply the term "risk factor", collected detailed data on cardiovascular outcomes and risk factors in a longitudinal cohort of individuals in Framingham, Massachusetts.

Analogous efforts are needed to permit intensivists to answer the following questions:
1) what is the incidence of important patient outcomes following ICU and hospital discharge?
2) what is the natural history of patient morbidity following ICU discharge?
3) what patient and ICU care factors are associated with these outcomes?
4) what is the optimal way to organize and deliver ICU care to optimize both short and longer-term patient outcomes?
5) what are some practical strategies that could be implemented at ICU discharge that might improve patient outcome?

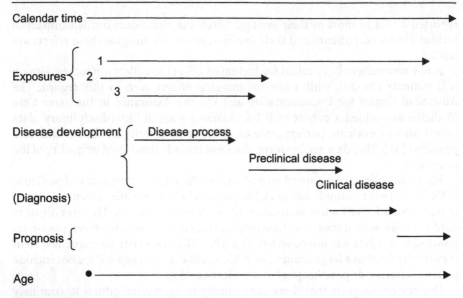

Fig. 1. Hypothetical etiologic exposure and phases of disease over time and age. Adapted from [35] with permission

To answer these questions, the most obvious research design would be that of an observational study; either a cohort or case control study. Both designs have advantages and disadvantages. In general, cohort studies that involve follow-up of persons over time are good for evaluating rare exposures and allow us to evaluate multiple outcomes. However, they are expensive to conduct, and require lengthy follow-up. Case control studies are useful to evaluate rare outcomes and allow for the evaluation of multiple exposure variables. Given the relatively limited knowledge regarding long-term outcomes of ICU care, we likely need information on multiple exposures and outcomes,: many of which will be uncommon.

A significant advantage of the cohort study over other observational designs is its' ability to incorporate time into the analyses [34]. In a cohort study, we can evaluate multiple axes of time of time, including calendar time, exposures, disease development and patient age (Fig. 1). Many of the exposure and confounding variables in the ICU vary over time, such as ventilator settings or the presence of respiratory failure. A cohort design that records events over time is required to evaluate this variation.

Moreover, a cohort design allows for time-dependent models to evaluate the association between exposures and risks. For most of ICU care, the association between exposure and outcome is unknown. Cohort studies may help us to further understand these relationships as well as how disease develops over time. For example, exposure can be related to outcome in any of the following ways:

• Risk can depend on cumulative exposure.
• Risk can depend on time since exposure.

- Risk can depend on exposure during a vulnerable period in the presence of a confounding variable.
- Risk depends on reaching a threshold of exposure.

The randomized, controlled clinical trial (RCT) is an alternative design that provides maximal internal validity to answer specific questions. In a clinical trial, the patient, the ICU, or a geographic region can be the unit of randomization and analysis. For example, patients could be randomized to receive a specific therapy, ICUs could be randomized to receive a new technology, or geographic reasons could be randomized to employ a specific nurse to patient ratio. This design provides the highest level of evidence for causal relationships between exposures and outcomes. However, this design is also costly, and randomizing patients is often problematic for logistic and ethical reasons.

A variation of a randomized design, intended to evaluate the effectiveness of a therapy with proven efficacy, is outlined in Figure 2. In this design, ICUs, or geographic regions, are randomized to receive an intervention (generally believed to be associated with improved outcomes), early versus late. All groups will receive the intervention yet in the process, we can evaluate the effectiveness, sustainability and generalizability of the intervention. Effectiveness can be evaluated by comparing the differences in outcomes for the two groups between the baseline period and assessment period 1. Sustainability can be evaluated by comparing outcomes between assessment periods 1 and 2 in the early intervention group. Generalizability of the intervention can be evaluated by comparing the difference in outcomes between assessment period 1 and 2 in the late intervention group. Because group assignment is not blinded, this design is most useful to evaluate therapies with proven efficacy. While these therapies are increasing in ICU care, they are still relatively scarce; the efficacy and or effectiveness of most ICU therapies are unknown.

Therefore, despite the benefits of randomized trials, we still need to understand the basic epidemiology of ICU practices, patient outcomes, and the relationships among them . The cohort study design can help us understand the epidemiology of patients with critical illness and their care, including the effects of factors that vary over time. Once the basic epidemiology of ICU care is better understood, clinical trials will be more useful to evaluate specific strategies to improve patient outcomes.

Designing a Study to Inform ICU Practice

Study Design

How might a cohort study of ICU practice and outcomes be designed? Because many of the outcomes of interest are uncommon and because we are also interested in how a hierarchy of factors such as ICU organizational characteristics may affect outcomes, a multicenter study would be helpful to increase the number of outcomes available for analysis, and to allow variability in organizational characteristics. Table 1 presents a framework for a hierarchy of factors that may influence

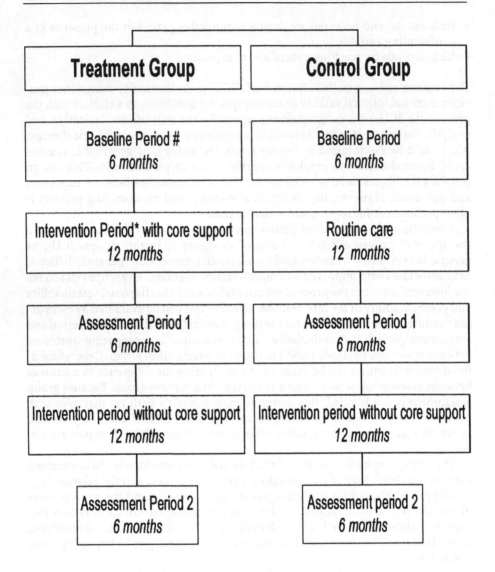

Fig. 2. Randomized study design for effectiveness study.

patient outcomes, including institutional, hospital, department or unit, work environment, team, individual and task related factors, as well as patient characteristics.

Because the extent and duration of exposure needed to predict outcomes is unknown, broad inclusion criteria should be applied initially. However, for reasons of practicality, it may be desirable to restrict the patient population to higher risk patients such as those hospitalized for a specified period of time (e.g., at least 24 hours) in the ICU.

Inclusion criteria to construct the cohort may vary for different questions. Data on survival are available for virtually all patients after admission to hospital or ICU.

Table 1. Hierarchy of influences on clinical practice and patient care outcomes

---

Institutional Context
    Societal and cultural pressures
    Legal and regulatory rules
    Economic influences

Hospital Context
    Financial resources and constraints
    Commitment and priorities of senior leadership
    Organization and activities related to performance improvement,
        infection control and risk management
    Organization and management of support services
        Medical records and management information system
        Pharmacy
        Laboratory
        Transport and messenger services
        Equipment maintenance and supply services

Department and Unit Context
    Structure of responsibility and accountability
    Operating policies and procedures
    Monitoring systems

Work environment
    Staffing levels and skills mix
    Workload and shift patterns
    Design, availability, and maintenance of equipment
    Administrative and managerial support

Team Factors
    Team structure
    Verbal and written communication patterns
    Supervision and availability of help

Individual (staff) Factors
    Knowledge and skills
    Motivation
    Physical and mental health

Task Factors
    Task design
    Availability and use of protocols
    Availability and accuracy of test results

Patient Characteristics
    Clinical condition (complexity and seriousness)
    Age
    Social Factors

However, examining additional outcomes might require that patients in the cohort survive until hospital discharge, or beyond.

Outcome Variables

Although the epidemiology of post-ICU outcomes is not well described, some outcomes are generic to all patients, and there are a number of adverse outcomes that are commonly observed. These can be categorized (Table 2) as clinical, patient-centered, and economic outcomes. Clinical outcomes include the occurrence of clinical events such as a cerebrovascular accident or fall, physiologic impairment such as renal insufficiency or pulmonary compromise, impairment of biological functioning such as hearing loss or swallowing disorders, or health status such as malnutrition. Some of these outcomes may be direct complications of therapy. Patient-centered outcomes include, at a minimum, physical functioning, social/ role functioning, psychological well-being, general health perceptions, and symptoms as well as satisfaction. Economic outcomes of interest to society include cost, health service utilization and productivity.

Exposure Variables

The exposures or risk-factors that may be related to these outcomes are even less well- defined. Determination of the relationship between an exposure variable and outcomes would require collection of a large number of potentially important variables and how these variables vary over time. Thus, this work is still largely exploratory.

For example, in examining patient sleep deprivation as an exposure variable that might predict adverse patient outcomes, we need to decide how the exposure relates to the outcome. Is there a threshold effect, or a cumulative dose, or an exposure rate that is associated with a specific outcome, such as post discharge dementia? Potential predictive factors and exposures are shown in Table 3. For example, sedative hypnotic medications may be related to post-ICU complications such as post-traumatic stress disorder. Sleep deprivation might be related to post- traumatic stress disorder. The method of ventilation might be related to future pulmonary functioning. Inadequate nutrition and lack of physical therapy in ICU might be related to poor physical functioning.

Data Collection

To obtain information on exposure variables, we would employ a battery of simple tools that could be deployed by multiple ICUs, such as a single page scanable sheet that could be collected daily or on ICU discharge, and a survey instrument that could be completed by ICU staff in 5-10 minutes. We have successfully pilot tested this approach to evaluate quality of care in 15 ICUs participating in an Institute for Healthcare Improvement project on the Idealized Design of the ICUs (IDICU).

Table 2. Types of outcomes to be evaluated

Outcomes	Examples	Data Sources / Measures
Mortality	ICU mortality Hospital mortality 30-day mortality 6-month mortality	National death index
Clinical Outcomes Clinical events Physiologic impairment Impairment of biologic functioning Health status	 Cerebrovascular accident Renal insufficiency Pulmonary compromise Hearing loss Swallowing disorder Malnutrition	Screening exam/ chart review/ patient or caregiver survey
Patient Centered Outcomes Physical functioning Social/role functioning Psychological well-being General health perceptions Symptoms Patient satisfaction	 Activities of Daily Living, Ability to perform vigorous activities Return to work Depression Vitality Pain Evaluation of the quality of ICU care, quality of communication	Patient / caregiver survey
Economic Outcomes Health care utilization Costs of care Care giver burden	 Readmissions Direct and Indirect costs Care giver quits work	Patient / caregiver survey, billing data

In this project, the charge nurse completed a daily information sheet that continued information on the vital statistics, nurse staffing, and length of stay for patients who were discharged. In addition the team making rounds in the ICU completed an information sheet that provided daily information regarding specific processes and complications of care such as peptic ulcer prophylaxis and pain scores on individual patients. From this information, we calculated 19 measures of quality of care, shown with their specifications in Table 4. The successful collection of these measures in the IDICU demonstrates the feasibility of employing simple standardized tools in a wide variety of ICUs during the care of ICU patients.

Given the large number of ICUs that would need to participate in the hypothetical cohort study we are designing, the central resources provided to individual ICUs

Table 3. Potential exposure variables for an ICU cohort study

Exposure	Potential data source
Patient characteristics Pre existing comorbidity Baseline functional status	Medical record/patient interview
Therapy provided to patient Medications Invasive treatment and monitoring Nutrition Sleep deprivation	Medical Record
Task characteristics Use of protocols	Survey of ICU staff
Individual provider factors Knowledge/skill Physical/mental health/fatigue	Survey of staff/observation
Team Factors Team structure Communication	Survey of staff/observation
Work environment Staff levels and skill mix Work load	Survey of staff/observation
ICU organization factors	Survey of staff/hospital leaders
Hospital or Health system factors	Survey of staff/hospital leaders
Regional characteristics Organization, finance, and delivery of health care	Area Resource File

by the coordinating center to assist with data collection would likely be minimal. As such, the probability of success of this data collection effort would ultimately require that it be made part of routine work processes. For example, we could design a data collection instrument that could also serve as the progress note. In addition to information currently reported about the patient's problems and event, the data collection would need to include specific variables that are explicitly defined and that are plausibly related to a specific outcome. For example, we may collect information on the total hours of mechanical ventilation. Because our understanding of the relationship between exposure and outcome variables is poor, a varying set of exposure variables may be collected over time and among ICUs.

Table 4. ICU quality indicators

Quality Indicator	Domains of Quality†	Definition of Indicator	Specifications
Outcome Measures			
ICU mortality rate	Safe Effective	% of ICU discharges who die in the ICU (no risk adjustment; to be used for comparison over time within an ICU)	*Numerator:* Total number of ICU deaths *Denominator:* Total number of ICU discharges (including deaths & transfers)
% of ICU patients with ICU LOS > 7 days	Safe Effective Efficient	% of ICU discharges with ICU Length of Stay (LOS) > 7 days	*Numerator:* All ICU patients with ICU LOS > 7 days *Denominator:* Total number of ICU discharges (including deaths & transfers)
Average ICU LOS	Safe Effective Efficient	Average ICU LOS	*Numerator:* Sum of ICU length of stay for all discharges *Denominator:* Total number of ICU discharges (including deaths & transfers)
Average days on mechanical ventilation	Safe Patient centered Efficient Effective	Average days on mechanical ventilation	*Numerator:* Total number of ventilator days *Denominator:* Total number of intubated/ trached patients who were mechanically ventilated
Suboptimal management of pain	Patient centered Effective Safe	% of "4 hour intervals" with a pain score > 3	*Numerator:* *Number* of "4 hour intervals" where the pain score is > 3 *Denominator:* Total number of "4 hour intervals"

Table 4. *(Continued)*

Quality Indicator	Domains of Quality†	Definition of Indicator	Specifications
Patient/family satisfaction	To be developed		
Access Measures			
Rate of delayed admissions	Efficient Patient centered Timely	Rate of delay admissions to the ICU	*Numerator:* Number of admissions that are delayed for >= 4 hours to ICU (exclude transfers from outside hospitals)
			Denominator: Total number of ICU admissions (excluding transfers from outside hospitals)
Rate of delayed discharges	Efficient Patient centered Timely	Rate of delay discharges from the ICU	*Numerator:* Number of discharges that are delayed for >= 4 hours from ICU
			Denominator: Total number of ICU discharges
Cancelled operating room (OR) cases	Equitable Efficient Patient centered Timely	Number of cancelled OR cases due to lack of ICU beds	*Numerator:* Number of cancelled OR cases due to lack of ICU bed
			Denominator: None (If total number of OR cases are available, than these data can be presented as a rate)
Emergency department (ED) by-pass hours	Efficient Equitable Patient centered Timely	ED by-pass hours per month due to lack of ICU beds	*Numerator:* Total by-pass hours per month that are due to lack of ICU beds
			Denominator: None

Table 4. *(Continued)*

Quality Indicator	Domains of Quality†	Definition of Indicator	Specifications
Complication Measures			
Rate of unplanned ICU readmissions	Safe Effective Efficient Patient centered	Rate of unplanned ICU readmissions	*Numerator:* Number of patients who had an unplanned ICU readmission w/in 48 hrs of ICU discharge
			Denominator: Total number of ICU discharges
Rate of catheter-related blood stream infections	Safe Efficient Effective	Rate of catheter-related blood stream infections (BSI) per 1000 catheter days	*Numerator:* Number of patients with catheter-related BSI as defined by CDC
			Denominator: Total number of catheter days in the ICU
Rate of resistant infections	Safe Effective Efficient Patient centered	Rate of "new onset" resistant infections per ICU patient day	*Numerator:* Number of patients who develop resistant infections in the ICU (defined as MRSA or VRE infections)
			Denominator: Total ICU patient days
Process Measures			
Appropriate use of blood transfusions	Safe Effective Efficient	The percent of packed red blood cell (PRBCs) transfusions for which the hemoglobin (Hgb) prior to transfusion is less than 8 gm/dl	*Numerator:* Number of PRBCs transfusions for which the Hgb immediately prior to transfusion was less than 8 gm/dl (include transfusions during episodes of massive bleeding {>=4 units per hour} assume that these transfusions all had Hgb <8).
			Denominator: Total number of transfusions

Table 4. (*Continued*)

Quality Indicator	Domains of Quality†	Definition of Indicator	Specifications
Prevention of ventilator associated pneumonia	Safe Effective Efficient	The percent of ventilator days where the head of bed (HOB) is elevated >= 30 degrees	*Numerator:* Number of ventilator days where the HOB is elevated >= 30 degrees *Denominator:* Total number of ventilator days
Appropriate sedation	Safe Effective Efficient Patient cantered	The percent of ventilator days where: 1) sedation was held for at least 12 hrs or until patient could follow commands OR 2) if patient follows commands without need to hold sedation	*Numerator:* Number of ventilator days in which 1) sedation was held for >= 12 hrs or until patient followed commands OR 2) patient followed commands without sedation held *Denominator:* Total ventilator days
Appropriate peptic ulcer disease (PUD) prophylaxis	Safe Effective Efficient	The percent of ventilator days where patient received PUD prophylaxis	*Numerator:* Number of ventilator days where patients received PUD prophylaxis *Denominator:* Total ventilator days
Appropriate deep venous thrombosis (DVT) prophylaxis	Safe Effective Efficient	The percent of ventilator days where patient received DVT prophylaxis	*Numerator:* Number of ventilator days where patients received DVT prophylaxis *Denominator:* Total ventilator days

† Domains of quality from the Aims of Medical care proposed by the IOM report "Crossing the Quality Chasm" [1]: Safe, effective, patient centered, timely, efficient, equitable

Outcome Variables

To obtain information on longer-term outcome variables, we would need to collect data using a set of simple deploy a number of simple instruments at multiple time points after hospital discharge. Although the optimal time after discharge to evaluate ICU outcomes is unknown, studies have examined outcomes for periods ranging from 30 days to years after hospital admission.

An innovative and clinically useful component of post-discharge data collection could be a nurse visit that would occur within two days of ICU and hospital discharge. This would permit a check on whether acute care plans were transmitted and being executed successfully, and the extent to which they are integrated with the chronic care plan.

Although a nurse visit would be ideal, some of these encounters could occur by phone, especially if the patient is relatively healthy. Additional post-discharge data collection would occur 6 months and 1 year after discharge. To better understand the natural history of patients exposed to ICU care, a random sample of patients could be followed for 5 years. Nevertheless, follow-up becomes increasingly difficult as duration increases. To improve follow up, at the time of hospital discharge we would want to obtain multiple contact points for use in the future.

These nurse visits would need to include explicit measurement of outcomes likely to be affected by ICU care. We have outlined some of these in Table 2. The nurse visit would include a structured history, physical and laboratory evaluation with referral for further evaluation as needed. We may be able to use information technology to facilitate collection of some of the outcomes. For example, patients or caregivers could respond to email or web based surveys. These surveys could be linked to the patient's primary care provider to allow for follow up. Alternatively, patients or caregivers could use telephone response systems to provide data.

We should not minimize the statistical expertise needed to analyze data collected as part of the effort described above. Longitudinal data, and data collected in multiple ICUs and institutions present challenges for analyses. The exposure variables vary over time; we will measure outcomes multiple times in the same patient (longitudinal data), and outcomes are likely clustered within ICUs and perhaps within health systems and countries. There are new and powerful ways to analyze this type of data, as demonstrated by recent analyses to evaluate the association between pollution levels in cities and mortality [36]. In any event, involvement of biostatisticians will be crucial.

Conclusion

Today's ICU providers have little ability to evaluate the long-term impact of their care. This severely limits their ability to improve ICU care. Moreover, relatively little is known about the long-term impact of ICU care on patients and how ICU care impacts those outcomes. We have outlined a cohort study that could provide insights into these questions and help to improve the quality of ICU care. The cohort design is ideal for such a study since it allows researchers to evaluate time-dependent models for the association between exposure and risk. Such mod-

Table 5. Ten new rules for 21st century health care. From [1] with permission

1. Base care in healing relationships (*not visits, only*)
2. Customize care to the individual patient (*avoiding unhelpful variation*)
3. Regard the patient as the source of all control (*rather than beginning with control in the system*)
4. Share knowledge and make information flow freely (*including unfettered access by patients to their medical records*)
5. Base decisions on evidence (*rather than habit*)
6. Improve safety as a system property (*rather than exhorting individuals*)
7. Embrace transparency (*not secrecy*)
8. Anticipate needs (*rather than reacting*)
9. Continually reduce waste (*of time, supplies, space, information, ideas, spirit, etc.*)
10. Cooperate (*as the highest professional value*)

els are necessary when evaluating ICU care, where exposure and confounding variables vary over time and when this variation may impact outcomes.

In addition to providing a framework for quality of care, the IOM report "Crossing the Quality Chasm" [1] also outlined some rules by which we could provide care (Table 5). These rules essentially state that we should view care through the patients' eyes and organize care to meet their needs.

Imagine a health care system that operates under these rules. We would not need to design a study to identify complications of ICU care, as it would be part of routine care. Different types of provider would share information with each other and their patients. Information systems would provide access to this type of data and information on the association between ICU care and outcomes. Some of these data will be available in real-time, while other portions can be used to help design ICU therapy. In this world, the daily practice of medicine would move closer to the methods and results restricted to formal clinical studies. In this setting, we will be able to promise patients who are admitted to an ICU that their care will be safe, effective, efficient, timely, patient centered, and equitable.

We have much to learn about the impact of ICU care on patient outcomes. We believe the suggestions outlined here could help inform practice in the ICU and lead to an improved quality of care.

Acknowledgement

This work was funded in part by an Agency for Healthcare Research and Quality grant number, U18HS11902-01.

References

1. Committee on Quality of Health Care in America, Institute of Medicine (2001) Crossing the Quality Chasm. National Academy Press, Washington
2. Becker GJ, Strauch GO, Saranchak HJ (1984) Outcome and cost of prolonged stay in the surgical intensive care unit. Arch Surg 119:1338–1342
3. Ridley SA, Wallace PG (1990) Quality of life after intensive care. Anaesthesia 45:808–813
4. Parno JR, Teres D, Lemeshow S, Brown RB, Avrunin JS (1984) Two-year outcome of adult intensive care patients. Med Care 1984 22:167–176
5. Covinsky KE, Wu AW, Landefeld CS, et al (1999) Health status versus quality of life in older patients: does the distinction matter? Am J Med 106:435–440
6. Wu AW, Yasui Y, Alzola C, et al (2000) Predicting functional status outcomes in hospitalized patients aged 80 years and older. J Am Geriatr Soc 48 (5 Suppl):S6–S15
7. Wu AW, Damiano AM, Lynn J, et al (1995) Predicting future functional status for seriously ill hospitalized adults. The SUPPORT prognostic model. Ann Intern Med 122:342–350
8. Chelluri L, Pinsky MR, Donahoe MP, Grenvik A (1993) Long-term outcome of critically ill elderly patients requiring intensive care. JAMA 269:3119–3123
9. Montuclard L, Garrouste-Orgeas M, Timsit JF, Misset B, De Jonghe B, Carlet J (2000) Outcome, functional autonomy, and quality of life of elderly patients with a long-term intensive care unit stay. Crit Care Med 28:3389–3395
10. Niskanen M, Ruokonen E, Takala J, Rissanen P, Kari A (1999) Quality of life after prolonged intensive care. Crit Care Med 27:1132–1139
11. Lipsett PA, Swoboda SM, Dickerson J, et al (2000) Survival and functional outcome after prolonged intensive care unit stay. Ann Surg 231:262–268
12. Konopad E, Noseworthy TW, Johnston R, Shustack A, Grace M (1995) Quality of life measures before and one year after admission to an intensive care unit. Crit Care Med 23:1653–1659
13. Capuzzo M, Bianconi M, Contu P, Pavoni V, Gritti G (1996) Survival and quality of life after intensive care. Intensive Care Med 22:947–953
14. Udekwu P, Gurkin B, Oller D, Lapio L, Bourbina J (2001) Quality of life and functional level in elderly patients surviving surgical intensive care. J Am Coll Surg 193:245–249
15. Kass JE, Castriotta RJ, Malakoff F (1992) Intensive care unit outcome in the very elderly. Crit Care Med 20:1666–1671
16. Trouillet JL, Scheimberg A, Vuagnat A, Fagon JY, Chastre J, Gibert C (1996) Long-term outcome and quality of life of patients requiring multidisciplinary intensive care unit admission after cardiac operations. J Thorac Cardiovasc Surg 112:926–934
17. Fakhry SM, Kercher KW, Rutledge R (1996) Survival, quality of life, and charges in critically III surgical patients requiring prolonged ICU stays. J Trauma 41:999–1007
18. McHugh GJ, Havill JH, Armistead SH, Ullal RR, Fayers TM (1997) Follow up of elderly patients after cardiac surgery and intensive care unit admission, 1991 to 1995. N Z Med J 110:432–435
19. Mahul P, Perrot D, Tempelhoff G, et al (1991) Short- and long-term prognosis, functional outcome following ICU for elderly. Intensive Care Med 17:7–10
20. Eddleston JM, White P, Guthrie E (2000) Survival, morbidity, and quality of life after discharge from intensive care. Crit Care Med 28:2293–2299
21. Zaren B, Hedstrand U (1987) Quality of life among long-term survivors of intensive care. Crit Care Med 15:743–747
22. Hurel D, Loirat P, Saulnier F, Nicolas F, Brivet F (1997) Quality of life 6 months after intensive care: results of a prospective multicenter study using a generic health status scale and a satisfaction scale. Intensive Care Med 23:331–337
23. Nasraway SA, Button GJ, Rand WM, Hudson-Jinks T, Gustafson M (2000) Survivors of catastrophic illness: outcome after direct transfer from intensive care to extended care facilities. Crit Care Med 28:19–25
24. Broslawski GE, Elkins M, Algus M (1995) Functional abilities of elderly survivors of intensive care. J Am Osteopath Assoc 95:712–717

25. Vazquez Mata G, Rivera Fernandez R, Gonzalez Carmona A, et al (1992) Factors related to quality of life 12 months after discharge from an intensive care unit. Crit Care Med 20:1257–1262

26. Rockwood K, Noseworthy TW, Gibney RT, et al (1993) One-year outcome of elderly and young patients admitted to intensive care units. Crit Care Med 21:687–691

27. Covinsky KE, Goldman L, Cook EF, et al (1994) The impact of serious illness on patients' families. SUPPORT Investigators. Study to Understand Prognoses and Preferences for Outcomes and Risks of Treatment. JAMA 272:1839–1844

28. Orlando R 3rd (2000) Quality of life in intensive care unit survivors: a place for outcomes research in critical care. Crit Care Med 28:3755–3756

29. Russell S (1996) Who knows where they go? Quality of life after intensive care. Aust Nurs J 3:20–22

30. Grady KL (2001) Beyond morbidity and mortality: quality of life outcomes in critical care patients. Crit Care Med 29:1844–1846

31. Metnitz PG, Vesely H, Valentin A, et al (1999) Evaluation of an interdisciplinary data set for national intensive care unit assessment. Crit Care Med 27:1486–1491

32. Fiser DH, Tilford JM, Roberson PK (2000) Relationship of illness severity and length of stay to functional outcomes in the pediatric intensive care unit: a multi-institutional study. Crit Care Med 28:1173–1179

33. Zimmerman JE, Wagner DP, Draper EA, Wright L, Alzola C, Knaus WA (1998) Evaluation of acute physiology and chronic health evaluation III predictions of hospital mortality in an independent database. Crit Care Med 26:1317–1326

34. Dawber TR, Kannel WB (1966) The Framingham study. An epidemiological approach to coronary heart diseae. Circulation 34:553–555

35. Samet JM (2000) Concepts of time in clinical research. Ann Intern Med 132:37–44

36. Sarnat JA, Schwartz J, Suh HH, Samet JM, Dominici F, Zeger SL (2001) Fine particulate air pollution and mortality in 20 US cities. N Engl J Med 344:1253–1254

Subject index

Printing: Mercedes-Druck, Berlin
Binding: Stein+Lehmann, Berlin